Lung Cancer

Making Sense of Diagnosis,
Treatment, and Options

Lung Cancer

Making Sense of Diagnosis, Treatment, and Options

Lorraine Johnston

O'REILLY®

Beijing • Cambridge • Farnham • Köln • Paris • Sebastopol • Taipei • Tokyo

Lung Cancer: Making Sense of Diagnosis, Treatment, and Options
by Lorraine Johnston

Copyright © 2001 O'Reilly & Associates, Inc. All rights reserved.
Printed in the United States of America.

Published by O'Reilly & Associates, Inc., 101 Morris Street, Sebastopol, CA 95472.

Editor: Linda Lamb

Production Editor: Ann Schirmer

Cover Designer: Kristen Throop

Printing History:

> May 2001: First Edition

Library of Congress Cataloging-in-Publication Data:

Johnston, Lorraine, 1950-
    Lung cancer: making sense of diagnosis, treatment, and options / Lorraine Johnston.
        p. cm.—(Patient-centered guides)
    Includes bibliographical references and index.
    ISBN 0-596-50002-5
    1. Lungs—Cancer—Popular works. I. Title. II. Series.

RC280.L8 J64 2001
616.99'424—dc21   00-065256

[M]

To my son Lou, for quitting smoking. May you never need this book.

Table of Contents

Preface

*A journey of a thousand leagues
begins with a single step.*

—Lao-tzu

A DIAGNOSIS OF LUNG CANCER is not an automatic death sentence. Because there are different kinds of lung cancers with different outcomes, the surgeon, oncologist, or institution you select must be the best qualified to treat your type and presentation of disease. The treatments chosen can have a profound effect on your disease, quality of life, and future. Correct and current information about lung cancer must find its way to you if you are to make appropriate treatment choices.

The goal of this book is to provide you with the tools you'll need to locate sound medical information about lung cancer. Many or most readers will eventually move well beyond this book in their ability to find reliable, current medical information. Advancing the reader's ability to do this is my goal. Did you know, for example, that:

- The current staging systems for lung cancer are not cast in concrete, and accurate prognostic forecasts cannot be made using stage (a determination of how far the cancer has spread) alone.

- The National Cancer Institute recommends that all lung cancer patients consider clinical trials of new substances to gain early access to better treatments.

- Biopsied tumor tissue should be archived so that emerging treatments requiring tumor analysis can be used if needed.

- With relative ease, you can find reliable information about the dosage, mode of action, and side effects of medications being recommended for your treatment.

- Second and subsequent opinions are a time-honored and expected venue that you should utilize, without guilt, to make the best treatment decisions.

- Reliable, peer-reviewed medical literature is easily accessed free of charge.

- Charitable groups exist expressly to fly you and your family, free of charge, to a distant cancer center where you might plan to be treated. The American Cancer Society and other networks can provide you and your loved ones with out-of-town accommodations free of charge.

- In all 50 states, laws exist to ensure your access to your medical records.

Who should read this book?

If you were diagnosed recently, this book can help you understand what tests and treatments you'll encounter in the following months. We discuss the emotional aspects of each experience: the shock and isolation of diagnosis and the reactions that follow, the fear of upcoming treatments, the anxiety associated with waiting to see if treatment is successful, the concern that smokers or ex-smokers might have regarding stigma or guilt for smoking tobacco.

If you're a long-term survivor of lung cancer, we provide the information you need to make sense of the possible long-term physical and emotional consequences of disease and treatment. You might still be coughing, for example; experiencing chest, hand, or foot pain; using oxygen daily; or experiencing continued fatigue. Some survivors might need information concerning the recurrence of disease and its treatment.

If you're a caretaker of someone with lung cancer, the insights from patients and the collective and pragmatic wisdom of others in this guide will enable you to make the most of your caretaking and advocacy efforts. It will assist you in relaxing and staying healthy so you can best care for your loved one, both emotionally and instrumentally. We can help you understand the reactions of your loved one and yourself and respond appropriately to the unique stress that a lung cancer diagnosis entails.

If you have not yet obtained a firm diagnosis of lung cancer, please do not read this guide until your doctors have clarified your circumstances. Symptoms that mimic lung cancer, such as shortness of breath or coughing, could be caused by several other disorders. You should seek appropriate treatment for these conditions from a qualified physician.

If you have other cancers affecting the lung, such as a lymphoma infiltrating the lung, neuroendocrine carcinoid non-lung tumors, mesothelioma, or lung metastases from breast, liver, or colon cancers, this book contains information that is not correct for your circumstances.

If you are primarily interested in preventing lung cancer, including quitting smoking, please see the literature provided by the Alliance for Lung Cancer Advocacy, Support, and Education (ALCASE) (*http://www.alcase.org*), because we discuss that topic only briefly.

How to read this book

Although the format of this book follows the path of your experience with lung cancer—symptoms, testing and diagnosis, surgery and hospitalization, and so on— we suggest you read only the material you need at a given point instead of reading cover-to-cover. We try to provide you with digestible amounts of information that you'll need at each stage. You might find it upsetting, for instance, to read about all symptoms, common and rare.

A few chapters will be useful to all readers. The chapters on researching your illness and clinical trials are intended to help you become an even better informed medical consumer who is able to find all the information needed to make sound decisions about treatment. A chapter is devoted to stress and its sometimes surprising effects on the immune system, offering a variety of ways to cope with stress and insights into making challenging experiences work in your favor. Two chapters on finding good medical care are worth your review.

Sources of information

The chief resources used in developing this book were the journals and texts of Western medicine, which we summarize and present to you in language understandable by those without a medical background. Appendix A, *Resources*, discusses references that can be accessed using the Internet, such as the National Cancer Institute's grand-daddy of all cancer information databases and Medline, the National Library of Medicine's database of more than eleven million published medical research papers.

Neither this nor any book can substitute for up-to-date oncology training and good medical care. You should always consult with lung cancer specialists before making decisions about your care.

Several chapters that are of interest to all cancer survivors, such as the chapters on stress and clinical trials, were reused from my earlier books about lymphoma and colorectal cancer, with appropriate changes made for lung cancer survivors.

About our patient stories

To me, the most riveting aspect of cancer literature is the story of the person living through the experience. These survivors serve as an anchor to reality and an inspiration for the rest of us. The experiences of patients and survivors, included throughout this guide, can help you learn what to expect in advance and where to find the best information for your circumstances—and to know that you are not alone. The italicized portions of the text are their own words.

Acknowledgments

As always, my first and greatest thanks go to my husband, Larry, who is taking a nap on the bunk beds with our cats as I write this preface. He has been, and continues to be, my role model for cancer survivors and for living in general.

Patients and caretakers

I extend humble thanks to the family of Anthony Capasso, especially to his sister Geri, for allowing me to include his story. Anthony, a never-smoker, fought bravely against lung cancer using both standard therapy and new treatments being tested in clinical trials. He passed away in August 2000. Seldom have I witnessed such love and bravery as exhibited by Geri in finding information and help for her brother. We should all be blessed with family like Anthony's. Truly love such as this will keep Anthony alive in the eternal sense.

Max Baldwin, a non-small cell lung cancer (NSCLC) survivor, allowed us to use his honest and brave story. Max used sound reasoning and intelligence to make good treatment choices, but he never forgot his humanity. He reviewed this guide before it was published and made suggestions for improvement.

Karen Parles, a young survivor of non-small cell lung cancer, created the Internet resource known as Lung Cancer Online (*http://www.lungcanceronline.org*). She reviewed this guide in its entirety, made many suggestions, revamped the Medline search section, suggested illustrations, directed me to oncologists who agreed to review the medical portions of this guide, and was emotionally supportive to me when I wasn't sure this book would get written. Karen's Lung Cancer Online site is one of the most reliable and comprehensive sites available for lung cancer patients and survivors.

Kathleen Houlihan, survivor of stage IIIB non-small cell lung cancer, wife of Jonathan Holt Truex, PhD, MD, and mother to several cats and dogs, opened her heart and her journal of lung cancer experiences for my use. Kathy refused to be blinded by science and statistics in seeking the treatment she felt was best for her. If I were to face lung cancer, I would want Kathy by my side.

Gilles Frydman, husband of a breast cancer survivor and creator and lifeblood of the nonprofit Association of Cancer Online Resources, Inc. (ACOR), has as always been stalwart and supremely ethical in supporting me and others who are dealing with cancer. Through his kindness and generosity, the one hundred ACOR cancer discussion groups provide a desperately needed means for cancer survivors and their loved ones to find emotional and instrumental support. Gilles gains nothing financially by providing this service. In the eyes of people like me, he's a hero.

The listowners of the ACOR LUNG-ONC cancer discussion group, in particular Larry Coffman, welcomed me warmly when I joined the group and did their best to assure lung cancer patients, survivors, and caretakers that they could trust me. Listowners, serving as volunteers in their free time, deal with the headaches of list management every day. They could have easily turned me away, but they did not. If you find the patient interviews in this book emotionally resonant and instructive, the listowners deserve the credit. You will find Larry's experiences as a five-year survivor of small cell lung cancer (SCLC) throughout this guide.

Several patients and survivors chose to contribute anonymously or to use first names only. Their hearts and common sense speak in a clear voice, even though their names are not used. Thank you.

And to lung cancer survivors everywhere who are exhibiting great courage in the face of fear, I thank you for keeping on, for seeking information, for becoming survivors.

The Patient-Centered Guides team

My editor Linda Lamb, breast cancer survivor and cofounder of the Patient-Centered Guides (PCG) series, continues to be far more than one could ask of a mentor and boss. Linda's insight into and trust of the patient's perspective are steadfast. Her keen ability to separate wheat from chaff, shaped by her own cancer experience, never fails. Writing for Linda is not work, it is fulfillment.

Shawnde Paull, editorial assistant, automagically transformed my writing and formatting into a real, live book. Every company has a person who really runs things behind the scenes; at the Patient-Centered Guides, Shawnde is that person. What she can do to a bibliography without trying very hard brings us lesser mortals to our knees. The other PCG authors and I whisper her name in awe.

Medical reviewers

Several oncology experts reviewed the medically intense chapters of this guide. If this book is a useful guide, it is so because of their efforts.

In daily life and in medical literature, medical experts do not always agree. When a consensus of opinion was clear, I included the agreed-upon facts; when not, I stated that differences of opinion exist on a given topic. Every effort was made to clarify obscure topics and provide correct and current information. Any errors that remain in this book are mine.

- **Stephen B. Baylin, MD.** Professor, Department of Oncology and Department of Medicine, Johns Hopkins University School of Medicine, reviewed both the chapter on prognosis and the appendix of experimental tumor markers, with special attention to the molecular indicators of tumor activity. Dr. Baylin's research laboratory at Johns Hopkins specializes in the molecular events important to steps in human tumor progression.

- **Steven Belinsky, PhD.** Director, Lung Cancer Program, Lovelace Respiratory Research Institute, Albuquerque, New Mexico, reviewed Chapter 5, *What Is Lung Cancer?*, and corrected information regarding the genetics and epidemiology of lung cancer. Dr. Belinsky's research on lung cancer is much needed and much appreciated; working with him was pleasant and fruitful.

- **Costas Giannakenas, MD, PhD.** Nuclear Physician, the University of Patras Medical School, Greece, recipient of the Eminent Scientist and Outstanding Scholar of the Year 2001 award, reviewed the chapters on treatment, with special attention to radiotherapy techniques. Dr. Giannakenas has as always shared not only his knowledge of oncology, but friendship and kindness as well.

- **Lynn Godmilow, MSW, CGC.** Director, Genetic Diagnostic Referral Service, University of Pennsylvania School of Medicine Department of Genetics, reviewed Chapter 5 with an eye to familial disease and the possibility of genetics counseling and intervention. Ms. Godmilow is among the best-informed genetics counselors I have had the pleasure of working with.

- Dr. Asnat Groutz, MD. A member of the Department of Obstetrics and Gynecology, Lis Maternity Hospital, Sackler Faculty of Medicine, Tel Aviv University, Israel, reviewed an earlier version of the chapter on sexuality and fertility that appeared in our guide for colorectal cancer patients. Much of this information also pertains to lung cancer patients treated with chemotherapy, and has been included in this guide. I again thank Dr. Groutz for this fine effort.

- David Harpole Jr. MD. Associate Professor of the Division of Thoracic Surgery, Duke University Medical Center, Durham, North Carolina, reviewed Appendix E, *Experimental Prognostic Markers*. This emerging field of study includes information that might soon appear on patients' pathology reports and thus be in need of discussion.

- Robert J. Kreitman, MD. Chief, Clinical Immunotherapy Section, Laboratory of Molecular Biology, National Cancer Institute, Bethesda, Maryland, reviewed Chapter 7, *Types of Treatment*, Chapter 8, *Treating Non-Small Cell Lung Cancer*, and Chapter 9, *Treating Small Cell Lung Cancer*. Dr. Kreitman has done copious research on the use of immunotoxins in cancer therapy.

- Charles Padgett, MD. Medical Oncologist, Good Samaritan Hospital, Baltimore, Maryland, reviewed Chapters 7 through 9, and the portion of Chapter 6, *Prognosis*, discussing bloodborne measures of tumor progression. He answered my many general questions on lung cancer, and my particular questions on recent advances in radiotherapy. His unbending integrity and the scrupulous care he applied to answering my questions reflect the high quality of his Johns Hopkins training and his subsequent empathic experiences with treating cancer patients.

- Roman Perez-Soler, MD. Associate Director for Clinical Oncology & Translational Research, Kaplan Comprehensive Cancer Center, New York University School of Medicine, New York, New York, reviewed the chapter on types of treatment, Chapter 7, and on the specific treatment of NSCLC. He offered many useful explanations of treatment, standard care, and experimental care. Dr. Perez-Soler is highly regarded by his patients, and we are fortunate to have his contributions.

- Jonathan Samet, MD, MS. Chairman of the Department of Epidemiology, Johns Hopkins School of Hygiene and Public Health, Baltimore, Maryland, reviewed Chapter 5 and suggested numerous improvements. I am especially grateful to Dr. Samet for his detailed, incisive review, the resources he recommended (including an excellent genetics text), and the many reprints of journal articles he gave me.

- **Penella Woll, MD**. Senior Lecturer in Clinical Oncology, Nottingham City Hospital, Nottingham, England, reviewed the chapter on adverse effects of treatment, tactfully offering numerous additions and clarifications. This chapter is critical to many lung cancer patients, on a par with treatment and prognosis, and Dr. Woll's careful review is literally priceless.

Finally, I thank medical researchers in the United States and elsewhere who, though often grossly underpaid and unrecognized, have devoted their lives to caring about our well-being and our outcomes. Thanks to the effort and altruistic collaboration of cancer researchers all over the world, we are witnessing and benefiting from robust progress in the understanding and treatment of cancer.

CHAPTER 1

Symptoms of Lung Cancer

The trouble with doctors is not that they don't know enough,
but that they don't see enough.

—Dominic J. Corrigan

MOST LUNG TUMORS PRODUCE NO SYMPTOMS in their earliest stages. In spite of this misleading indicator of good health and the high incidence of lung cancer worldwide, accurate and affordable early screening for lung tumors remains elusive. This means that individuals must persist on their own in evaluating their lung health—with or without symptoms. Unfortunately, the symptoms of lung cancer can be both straightforward and confusing, because multiple organs might be affected.

If you or your loved one is having symptoms that you suspect might be lung cancer but diagnosis has been elusive, contact the National Cancer Institute for the name of a nearby lung cancer specialist. Contacting an experienced practitioner is particularly important if the person experiencing symptoms has a family history of lung cancer, pursues an occupation at increased risk for lung cancer, or has ever smoked.

Symptoms and syndromes

One's experience with lung cancer symptoms can be unique. You might have a lengthy series of diagnostic tests triggered only by a stubborn cough or chest pain, a symptomless early lung lesion appearing on a routine x-ray, a frightening amount of blood expelled during a coughing spell, or a series of odd symptoms such as a toothache, an earache, or weight loss that seemed unrelated to lung function. Larry Coffman, a five-year survivor of small cell lung cancer, describes his acute symptoms:

> *During a jam session in December, I began coughing uncontrollably*
> *and couldn't stop. I coughed so long and hard that I had what is termed*
> *"respiratory arrest," and passed out, falling off my drum stool. I didn't*
> *even know I was out until my brother and friend were picking me up off*
> *the floor.*

I was diagnosed with SCLC (small cell lung cancer) located in the right upper lobe on January 5. The doctor making the initial diagnosis told me to "go home and get your affairs in order," and gave me a one in twelve chance for survival.

Definition of syndrome

In the course of getting a diagnosis, you may hear reference to a particular syndrome. A syndrome is a collection of simultaneous symptoms with a common cause, observed often enough in patients with a given disease to characterize that disease.

The lists of symptoms in the sections that follow may seem complex, confusing, or ominous. Symptoms and syndromes are listed here to indicate to you the range of things your doctors may look for, to help give some reason behind a diagnostic test or exam that may at first seem odd, or to give you an idea of the range of symptoms that lung cancers may present. As you can see, symptoms vary tremendously. Discuss any symptoms with your doctor.

Pulmonary symptoms

The symptoms of lung cancer that are clearly and directly related to lung function are:

- Coughing, the most common symptom (74 percent of patients)
- Bloody or dark phlegm (sputum; 57 percent)
- Shortness of breath (37 percent)
- Chest pain (25 percent)
- Hoarseness (18 percent)
- Paralysis of the diaphragm, either symptomless or as shortness of breath
- Wheezing or vibrating breathing noises (stridor)
- Recurrent pneumonia or bronchitis
- Difficulty swallowing (dysphagia)
- Excess mucus production (bronchorrhea)

The illustration of the lungs in Figure 1-1 can help you determine where your tumor has been found and what other nearby organs it might affect.

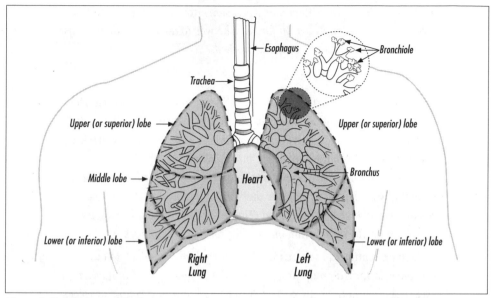

Figure 1-1. Structure of the lungs

Kathy, the wife of a lung cancer survivor, describes her husband's painful, but confusing symptoms and several misdiagnoses. His health problems began with a heart attack:

> *I think everything began for us in early 1998, when Marty came in from working hard outside, where we were building a concrete patio. We live in Florida, so my first thought was heat exhaustion, but he didn't cool off, so I contacted our neighbor who knew something about nursing. We ended up calling 911.*
>
> *When I got to the hospital, they said the doctor wanted to talk to me, and escorted me to the emergency room doctor, who told me Marty's heart had stopped. I was stunned. Then he said, "But we shocked him twice and we got him back." He had a stent implanted in his artery that same day.*
>
> *This whole experience was traumatizing for our family. Christy, then eleven, blamed herself for her dad's heart attack. Emily, then three, got very aggressive with her teachers and was almost suspended from preschool (if you can imagine), and I had to face the thought of losing my husband. Marty and I were not in the best position in our marriage; we had problems that I was on the brink of addressing with Marty when he had the heart attack. We struggled through the next six months, with*

Marty returning to the ER on many occasions from fear that he was having another heart attack. In January, he was told to take a double dose of Prevacid for acid reflux, and that worked.

The next year, he began having pain:

He felt good until April 1999, when he began to get earaches. He went to two doctors who said nothing was wrong. On May 4, 1999, he went to our family doctor, who wasn't on our insurance plan. He said Marty had an ear infection and put him on antibiotics. While there, Marty mentioned a pain he was having in his side, like bruised ribs. The doctor thought it was something with the diaphragm and I think the antibiotic was to have taken care of that, too. The ear got better, but the side pain did not, so the doctor put him on another round of antibiotics.

The pain continued to increase. Now Marty had to go back to our insurance doctors, a group practice, in order to have x-rays and other tests. They sent him for an x-ray, which he had to wait a couple of weeks to get because our insurance company (which had been sold the prior year) would allow us to only go to one imaging/diagnostic center. Marty couldn't take the wait, so he went to the emergency room, where they did a sonogram, x-ray, and abdominal CT scan. The findings were that he was extremely constipated, and they sent him home. I think he was back the next day because the pain was so bad and the Darvocet was not enough. This was the end of May. He did finally have a substantial bowel movement, but the pain was still there and increasing.

Marty's report of pain was generally discounted, or blamed on emotional problems:

I was getting very testy because I felt that he needed to be more patient with the doctors and with the fact that it took so long to get diagnostic tests done. The doctors did not take him seriously because he had had so many pseudo-heart attacks from the acid reflux the year before, and I think they thought, like I did, that he was being a baby. In June, we went through the same thing, tests scheduled, going to the emergency room, too much pain, and so on.

By the end of June, he was frustrated and he went back to our family doctor (no insurance). Now the pain had gotten so bad that his spine was curved and he couldn't stand up straight. The doctor knows us, and he believed Marty was truly in pain, so he called the insurance doctors to talk to them. The pain was getting so bad that Marty got himself admitted

*to the hospital where they did an MRI and chest CT. Both came up
normal. Our doctor couldn't believe that Marty's spine looked normal on
the MRI. The pulmonary doctor called me at work to ask me about
Marty's emotional stability. I was so frustrated at this point that I didn't
know what to say. I called our doctor, who told me I shouldn't discount
Marty's pain, that he believed Marty was truly in pain. So I picked Marty
up from the hospital, nothing accomplished.*

*He managed on pain killers for a few weeks. I was totally impatient
with him.*

When the pain could no longer be discounted, Marty was admitted to the hospital:

*On July 13, 1999, Marty's work called me to ask that I come get him
because he was in so much pain. I called the neurologist's office, and they
agreed I could bring him straight there. We sat in the waiting room for the
longest time. While we were, there a woman asked me what was wrong
with my husband; I just said, "I don't know." The woman said he looked
like he was in a great deal of pain. We waited a long time at the office and
I had to keep asking for help because he was in so much pain and I didn't
know what to do. Once we got into the room, the nurse (or physician's
assistant) kept coming in, then leaving. I had to leave the room to ask for
help because Marty was getting so upset, which made him feel worse.
Finally the doctor arrived, and he said he was having Marty admitted to
the hospital.*

Symptoms in nearby organs

Nonrespiratory symptoms associated with lung cancer might be associated with pressure of a tumor on another organ, or with spread of disease (metastasis) outside the lungs or bronchial tubes.

This man tells of an unexplained fever that led to the discovery of a tumor in his lung and to surgery:

*It started off with a low-grade fever that went on for quite some time
—for weeks. I finally went in to see the doctor at a first-aid clinic at the
local hospital.*

He took a few tests. My blood sugar was way out of whack, 400 or something. Later the doctor said, "You can't really get a sugar reading when someone has a fever." That was the first time I found out about the diabetes I have.

The doctor put me on an antibiotic to try to knock the fever. It didn't work.

Then I went into the regular doctor's office and had a chest x-ray. It showed the tumor in the lung. (They said from the beginning that it was a tumor, but not that it was necessarily cancer.) It was good-sized, a little bigger than a golf ball. Even I could see it plainly on the x-ray. They were going to treat it. First they treated it with another antibiotic—a new, expensive antibiotic—to see if they could do anything with it, that way.

That didn't work. It didn't respond to any antibiotics.

The following symptoms have been associated with the spread of disease in many patients. Unlike the list for pulmonary symptoms, the order of this list is not indicative of frequency of occurrence. In some cases, several of these symptoms might occur together:

- Headache

- Weakness, numbness, or paralysis

- Dizziness

- Partial loss of vision

- Bone or joint pain

- Abdominal pain upon probing

- Unexplained weight loss

- Loss of appetite

- Unexplained fever

- Yellowing of the skin (jaundice)

- Pain or shortness of breath caused by fluid in the chest (effusion)

- Cardiac symptoms, including irregular pulse and difficulty breathing

- Swelling of the face, arms, and neck, possibly with visible veins on the skin of the chest caused by superior vena cava syndrome (SVCS), pressure of a tumor on the large chest vein known as the superior vena cava.

- Pancoast syndrome, caused by a tumor that presses on a nerve in the superior sulcus, a groove in the upper lung and its sac through which a major artery runs. Symptoms of Pancoast syndrome include Horner's syndrome, with symptoms such as a weak or drooping eyelid, lessened or no perspiration on one side of the face, and a smaller pupil in one eye; pain in the shoulder or upper chest; weakening of hand muscles; or bone pain or fracture. An accumulation of fluid in the pleural space (shown in Figure 1-2), can cause symptoms of several different types of cancer.

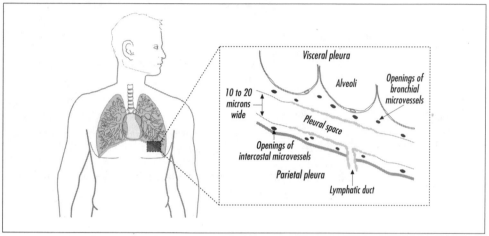

Figure 1-2. Pleural structures of the chest and lungs

Common sites of distant spread

Lung cancer tends to spread to certain organs more often than it does to others: liver, brain, spine, pelvis, nearby lymph nodes, and the adrenal glands. These organs are depicted in Figure 1-3.

Rare symptoms of metastasis

Rare symptoms of metastasis include:

- Lumps in or beneath the skin
- Protrusion of the eyes
- Eyelid tumors
- Perforation of the bowel experienced as severe abdominal pain with fever

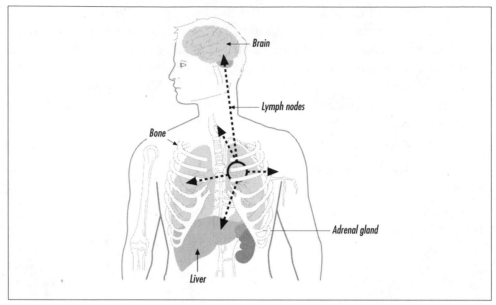

Figure 1-3. Common sites of metastasis

- Acute pancreatitis experienced as severe abdominal pain and swings in blood sugar levels

- A lump in a salivary gland

- A lump in one tonsil

- A breast lump

- Bleeding in the gastrointestinal tract detectable with fecal occult testing

Kathleen Houlihan describes her earliest symptoms and the misdiagnoses that followed:

> *Last summer in July, my left shoulder started hurting. When it still hurt after a couple of weeks, I went to my doctor. He recommended ibuprofen and several exercises. When it still hurt a month later, he recommended physical therapy. A month later, I saw an orthopedic surgeon, who said I did not need surgery, but just to wait it out: "That's why they call it a pain in the neck, because it takes a long time to heal." He also recommended an x-ray. But I have $5,000 deductible insurance, so I didn't want to waste money on an x-ray for a muscle problem!*
>
> *Then came the holidays, then tax training class in January. Then back to the doctor in February. He recommended either MRI, a neurologist, a*

different orthopedic doctor, or more physical therapy. I didn't want to spend money on any of them, but I was considering the options when I started coughing up a little blood. My husband Holt and I were taking a long weekend trip that weekend, and I was trying to ignore it, so I didn't call the doctor until eight days later. He said I really should get an x-ray, but to conserve money, I could take a tuberculosis test first.

That evening, I came down with a fever and started feeling sick. The next day I went in to the doctor. The regular doctor was out, but the associate diagnosed me with a sinus infection, even though I didn't have any sinus pain. She said she could see yellow junk in my sinuses, and the coughing of blood would be consistent with a sinus infection—drainage and coughing up. She gave me an antibiotic. My activity level went down and the coughing of blood stopped for several days; as I got more active, it resumed. But Holt was about to leave town and we were getting ready for that, so there was another delay of about a week.

The day after he left, I finally went for a chest x-ray, where this tennis ball tumor (7 × 8 centimeters) showed up. That's what had been causing the pain. I had a CT scan the same day. I got the results that afternoon that it could be malignant, or fungal, or tuberculosis. They couldn't really tell without a biopsy.

Holt flew back from West Virginia the next day, and we saw a different doctor on Monday. On Tuesday, he scheduled a biopsy for the following Tuesday. On Wednesday, we got the results that it is an adenocarcinoma of the lung (non-small cell lung cancer).

Symptoms in tumor-free organs

Ten to twenty percent of lung cancer patients experience symptoms or groups of symptoms (syndromes) in organs that are neither invaded by nor obstructed by the tumor. These findings are known as paraneoplastic syndromes. In some instances they appear early in the development of lung cancer and might trigger early diagnosis.

Investigators believe paraneoplastic syndromes are caused by various substances released by tumors (such as hormones; hormone-like proteins; bioactivators called cytokines; and proteins released by white blood cells called antibodies) or by differences in the availability of critical metabolic substances, such as iron.

Some paraneoplastic syndromes are rare. Some can be caused by other cancers or other illnesses in addition to lung cancer. Not all subtypes of lung cancer are capable of causing all of the paraneoplastic syndromes.

The most common paraneoplastic syndromes in non-small cell lung cancer patients are:

- Hypercalcemia (high blood calcium levels). Overstimulated parathyroid glands or cytokines released by the tumor (such as tumor necrosis factor, interleukin-1, or transforming growth factor alfa) and some prostaglandins might recruit too much calcium from bone into the blood. Another possible cause of hypercalcemia is invasion of bone by a tumor. The many symptoms associated with hypercalcemia are described in the section "Hormonal (endocrine) syndromes."

- Excess growth of certain bones, especially in fingertips (hypertrophic osteoarthropathy).

- Blood clots.

- Excess breast growth in men (gynecomastia).

The most common paraneoplastic syndromes in small cell lung cancer patients are:

- Syndrome of inappropriate antidiuretic hormone (SIADH), causing low blood levels of sodium. SIADH is caused by secretion of antidiuretic hormone by the tumor. Antidiuretic hormone, also called vasopressin, acts on the kidney to lower levels of sodium in the blood (hyponatremia). The many symptoms associated with SIADH are described in the section "Hormonal (endocrine) syndromes."

- Blood clots.

- Loss of balance and unsteady arm and leg motion (cerebellar degeneration).

The sections that follow, organized by body system, describe these and other paraneoplastic syndromes in detail.

Blood (hematologic) syndromes

Certain lung cancer tumors produce hormones, antibodies, or cytokines that can disrupt the normal growth and activity of red blood cells, white blood cells, or platelets. In other instances, blood imbalances might be caused by iron deficiency or chemotherapy. These imbalances might manifest as:

- Excessive numbers of platelets (thrombocytosis), causing blood clots

- Too few or poorly functioning platelets, causing bruises and tiny "blood blisters" (thrombocytopenic purpura)

- Irregular growth, appearance, or untimely destruction of red blood cells (polycythemia, hemolytic anemia, or red-cell aplasia), causing fatigue

- Abnormal levels or functions of blood proteins (dysproteinemia), causing fatigue, headache, or dizziness

- Abnormal white blood cell production or function (leukemoid reaction or eosinophilia), causing fevers, fatigue, or perhaps no symptoms at all

Vein and artery (vascular) syndromes

Certain types of lung tumors can affect the circulatory system as follows:

- Thrombophlebitis, an inflammation in an artery or vein caused by a blood clot

- Arterial thrombosis, a blood clot in an artery

- Nonbacterial thrombotic endocarditis (NBTE), a deposition of material onto the valves of the heart

Skin (cutaneous) syndromes

Various skin conditions are associated with some cases of lung cancer. These conditions are thought to be caused by aberrant behavior of white blood cells and their antibodies, reacting either to the tumor or to substances produced by the tumor:

- Chronic inflammation of the skin (dermatomyositis), which often occurs in conjunction with muscle and subcutaneous tissue inflammation.

- Gray-black warty patches on the elbows, knees, armpits, or groin (acanthosis nigricans).

- Itching (pruritis).

- Chronic red patches (erythema multiforme).

- Dark patches (hyperpigmentation).

- Hives (urticaria).

- Scaly patches (scleroderma).

- New tissue growth in fingertips (digital clubbing)—a widening and rounding of the fingertips and nails, and, when fingers are viewed from the side, a loss of normal indentation where the fingernail emerges from the skin. Clubbing, shown in Figure 1-4, is sometimes classified as a musculoskeletal change.

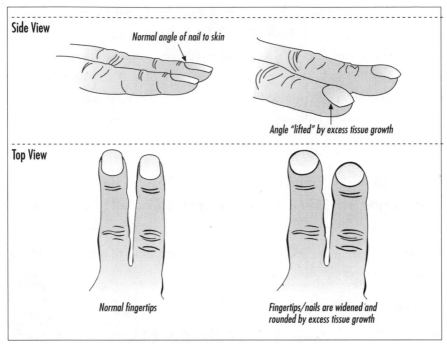

Side View

Normal angle of nail to skin

Angle "lifted" by excess tissue growth

Top View

Normal fingertips

Fingertips/nails are widened and rounded by excess tissue growth

Figure 1-4. Clubbing of digits

Muscle and skeleton syndromes

Certain lung tumors can cause the following symptoms by producing hormones or causing unusual tissue growth:

- Inflamed muscles, skin, and subcutaneous tissue (polymyositis-dermatomyositis). Thought by some researchers to be a paraneoplastic syndrome. Some researchers believe this finding justifies intensive testing for presence of malignancy; other studies have found no link between malignancy and this syndrome.

- Abnormal bone growth in certain bones, especially fingertips (hypertrophic osteoarthropathy). This abnormal bone growth is visible on x-rays and bone scans, and might be associated with bone or joint pain.

- Softening of the bones (osteomalacia) or occurrence of fractures.

- Various painful or dysfunctional muscular symptoms (myopathy).

Nervous system (neurologic) syndromes

Some or most of the paraneoplastic syndromes that affect the nervous system appear to be caused by an attack of antibodies against healthy tissue. Antibodies are white blood cell proteins that normally sequester and immobilize foreign tissue, such as viruses or bacteria. Neurologic syndromes include:

- Cerebellar degeneration, causing problems with balance or unsteady arm and leg movements

- Lambert-Eaton myasthenic syndrome (LEMS), characterized by muscle weakness and dysfunction, especially in the pelvis and thighs; and at times joint soreness, difficulty swallowing, and other symptoms resembling myasathenia gravis

- Peripheral neuropathy, evidenced by pain, tingling, or numbness in hands or feet

- Encephalopathy, an infection or inflammation in the brain

- Myelopathy, presenting as back pain or tenderness or bone marrow dysfunction

- Psychosis, mimicking such mental illnesses as schizophrenia or bipolar disorder

- Dementia

- Pseudo-obstruction of the bowel, including nausea, vomiting, abdominal pain, and changed bowel habits

- Rarely, visual changes (retinopathy)

- Flushing or sweating on one side of the body (Harlequin syndrome)

Hormonal (endocrine) syndromes

Certain types of lung cancers are capable of producing hormones that act on organs within the brain (the pituitary and hypothalamus) or upon other organs, such as the kidneys, adrenal glands, thyroid, ovaries, or testes. Some lung cancers, particularly SCLC, can affect the endocrine glands (as seen in Figure 1-5), producing unusual symptoms.

These hormones may cause the following conditions to occur:

- Syndrome of inappropriate antidiuretic hormone (SIADH), resulting in low levels of sodium in the blood. Often associated with small cell lung cancer and sometimes with bronchial carcinoid tumors. Symptoms include:
    - Fatigue
    - Loss of appetite

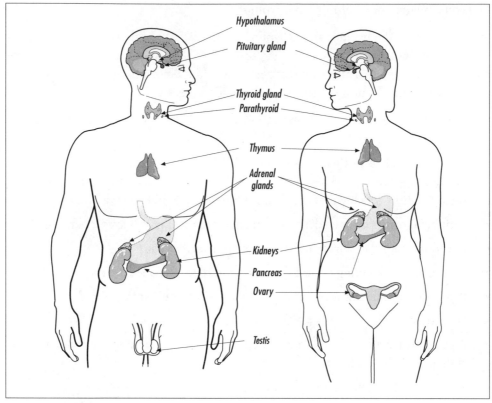

Figure 1-5. The endocrine glands

- – Muscle cramps or weakness

- – Nausea

- – Vomiting

- – Restlessness and confusion

- – Seizures

- – Coma

- – Respiratory arrest

- High blood calcium levels (hypercalcemia). Symptoms are:

  - – Loss of appetite

  - – Nausea and vomiting

  - – Lethargy and weakness

  - – Irregular pulse

- Irritability
- Frequent urination
- Excessive thirst
- Confusion and coma
- Dehydration
- Constipation

- Cushing's syndrome, an overproduction of adrenal hormones by cancerous tissue. The most common symptoms in lung cancer patients are weight loss, fluid retention (edema), muscle weakness (myopathy), and high blood pressure (hypertension). Less common Cushing's symptoms in lung cancer patients are stretch marks (striae), obesity in the trunk with thinning of arms and legs, a moon-shaped face, a fatty hump on the back of the neck ("buffalo hump"), bone loss, diabetes, and moodiness.

- Carcinoid syndrome, characterized by skin flushing, diarrhea, and wheezing or asthma symptoms.

- High or low blood sugar (hyper- or hypoglycemia).

- Breast growth in males (gynecomastia).

- Discharge of milk from the nipple (galactorrhea).

- Excess levels of growth hormone, possibly linked to excessive bone growth or clubbing of fingers.

- Excess calcitonin secretion, usually symptomless.

- Excess levels of thyroid-stimulating hormone, possibly causing symptoms of hyperthyroidism. These symptoms include high blood pressure, heat intolerance, hair loss, moodiness, and weight loss.

Miscellaneous syndromes

Several syndromes sometimes associated with lung cancer are not classified within other groups:

- High levels of uric acid in the blood (hyperuricemia), causing joint pain
- Nephrotic syndrome, heralded by fluid retention in various body parts, weight gain, high blood pressure, and poor appetite
- Weight loss in spite of adequate nutrition (cachexia)
- Fever

Summary

Lung cancer symptoms can range from absent to profound. Many patients have difficulty finding doctors who can recognize the more unusual symptoms of lung cancer. Knowledge and persistence are needed to obtain a correct diagnosis in a timely manner.

CHAPTER 2

Diagnosis and Staging

To learn how to treat a disease, one must learn
how to diagnose it. The diagnosis is the best trump
in the scheme of treatment.

—Jean Martin Charcot

THERE ARE MANY DIAGNOSTIC TESTS used to detect lung cancer and its spread. This chapter enumerates these complex tests and their purposes and describes the very critical and detailed staging process. Experiencing these complex tests is described in Appendix B, *Tests and Procedures*.

Before we discuss diagnosis and staging in detail, it's important to note that the process of discovering cancer is, by most people's accounts, associated with great emotional upheaval. At the end of this chapter we discuss the emotional tumult associated with diagnosis and the range of responses that one might have.

General information

Several issues arise with almost all medical tests and should be considered beforehand.

Pain control

It's not unusual to feel nervous about tests. You have the right to ask for and receive pain medication before any potentially painful test is administered. Various pain-controlling medications can be requested in advance, such as the injected sedative Demerol; the sedative and brief amnesiac Versed, also injected; the topical cream EMLA, which contains the drug Xylocaine, familiar to us from dental care; throat sprays and gargles; or the short-acting antianxiety tablet Ativan.

Many tests done today require that you lie on a table for extended periods while cameras and x-ray machines do imaging. Get comfortable for this opportunity to nap by asking for extra blankets and finding a position that you can maintain pain-free for long periods. Ask for pillows to support your back and knees if you suffer from back pain.

Unnecessary testing

Become aware of alternatives to testing. For tests about which you feel unaware or uneasy, ask the following:

- Why is this procedure or test necessary? Will it change my treatment plan?

- Is there a safer or more comfortable alternative?

- What are the risks and side effects?

- How will pain be controlled?

- Can you please explain this procedure to me or provide me with literature that describes it thoroughly?

- How experienced is the technician or doctor performing this procedure?

Inform and be informed

Never assume that hospital staff members are fully aware of your circumstances. Always tell the technicians doing tests that you are a lung cancer survivor. Tell them of any other health problems or allergies you have, such as previous allergic reactions to the iodine in shrimp; of any prescribed or over-the-counter medications you are taking; and of your previous surgeries.

Timely results

To spare yourself agonized waiting, you should discuss in advance with your treatment team how test results will be relayed to you. Some patients mistakenly assume that their doctors will take the initiative and contact them, when in fact it may be the doctor's policy that the patient should take the initiative and call for results. Be aware that some physicians are reluctant to leave test results on an answering machine without assurance from you that this is not a violation of your privacy. In addition, many ancillary doctors involved in your testing may choose, for ethical reasons, to communicate only with your primary oncologist or surgeon unless instructed otherwise.

Physical examination

A thorough physical examination is always performed as part of diagnostic testing for lung cancer. Vital statistics and a full patient history of lifestyle choices and symptoms are recorded.

Diagnostic tests

The first test normally done when lung cancer is suspected is a chest x-ray. As the diagnostic process unfolds, subsequent tests might be chosen or discarded based on results of prior tests.

A lung cancer survivor recalls the process of his diagnosis:

> In 1997, I had pneumonia and was hospitalized for fourteen days. At the end of that time, I still wasn't breathing right. The pulmonary doctor sent me in for a CT scan and put a needle in my lung. He felt something going on. When the needle hit the mass, blood came out of my nose and mouth. However, he didn't find any malignancy.
>
> Next winter, I went to Tucson and noticed I spit up small amounts of blood. I went back to pulmonary specialist—a different one. I had been losing energy, had less breathing capacity, and was coughing.
>
> In June, the doctor went down my throat to look at the mass. He said that he was afraid to touch the mass because of the risk of bleeding. Said that I might suffocate in my own blood. Said that he didn't see any other options but surgery. He didn't know if the mass was cancerous or not.

Body fluid analysis

As of this writing, sputum is the body fluid most often tested for lung cancer. Sputum analysis involves the collection of mucus and fluid from the lungs for microscopic examination seeking tumor cells. This technique is not always sensitive enough to detect lung cancer, however, because some lung tumors do not shed cells into sputum (false negatives) and other bodily processes can cause the contents of sputum to appear cancerous (false positives).

Markers for cancer called *tumor markers*, detectable in blood or other body fluids, are being studied. The goal is to identify very early markers for lung cancer that are found in easily collected body fluids.

Imaging studies

Imaging studies exploit the fact that tumors differ in appearance from normal tissue under certain conditions. Imaging studies include:

- **Radiographic studies (x-rays).** A chest x-ray is usually the first test done to diagnose lung cancer.

- **Computed tomography (CT).** Numerous thin x-ray images are assembled into a detailed image by computer. A new form of CT, called spiral or helical scanning, that more accurately images three dimensions, has in some studies found very early lung cancers.

- **Magnetic resonance imaging (MRI).** An imaging of tissues that respond differently to magnetic waves. Anomalies in soft tissue, such as brain tissue, are often seen better with MRI than with CT.

- **Positron emission tomography (PET).** An assessment of the uptake of mildly radioactive glucose, ammonia, water, methionine, or other metabolic agent bytissue suspected to be cancerous. Cancerous tissue often metabolizes these agents more rapidly than does healthy tissue.

- **Bone scan.** This is done with or without contrast agents, using a camera sensitive to bone density or to scintigraphic contrast agents.

- **Antibody scanning (radioimmunoscintigraphy) and other nuclear scans.** The concentration of the contrast agent in specific areas of the body can be detected with special imaging devices, such as CT, single proton emission computed tomography (SPECT), or a gamma camera.

- **Ultrasonography (ultrasound).** The mapping of organs, using echoes from sound waves, might be performed on the thyroid, adrenals, liver, kidneys, chest wall, or other organs to determine the cause of unusual symptoms and delineate the spread of disease.

Endoscopy

Endoscopy is the use of very small cameras, fiber optics, microscopes, and biopsy instruments to view and sample tissue in internal organs. These instruments are guided through natural body openings or very small incisions, then manipulated within the body remotely via controls channeled through a narrow tube.

Typical endoscopy techniques for lung cancer include:

- **Bronchoscopy.** The endoscope is passed through the nose down into one of the two bronchial tubes. Injectable fluorescent substances, exploitation of auto-fluorescence of cancerous tissue, tissue sampling, needle biopsy, bronchial washing, or ultrasound might be performed with bronchoscopy.

- **Thoracoscopy or video-assisted thoracic surgery** (VATS). Lung tissue is visualized using an endoscope inserted through a small incision in the chest wall. Tissue can be removed for analysis using either a stapler or a laser.

- **Mediastinoscopy.** To sample lymph nodes in the mediastinum (the central portion of the chest between the lungs that contains all other chest organs), an endoscope is inserted through an incision just below the collar line.

Note that lung cancer specialists do not always agree on the map of lymph nodes and the tissues they drain. Some specialists might consider involvement of certain mid-chest lymph nodes (shown in Figure 2-1) to indicate one-sided disease, whereas others would consider it to indicate both sides of the chest.

Kathy recalls the tests and waiting when her husband Marty was admitted to the hospital to find the cause of his pain:

> It was our understanding that the admission was for 24-hour observation and some tests. The doctor made some comment to us about not wanting to get into trouble with the insurance company, so he had to figure out what was wrong within that time. They did an MRI and nothing showed up, but they also did a chest CT, and this time a thickening appeared, which they said was a pleural effusion. So they had reason to keep him in the hospital and they brought in the pulmonary doctor who had seen him when he was in the hospital at the end of June. They tested him for a blood clot in the lung, but found nothing.
>
> Then they did a bronchoscopy, looking for cancer. The pulmonary doctor said he took out a lot of tissue and stuff to do biopsies on. We had to wait until Monday for the results. That was a long weekend.
>
> During this whole time, our family doctor (not the insurance doctors) came to check on Marty every day except the weekend. I don't even know if our insurance doctors knew he was in the hospital. The neurologist remained as the admitting doctor, and I suspect he was pushing the insurance company to keep Marty there. He was in so much pain that releasing him would have been ridiculous, and we couldn't have gotten the testing done as quickly.

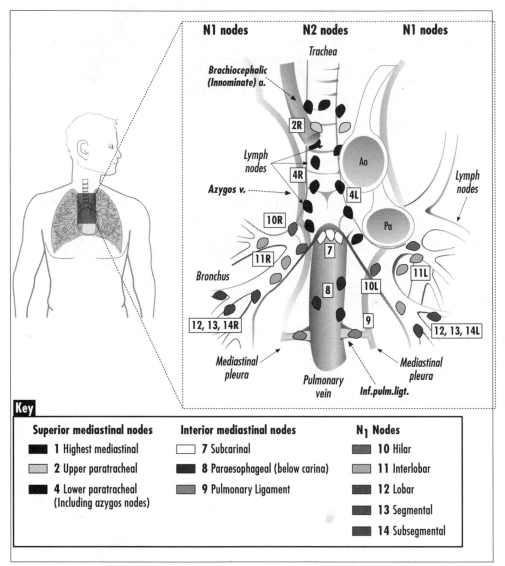

Figure 2-1. Locoregional lymph nodes of the lungs, copied with permission from Clifton Mountain, MD. (N2 lymph nodes (highest mediastinal), 3 (prevascular and retrotracheal), 5 (subaortic), and 6 (para-aoritic) are not shown in this diagram.)

When the biopsy came back negative, exploratory surgery was done:

> *On Monday, the pulmonary doctor told us all the biopsies were negative. I could tell he was still thinking and I don't remember what he said, but I knew there would be more tests. I guess at this point I started*

to believe that maybe this was just an infection because the biopsies were negative. Of course, every day I was on the Internet trying to get information about pleural effusions, which were caused by congestive heart failure, cancer, or infection.

Tuesday morning, the pulmonary doctor tells us he has arranged for a thoracic surgeon to do exploratory surgery of the outside of the lung, a thoracoscopy. He told me he had to talk the surgeon into doing the surgery because the surgeon didn't think the surgery would work. The surgeon thought the lung would be adhered to the chest wall. I didn't ask why he thought that, and I didn't quite understand why that was a possibility. We waited all day to go to surgery. Finally, at 4:30 they came for Marty.

I waited by myself in the waiting room. There was another family (at least six of them) waiting anxiously for the mother (sister, daughter, whatever) to get out of emergency gallbladder surgery. They were bothersome to me; they talked too much, they were so worked up over gallbladder surgery, but I kept telling myself that at that time, they didn't know that other people were having surgery for much worse reasons and to them, this was a terrible situation.

At 8:00, the surgeon comes in to talk to me. In the little consultation room, he tells me the lung collapsed like it was supposed to, and he could clearly see everything, and it was malignant. I just looked at him. I'm thinking, "It's supposed to be an infection." I said, "Are you sure?" He said yes, he was sure, he had seen it before many times and he was sure, but he took samples to be biopsied to see if it was treatable or not. I asked him not to tell Marty until the biopsies came back in two days.

Blood testing

Blood drawn from an arm vein is analyzed as part of the diagnosis of lung cancer. Tests performed are:

- Liver function
- Lactate dehydrogenase
- Alkaline phosphatase
- Kidney function
- Blood cell counts
- Hormone levels

- Antibody levels

- Electrolyte counts

Normal values are described in Appendix C, *Test Results*.

Needle biopsy (fine needle aspiration)

Needle biopsy is a technique for removing part of a suspicious mass or fluid to determine if cancerous cells are present. Often, a CT scan or ultrasound is used simultaneously to view the mass so targeting is accurate. Needle biopsies collect samples only—they do not remove all cancerous cells and are not intended to cure disease. For lung cancer, the following needle biopsies are common:

- **Transbronchial needle aspiration.** Inserting a thin needle into lymph nodes near the lung via a bronchoscope, as discussed previously. The sampling of lymph nodes nearest the tumor, but outside the lung, allows more accurate staging of disease without invasive surgery.

- **Percutaneous needle biopsy.** Inserting a thin needle into a suspicious mass through the skin of the chest wall (transthoracic) or abdominal wall and withdrawing a small portion of the mass.

- **Bone marrow biopsy.** Removing a small core of bone and marrow, usually from the back of the hip, using a hollow needle.

- **Liver biopsy.** Inserting a thin needle into the suspicious mass through the abdomen and withdrawing a small portion of it. Liver biopsy is a form of percutaneous needle biopsy.

- **Needle aspiration.** Aspirating fluid in the abdomen or chest (pleural effusion or ascites) to search for cancer cells.

- **Lumbar puncture (spinal tap).** Obtaining spinal fluid for analysis, if spread of cancer to the central nervous system is suspected.

Thoracentesis

If you have fluid collecting between the lungs and the chest wall, your doctor will probably want to examine it to see if it contains cancerous cells. A procedure resembling needle biopsy, called thoracentesis, will be performed to extract some fluid for laboratory analysis.

Pathology

Cancer cells are not uniform, although cancer cells of the same type of lung cancer might have some similar characteristics, such as size. Cancer cells can have different behavioral characteristics, such as aggressiveness; that is, the number of times they divide in a given period of time. Pathologic analyses enable doctors to diagnose the cancer's type precisely and determine characteristics of the cancer, both of which contribute to informed recommendations for effective treatment. There are several methods for examining cancer cells to determine their type, behavior, and potential response to treatment:

- **Cytology.** The examination of internal components of cells under a light microscope or electron microscope. For lung cancer, sputum cytology is used to find cancerous cells in phlegm to determine their type and other characteristics, such as aggressiveness.

- **Immunocytology.** The determination of which of several characteristic immune system markers the cell carries on its surface. This information is useful in predicting how the cell might respond to some of the newer therapies (many of which are still in clinical trials) or how aggressive the cancer might be.

- **Histology.** The examination of many intact cells in a cluster under a light microscope or electron microscope. When large enough samples of cells are obtained, as is the case with most endoscopic procedures or surgical excision, histologic analyses are performed. Histology is useful because a cell's behavior often correlates with its overall appearance, but many investigators believe that newer technologies, such as immunocytology and cytogenetics, will provide more meaningful information in the future.

- **Cytogenetics.** Many genetic changes occur in lung cancer cells. The direct examination of genetic material in cancer cells retrieved by sputum collection or biopsy is called cytogenetics. The goal is the recognition of these changes early enough in the development of disease to effect a cure. Please see Chapter 5, *What Is Lung Cancer?,* for progress in analyzing genetic changes that might enable early detection. See Appendix E, *Experimental Prognostic Markers*, for genetic changes that might affect the outcome of disease and treatment.

Diagnosis without open surgery

Several tests used in diagnosis, particularly endoscopic biopsies, can offer very sound information about how far disease has spread and what kind of cancer exists. Minimally invasive endoscopic biopsies of suspected lung cancer are performed whenever feasible.

If imaging studies and endoscopic biopsies indicate that additional surgery would not be useful in your case, the staging done based on these tests is considered conclusive and is used to plan your treatment. Preliminary tests might indicate that further surgery is necessary for diagnosis, though.

Diagnostic surgery

Chest surgery known as thoracotomy might be performed to obtain tissue samples for diagnosis or with curative intent. Thoracotomy is considered the least invasive of the open-chest surgeries used for lung cancer.

Open-chest surgeries that are more extensive than thoracotomy usually are not done simply for diagnosis. When they are performed as part of a plan for a cure, additional biopsy material will be collected during surgery so the type and stage of cancer can be determined as accurately as possible. Appropriate uses of thoracotomy and other surgical procedures as treatment are discussed in Chapter 7, *Types of Treatment*.

Surgical pretesting

Chest surgery is a significant medical procedure that taxes your heart and lungs during and after surgery. If your doctor determines that thoracotomy is necessary to diagnose your illness, you will be given additional tests to determine if your heart and one or both lungs can withstand surgery and function adequately after surgery.

These tests are detailed in Appendix B, *Tests and Procedures*.

- Spirometry and other lung volume tests

- Measures of lung gas exchange

- Perfusion/ventilation radionuclide tests

- Exercise testing (stress EKG)

Postoperative diagnosis

If you require surgery to diagnose lung cancer, the surgeon's close examination of all surrounding tissue and the retrieval of additional biopsy material will contribute additional information for either confirming or correcting your diagnosis and stage. For example, lymph nodes near the lung that appeared enlarged on imaging studies might upon pathologic examination be unaffected by tumor infiltration. Thus, staging in this rare instance might be revised downward to an earlier stage.

A male survivor of lung cancer describes his surgery and staging:

> I went in for surgery in July. The tumor was in my right lung. I saw the x-rays and CT scan. Before I gave the surgeon the go-ahead to go in, I questioned him about how far he was going to go. He said I'd have to leave it to his best judgement; he wasn't able to promise me anything until he saw what he was up against. I asked if he was the best surgeon in Omaha for the job; he said he was.
>
> The surgeon ended up taking three-quarters of my lung. He also took 12 lymph nodes; 4 were malignant. They were concerned about some mediastinal nodes that they couldn't remove. They used chemotherapy and radiation to go after those nodes.

Type, stage, and grade

After a lung cancer is confirmed, there may be some question about which type of lung cancer exists; how far it has spread, called stage; and how aggressive it is, called grade.

It is extremely important that your disease be identified correctly and staged so the best treatment can be planned. All biopsies of tumor tissue should be reviewed by an experienced pathologist to be certain that tumor type is identified correctly. If your biopsy material is reviewed by a pathologist in a community hospital, have a second review done by a pathologist at a university hospital, at a National Cancer Institute-designated regional cancer, or at the National Cancer Institute (NCI) in Bethesda, Maryland.

WHO/IASLC classification system

Knowing your lung cancer type gives you a way to compare your diagnosis and recommended treatments to reports in the literature and descriptions of clinical trials. It also gives you the vocabulary you need to speak unambiguously with medical professionals who might not already be familiar with your case. Be certain to obtain copies of all medical records, especially pathology reports. Note that occasionally a person will be diagnosed with a mixture of subtypes, or with simultaneous small cell and non-small cell lung cancers.

The most recent World Health Organization/International Association for the Study of Lung Cancer (WHO/IASLC) classification system describes lung cancers as follows:

- Preinvasive Lesions

    - Squamous dysplasia/carcinoma in situ

    - Atypical adenomatous hyperplasia

    - Diffuse idiopathic pulmonary neuroendocrine cell hyperplasia

- Squamous cell carcinoma

    - Variants: papillary, clear cell, small cell, and basaloid

- Small cell carcinoma (older name: oat cell)

    - Combined small cell carcinoma

- Adenocarcinoma

    - Acinar

    - Papillary

    - Bronchioloalveolar carcinoma: nonmucinous, mucinous, mixed mucinous and nonmucinous, or indeterminate

    - Solid adenocarcinoma with mucin

    - Adenocarcinoma with mixed subtypes. Variants: well-differentiated fetal adenocarcinoma, mucinous (colloid) adenocarcinoma, mucinous cystadenocarcinoma, signet ring adenocarcinoma, and clear cell adenocarcinoma

    - Large cell carcinoma. Variants: large cell neuroendocrine carcinoma, combined large cell neuroendocrine carcinoma, basaloid carcinoma, lymphoepithelioma-like carcinoma, clear cell carcinoma, or large cell carcinoma with rhabdoid phenotype

    - Adenosquamous carcinoma

    - Carcinomas with pleomorphic, sarcomatoid, or sarcomatous elements: carcinosarcoma, pulmonary blastoma, other, and carcinomas with spindle and/or giant cells: pleomorphic carcinoma, spindle cell carcinoma, or giant cell carcinoma

- Carcinoid tumor: typical carcinoid or atypical carcinoid
- Carcinomas of salivary gland type: mucoepidermoid carcinoma, adenoid cystic carcinoma, and others
- Unclassified carcinoma

Staging lung cancer

Staging is a way of describing how far cancer has spread from the original tumor so correct treatment can be chosen for the best outcome. Staging via surgery (pTNM) is considered more accurate than staging using symptoms and imaging studies (cTNM), but lung cancer patients with clear presurgical evidence of widespread disease usually are not staged via surgery that would contribute little new information to staging information or to cure.

Staging of small cell and non-small cell lung cancer is accomplished using two distinct systems, each discussed more fully in the following sections.

For both small cell and non-small cell lung cancer, the staging systems currently in use are considered by some researchers and oncologists to be largely useful, but still less than perfect. Many cancer specialists incorporate additional clinical measures—age, other health problems, or the ability to do everyday things—to discuss the effect of disease and its probable outcome more accurately. In the discussion that follows, these differences are noted.

Staging non-small cell lung cancer

In 1997, the American Joint Committee on Cancer and the Union Internationale Contre le Cancer adopted the Revised International System for Staging Lung Cancer to assign patients to more specific categories so treatment, prognostic information, and statistics would be more accurate.

Non-small cell lung cancer is staged at levels I through IV, with higher levels connoting more widely spread disease. Spread is assessed using three gauges: primary tumor characteristics (abbreviated T), lymph node involvement (N), and metastasis (M) to other organs. A value is assigned to each of these characteristics. The cancer is then described as a combination of these characteristics (for example, T2, N1, M0), and an overall stage is assigned based on the combination.

The levels of staging used for non-small cell lung cancer are only guidelines, subject to reinterpretation and modification by your treatment team, based on the unique characteristics of your illness and the team's training and experience.

Proximal, distal, ipsilateral, and contralateral

In the sections that follow, you'll see the words proximal, distal, ipsilateral, and contralateral. Ipsilateral means "same side"; contralateral means "opposite side." Proximal and distal mean *near* and *far*, respectively, but their meaning in a given instance is determined by context. For instance, if a bronchial tumor is described simply as proximal, the intent is that it is located closer to the top of your body where the bronchi branch away from the trachea. If a tumor is described as proximal or distal to some other lung structure, though, the described location is not relative to the top of your airway, but to that other lung structure.

TNM staging definitions

The following 1997 tumor/lymph node/metastasis (TNM) staging definitions have been adapted from the second edition of Harvey Pass's book *Lung Cancer: Principles and Practice* (Lippincott, 2000) and the National Cancer Institute's June 1999 version of the physicians' treatment statement for non-small cell lung cancer, available at the NCI's web site, *http://cancernet.nci.nih.gov/clinpdq/soa.html*. You might find Figure 1-1, in Chapter 1, *Symptoms of Lung Cancer*, helpful in understanding these terms.

T: primary tumor

The characteristics of the primary tumor are defined as TX, T0, Tis, T1, T2, T3, or T4, depending on size and where it is found:

- TX (occult stage). The primary tumor cannot be assessed, or the tumor has been proven only by detecting malignant cells in sputum (phlegm) or in bronchial washings, but the tumor is not visible with imaging or bronchoscopy.

- T0. No evidence of a primary tumor can be found.

- Tis (carcinoma in situ). A lung tumor that has not yet invaded other tissue has been found contained within a few layers of localized cells.

- T1. A tumor that is 3 centimeters or smaller in its largest dimension was found, surrounded by normal lung tissue or normal tissue of the sac that lines the lung (the visceral pleura). There is no bronchoscopic evidence of invasion closer to the main bronchial tube than the lobar bronchus, a branch of the main bronchus. A rare superficial tumor of any size, however, with its invasive portion limited to the bronchial wall, and that might extend upward toward the main bronchus, also is considered T1. (Note that some researchers consider 5 centimeters rather than 3 to be critical size.)

- T2. A tumor with any of the following features of size or extent:
  - Larger than 3 centimeters in its largest dimension. (Note that some researchers consider 5 centimeters rather than 3 to be critical size.)
  - Involving the main bronchus, at least 2 centimeters away from (distal to) the carina, a ridge-shaped formation of the trachea where it branches in two to become the bronchial tubes.
  - Invading the sac that lines the lung (the visceral pleura). Some researchers say that invasion of the innermost elastic pleura or the next layer, parietal pleura, should not be considered automatic designators for T2 or T3 status, as they are today. Worse prognosis is associated with deeper invasion; they believe these shallower tumors should be classified as T1 and T2, respectively.[1]
  - Associated with lung collapse (atelectasis) or with obstructive pneumonitis that extends to the hilar region (the opening on the surface of the lung through which the bronchus, nerves, and blood vessels pass), but does not involve the entire lung.

- T3. A tumor of any size that:
  - Is in either of the main bronchi (the two tubes that lead from the trachea into the lungs) that is less than 2 centimeters away from (distal to) the carina (a ridge-shaped formation of the trachea where it branches in two to become the bronchial tubes), but without involvement of the carina; or
  - Is associated with lung collapse (atelectasis) or obstructive pneumonitis of the entire lung; or
  - Directly invades any of the following: the chest wall, including tumors that form in the groove in the upper lung and its sac through which runs a major artery (superior sulcus tumors); the muscle separating the chest and abdomen (the diaphragm); the parts of the two sacs containing the lungs that lie in the center of the chest (mediastinal pleura); the thick outer wall of the sac containing the heart (parietal pericardium); the phrenic nerve, if a direct extension of the primary tumor and no T4 criteria are met; or the main arterial and venous trunks that are not the "great vessels" (see T4).

- T4. A tumor of any size that:

  - Invades any of the following: the center of the chest between the two sacs containing the lungs; that is, the part of the chest in which all organs other than the lungs are located (the mediastinum)—some researchers consider invasion of fat only to indicate lower stage; the heart; the great blood vessels of the chest (aorta, superior vena cava, inferior vena cava, main pulmonary artery, intrapericardial portions of the trunk of the right and left pulmonary arteries, and intrapericardial portions of the superior or inferior right or left pulmonary veins); the windpipe (trachea); the esophagus; the spine (vertebral body); the ridgelike connection between the trachea and the two bronchial tubes (carina); or the portion of the vagus nerve known as the recurrent laryngeal nerve.

  - Has separate "satellite" tumor nodules in the same lobe of the lung.

  - Is a tumor releasing fluid that contains cancer cells (malignant pleural effusion) into the chest. Most pleural effusions associated with lung cancer are cancerous. There are a few patients, though, in whom repeated examination of this fluid shows no evidence of cancer cells. When these findings and the doctor's opinion indicate that the effusion is not related to cancer, pleural effusion might be excluded as a staging element and the patient might be staged as T1, T2, or T3.

- Some researchers include tumors invading the superior sulcus that trigger Pancoast syndrome to be T4, not T3.

N: regional lymph nodes

Lymph nodes are part of the lymphatic system, a fluid-filled series of ducts and nodules that parallel the bloodstream and trap foreign bodies and infectious agents so the immune system can destroy them. The spread of many (but not all) cancers includes spreading via lymphatic ducts. Consequently, for many cancer types, key lymph nodes or all lymph nodes in a region are examined using a variety of tools to determine if they harbor cancer. Note that some researchers believe that mapping of chest lymph nodes and the areas they drain as used today is inadequate to truly determine N status:

- NX. Regional lymph nodes cannot be assessed.

- N0. No spread (metastasis) of the lung tumor to regional lymph nodes.

- N1. Metastasis to same-side (ipsilateral) lymph nodes near the bronchial tube and/or to ipsilateral hilar lymph nodes (nodes near the opening on the surface of the lung through which the bronchus, nerves, and blood vessels pass) and to intrapulmonary nodes, including involvement by direct extension of the primary tumor.

- N2. Metastasis to same-side (ipsilateral) mediastinal and/or subcarinal lymph node(s).

- N3. Metastasis to opposite-side (contralateral) mediastinal, contralateral hilar, ipsilateral or contralateral scalene, or supraclavicular lymph node(s).

M: distant metastasis

Distant metastasis is the growth of one or more tumors into organs relatively far from the lung. For lung cancer, the liver, brain, adrenals, and bone (spine, ribs, and legs) are the most common sites of metastasis. Some researchers believe that a subcategory should be created to describe a single metastasis to just one organ. The stages are:

- MX. Distant metastasis cannot be assessed.

- M0. No distant metastasis.

- M1. Distant metastasis present. M1 includes separate tumor(s) in a different lobe of the lung, same side (ipsilateral), or opposite side (contralateral) to the tumor. Some researchers include distinct tumors that have passed through the parietal pleura as M1.

Abbreviations for spread to specific organs

M notations might contain abbreviations for the organs involved:

Abbreviation	Organ
BRA	brain
EYE	eye
HEP	hepatic (liver)
LYM	lymph nodes
MAR	bone marrow
OSS	osseous (bone)
OTH	other
OVR	ovary
PER	peritoneal (abdomen)
PLE	pleura
PUL	pulmonary (lung)
SKI	skin

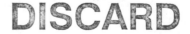

Stages of non-small cell lung cancer

Please refer to the earlier section "TNM staging definitions" to understand these stages. For example, if the values you were assigned were T1 for tumor characteristics, N2 for regional lymph nodes, and M0 for distant metastases, your cancer would be considered Stage IIIA. If you have multiple tumors, the one with the highest stage is used to plan your treatment:

- Occult carcinoma. TX, N0, M0

- Stage 0. Tis, N0, M0

- Stage IA. T1, N0, M0

- Stage IB. T2, N0, M0

- Stage IIA. T1, N1, M0

- Stage IIB. T2, N1, M0 *or* T3, N0, M0

- Stage IIIA. T1, N2, M0 *or* T2, N2, M0 *or* T3, N1, M0 *or* T3, N2, M0

- Stage IIIB. Any T, N3, M0 *or* T4, Any N, M0

- Stage IV. Any T, Any N, M1

Staging small cell lung cancer

The staging of small cell lung cancer does not adapt readily to the TNM staging system described previously. Because small cell lung cancer is most often diagnosed in later stages, extensive surgery is seldom recommended as treatment. This means that lymph nodes and other organs cannot be assessed in detail, as is required for determining staging levels I through IV based on TNM. Consequently, findings from diagnostic tests other than extensive open surgery are used.

Two stages are used to describe the extent of small cell lung cancer. The National Cancer Institute describes them as follows, using the Veterans Administration Lung Cancer Study Group criteria:

- Limited stage small cell lung cancer describes a tumor or tumors confined to areas that can be irradiated "tolerably"; that is, areas small enough to produce only radiation side effects that the patient can tolerate. These limited areas include:

  - The half of the chest (hemithorax) in which the tumor originates

  - The middle of the chest between the lungs (mediastinum)

- Lymph nodes closely adjacent to the lung (supraclavicular nodes)
- Extensive stage small cell lung cancer describes any tumor or tumors that are too widely spread to fit the definition of limited stage disease.

The NCI notes that "there is no universally accepted definition" of the term limited stage. They note that patients who have fluid in the chest, a very large lung tumor, or supraclavicular nodes on the opposite side of the chest from the tumor "have been both included within and excluded from limited stage by various groups." One research group has found that an additional stage known as "very limited disease" emerges as a prognostically meaningful subset if no evidence is found of mediastinal or supraclavicular lymph node involvement, an obstructing tumor, or pleural effusion.[2]

Other investigators believe that patients who have small cell lung cancer for whom open surgeries are justified can indeed be staged using the TNM system and that the information gained by doing so is more predictive of the outcome of treatment than the two-system staging described previously.

Grading (tumor aggressiveness)

A separate grading indicator is not always used for lung cancers because tumor type is in itself a measure of aggressiveness, with SCLC considered among the most aggressive of all cancers. Nonetheless, you might see specific grading information included in your biopsy report for NSCLC along with the TNM designation. The American Joint Commission on Cancer recommends the following terminology for grading tumors:

- GX. Grade cannot be assessed (undetermined grade)
- G1. Well-differentiated (low-grade)
- G2. Moderately well-differentiated (intermediate grade)
- G3. Poorly differentiated (high-grade)
- G4. Undifferentiated (high-grade)

Well-differentiated or low-grade tumors are the least aggressive; undifferentiated or high-grade tumors are the most aggressive.

Restaging

Disease that was first staged using only imaging studies and clinical measures (such as symptoms) might be restaged at a higher level later if surgery reveals more disease. Disease that is pretreated with chemotherapy before surgery might be restaged at a lower stage after surgery.

Cloudy diagnostic issues

Several issues can make diagnosis of lung cancer difficult. Your wishes to pursue diagnosis and your doctor's experience and training will determine what action is taken in these cases:

- Benign chest lesions can be mistaken on x-ray for malignant lesions. Solitary pulmonary nodules (SPNs) that resemble lung cancer on imaging studies, for example, can be caused by other disease processes, such as coccidiodomycosis. X-rays repeated at intervals might show no growth or very slow growth of these lesions. Some researchers regard a lung nodule that appears stable on x-ray for two years to be benign, but one study of bronchioloalveolar carcinoma (BAC) has shown that this subtype of lung cancer can appear unchanged for up to seven years on imaging studies.[3]

- X-ray studies might show a pattern of (usually benign) calcification or fat that is difficult to interpret, requiring further testing. CT scans sometimes show clear, dense chest lesions that are ambiguous.

- If radiologists do not vigorously seek and scrupulously compare old x-rays to new ones, malignant changes can be missed. One study found this neglect to be the most common cause of missed diagnoses.[4]

- Multiple primary lesions can appear in a percentage of patients, making it difficult to determine if and what kind of cancer exists.

- Mucinous bronchioloalveolar carcinoma (BAC) can appear as pneumonia on imaging studies.

- Sputum tests can be positive when x-rays and imaging studies are negative. Repeated bronchoscopy every three months for up to five years may be recommended to rule out lung cancer.

- Fine needle biopsy may miss the tumor and retrieve only healthy cells. A biopsy with wider-gauge needles can provide more complete, intact cellular material for a more accurate analysis than do narrower-gauge needles.

- Sputum containing cancer cells can be dragged into the cellular material retrieved during needle biopsy, making the target tissue appear malignant when it is not. Experienced pathologists can recognize a few free-floating tumor cells amidst dense tissue as possible contamination.

- Results of PET scanning to measure tissue metabolism can be ambiguous. Tissue that is not cancerous, such as that affected by tuberculosis or aspergillosis, can at times exhibit the higher metabolic rate of cancerous tissue. At times, BAC tumors might not take up metabolic agent or may appear weblike and diffuse, or like ground glass, confusing the radiologist.

- Newer multipurpose scanners that can do both PET and other radionuclide studies might not be as accurate as a scanner dedicated to PET.

- White blood cells known as lymphocytes can be present in the lungs when an infection is being resolved. These cells can be mistaken for small cell lung cancer. Reactive white blood cells associated with mediastinal Hodgkin's lymphoma or non-Hodgkin's lymphoma can be mistaken for small cell lung cancer.

- Normal lung cells sometimes assume unusual shapes or clusters in the process of repairing damage caused by irritants, asthma, bronchitis, or the like. These cells can be mistaken for lung cancers.

- What appears to be an enlarged or abnormal adrenal gland or liver lesions should be biopsied; benign processes or previous chemotherapy can cause these lesions.

- Pathologic analysis of biopsied lung cancer cells is not without error. NCI says:

  Electron microscopy, which can detect neuroendocrine granules, may help to differentiate between small cell and non-small cell cancers [...] Careful diagnosis is important, however, since the differential pathologic diagnosis from small cell lung cancer may be difficult.

Getting the best diagnosis

Regardless of your diagnosis, it would be wise to seek one or more second opinions about diagnosis, staging, and treatment options from a regional cancer center or university hospital. The oncologist you're already seeing may be affiliated with one of these groups, and thus may have the necessary qualifications. The best way to determine this, though, is to obtain second or third opinions.

Emotions at diagnosis

The events at diagnosis and those that follow over the next months or years are very likely to take an emotional toll. There are as many reactions to cancer as there are people, and you can't always be sure how you or your loved ones will react in stressful, frightening circumstances.

Fear

If you had any hint that your symptoms might be cancer-related, you are probably already familiar with tremendous, overwhelming feelings of fear and their aftereffects. The initial physiology of fear is such that your body prepares you very specifically for either battle or retreat. Humans have evolved to note and react quickly to changing stimuli during a fearful encounter. This evolution may explain why many people, when first diagnosed with cancer, want immediately to start a treatment—any treatment—just so they're doing something to fight back.

Unfortunately these bodily preparations for action, such as increasing your pulse rate and redirecting blood flow from your limbs to your heart, brain, and other internal organs, are not the ideal biological events to prepare you for understanding and remembering your doctor's explanations. The moment that fear hits and adrenaline pumps, senses become heightened in preparation for lifesaving action. The sensation that you can somehow see everything around you with remarkable clarity, however, is not necessarily going to help you remember the doctor's description of two tests that need to be done (and a third test only if the first two are inconclusive) and where your doctor said she prefers these tests be done. Instead, you may remember exactly where you were sitting, the color of the doctor's office walls, and that stray hair of the doctor's that wouldn't stay put.

Shock and numbness

Your cancer diagnosis will very likely seem unreal to you at first. You might awake from sleep feeling fine, for example, then remember after thirty seconds or so that you've had extensive surgery for cancer. You might not hear people who speak to you; you may have difficulty concentrating on routine normal tasks; you might feel as if you're walking underwater; you might have to remind yourself to look both ways when crossing the street and to use special care when driving. Some cancer survivors or their loved ones report becoming paralytic for days, unable to sleep, rise, eat, or work.

Kathy tells of her first reaction to the surgeon's news after her husband Marty's thoracotomy:

> I was in a daze. I went to find the phone in the waiting room, and of course the other family who had been annoying me are now sitting in the chairs by the phone. They are not using it, so I walk over, pick up the phone, called my mother who was at my house with my kids, and I tell her, "It's malignant."
>
> The other people slowly walked away and were very quiet then. My mother immediately called my sister to come to the hospital. I sat just stunned. A woman waiting on someone else started to talk to me. She said she could tell I had gotten bad news. She was so very kind to sit with me until my sister got there.
>
> After the doctor told me about the cancer, I told the doctors not to tell Marty anything until they had done the biopsies—this gave me time to compose myself and ensure there was no doubt. The pulmonologist told me about the biopsies, and I was the one who told Marty.
>
> I felt like I was in a daze. Marty hardly asked any questions and didn't want to talk about the cancer. He couldn't say the words, "I have lung cancer" without falling apart.

Mental slowness

Many cancer patients and their loved ones, most being intelligent and competent people—even some doctors diagnosed with cancer—report not being able to remember anything of the doctor's explanation after hearing the word cancer.

If you will be meeting the doctor in person to discuss test results and treatment choices, be prepared to have difficulty absorbing what is said. For example, you could be prepared to take notes, or take a friend or a tape recorder with you. Tell the doctor that you will be calling back with a list of questions after you have had time to absorb this information. If she expresses impatience or reluctance to help you, consider finding another doctor.

Detachment

Many people note that, upon learning of their diagnosis, they were completely objective and calm and felt nothing at all, as if they were outside of their body observing this happening to someone else. This is called dissociation. Dissociation temporarily allows you to absorb information without emotional pain.

Childlike or nonsensical behavior

Some people note that they said and did things that made no sense, sometimes quite childlike things. This behavior can be a seeking of comfort in happier times, technically called regression. The wife of a cancer survivor recalls:

> When my husband phoned to say his CT scan showed what was almost certainly cancer, I left my office immediately. Once at home I found that, although I was forty years old, all I wanted to do was reread my old girlhood Nancy Drew books.

Denial

Some people respond to the news of their diagnosis with the belief that there is an error in the laboratory test, or that their results have been confused with someone else's. This reaction, called denial, is a protective reaction that allows you to absorb an onslaught of information more slowly. Denial can be used successfully to help you forget about cancer between treatments and return to your productive life. Denial can be a dangerous adaptive strategy, however, if you forget medical appointments, neglect care, or become convinced that your health will improve spontaneously with no treatment.

Displacement activity

Some people respond to the bad news of diagnosis by becoming very organized, plunging into the intellectual aspects of the problem, organizing all insurance information and doctors' appointments, and so on. This defensive behavior is called displacement activity and, like other defensive behaviors, it serves to push pain out of the mind. It also can serve the very useful purpose of getting everything in order for upcoming treatment and ensuring that the patient and her family will have the information they need to make treatment choices.

After her husband's diagnosis, Kathy says:

> I went into overdrive, doing everything and taking care of everyone's feelings.

Others engage in displacement activities, such as hobbies. Again, these behaviors are not wrong—in fact they are likely to be healthy—as long as treatments and doctor appointments are not missed.

Anger

Although many people develop focused feelings of anger some time *after* their diagnosis, others may feel a generalized anger at the time of diagnosis. They may lash out at the doctor who was the bearer of bad news about the cancer diagnosis, or at loved ones for seemingly meaningless reasons. If you're a smoker or an ex-smoker, you might feel anger directed at yourself, your environment, or the tobacco industry. If a toxic industrial exposure is considered the source of your disease, you might feel anger that regulatory agencies did too little too late, or nothing at all, to protect you.

Sometimes anger is a form of projection, a displacement of painful feelings within the self outward onto others. As such, projection serves to reduce unbearable levels of pain. At other times, the angry person may simply feel overwhelmed by having to face all of the stresses and responsibilities of normal life, plus a cancer diagnosis. Yet others feel that being angry is more socially acceptable than feeling sad. Anger can be a useful emotion if targeted properly and harmlessly, but it can also signal the beginning of depression and can drive away others whose support you will almost certainly need.

Sadness

Many people report that they cry or otherwise express great sadness about their illness and that they feel better after doing so. Sadness is of course an entirely normal reaction to a cancer diagnosis.

Max Baldwin tells us:

> I was initially diagnosed as a stage 3 that was operable, but a second opinion from a specialized cancer hospital showed it to be a stage 4 and inoperable. My reaction to hearing this? It felt like someone slapped me up the side of my head with a 2 × 4 piece of lumber. Maybe that is a poor description, but it sure got my attention. As you can imagine, my thoughts went to the depths of despair.
>
> However, since I live alone and do not have a wife for support, I had to get tough quickly. As I write this months later, I have adjusted to hoping for the best, but planning for the worst.

Guilt

Guilt is the burden we carry for things we feel we could have handled differently. Survivors of lung cancer who once smoked might feel that, had they lived differently, they would not have developed cancer. This feeling haunts many survivors of several different types of cancer, but for lung cancer survivors it's especially painful because the medical community in the US strongly stresses prevention via avoiding smoking, and the public is well aware of this.

Shame

Unlike guilt, shame is the burden we carry for things we can't do anything about. Unlike survivors of cancers that affect the kidney or the thyroid, for instance, some lung cancer survivors might be reluctant to discuss their condition with others, fearing their negative reaction, even if he or she has never smoked.

Blame

Like anger, blame can be a form of projection. If someone has been blaming herself for her own or another's cancer, the feelings may become unbearable and she may begin looking elsewhere for an explanation. Unfortunately, some people decide that the best solution is for another person to carry this blame. Those who have been coping with stress in this way for many years sometimes skip the self-blame phase and go directly to blaming others.

If someone in your life appears to be blaming you for cancer, you might try discussing the pointlessness of blame with her. If discussion doesn't improve the relationship, it might be best to remove this person from your immediate circle of activities temporarily and deal with her only when you feel most able.

Withdrawal

Others report that they or their loved ones initially seemed detached, withdrawn, or uncaring. Those who withdraw may do so for many reasons: as a habit formed during earlier stressful experiences, as a means to avoid shameful feelings about expressing emotion, in an attempt to keep emotional levels low so that others won't become upset, as an attempt to reduce exposure to painful ideas, and so on.

Perspective on emotions

All of these reactions, and many others, are normal, albeit painful. You may feel that these feelings are useless or counterproductive, but like all defensive behaviors, they serve to protect your mind from harm until you can assimilate this experience and begin to build a frame of reference from the facts. Don't berate yourself if you're not feeling like the poster child for mental health week.

A gentleman diagnosed via surgery and treated with chemotherapy and radiotherapy tells us:

> Have patience with yourself. About six to eight weeks after I got out of the hospital, I was bawling and crying. My nerves were shot. I had to ask people not to come visit. You have to get over that initial response to the word "cancer," but you can learn to live with it.
>
> And find a support group. The more you can talk to people in the same situation, the better you'll get through this experience.

In addition to testimonials from survivors, objective scientific studies also have shown that support groups and counseling make a difference in one's comfort and ability to deal with cancer.

Summary

The information in this chapter is intended to remove the edge from the fear you're feeling. Knowing that delays you may have experienced obtaining a diagnosis are common; that multiple diagnostic tests are sometimes needed; that the diagnostic process can unfold in stages with increasing levels of certainty, perhaps entailing changes in your treatment plan or your choice of doctors; that you're not alone; that what you're feeling is normal—these are the first steps of the journey.

CHAPTER 3

Finding the Right Treatment Team

There are in fact two things, science and opinion; the former begets knowledge, the latter ignorance.

—Hippocrates

CHOOSING THE RIGHT SURGEON and the best oncologists for any treatment you need are the most important decisions you'll make during the early days of your diagnosis.

Unless you have symptoms that warrant emergency treatment, generally you can take a week or two to locate the best doctors for your circumstances without compromising the outcome. If you're pressed for time, though, or are feeling too anxious just now to pursue this issue with the necessary tenacity, you can limit your search to contacting the nearest university medical school or to contacting the National Cancer Institute (NCI) at (800) 4-CANCER and asking for the names of several surgeons and oncologists at their institution or in your area.

In this chapter, we first look at the various types of surgeons and oncologists and how to locate qualified candidates. Then we discuss considerations in deciding on the right surgeon and oncologists for you, including currency of medical background, affiliated treatment centers, and manners of conducting practice.

Certain lung cancers are treated with chemotherapy or radiotherapy before or after surgery, some are treated with surgery alone, and some are treated with chemotherapy alone. There are also experimental treatment options available through clinical trials. If your condition allows, you should feel comfortable seeking second and third opinions at an NCI-designated cancer center before starting treatment. Additional medical opinions allow you to resolve conflicting treatment recommendations and to gain peace of mind about your treatment plan. It is important that you know you are getting the best care available.

Types of surgeons

The surgeon specifically trained to perform surgery when lung cancer is suspected is a thoracic or cardiothoracic surgeon, board-certified by the American Board of Medical Specialties (ABMS). Thoracic surgeons have been shown to achieve better results for lung cancer than general surgeons.

Types of oncologists

There are two types of oncologists who treat lung cancer (any oncologist you choose should be board certified):

- The medical oncologist, trained in the use of chemotherapy. The medical oncologist is usually simply called an oncologist. Board certification for this discipline is called medical oncology. At large cancer centers, expect to find a thoracic oncologist who specializes in treating lung cancer.

- The radiation oncologist, trained in the use of radiation therapy. Your radiation oncologist will coordinate treatments you may need with your medical oncologist and your surgeon. Choose a radiation oncologist who is board certified in radiation oncology.

Surgical and oncologic specialists are usually associated with university medical schools. If you cannot find a suitable specialist in your area to provide your treatment, you should plan to travel for at least one second opinion from a specialist during the course of your treatment.

Geri Capasso describes her brother Anthony's visit to a specialist:

> I went with my brother to see a new doctor today at St. Vincent's in New York. He reviewed everything, and since my brother's treatment is still showing improvement, he suggested that we stay with it. He did, however, suggest that my brother get a Port-A-Cath. He stressed titanium, not plastic, because of the risk of infection. He said it's risky to get cisplatin through the veins: if it leaks, it can be very damaging. If my brother weren't on a protocol (AG3340), this doctor's method is to do a needle biopsy and remove cells and send them to a lab in California. This lab tests different chemos and combinations to see which one works most successfully on the individual's cancer cells. I liked him and his approach. His positive attitude was refreshing.

General points for finding good doctors

You should search carefully for a surgeon and oncologists who have a great deal of experience with your illness and who stay informed of the latest breakthroughs in lung cancer diagnosis and treatment, because treatments are evolving with vigor. It's better to make a good choice at first rather than later, and it's especially important to find the right doctor before you decide to proceed with surgery, and perhaps chemotherapy or radiation therapy.

A surgical patient describes his experience with misdiagnosis:

> The doctor thought they should take a biopsy of it. I went to a lung doctor and had a bronchoscopy. It goes up your nose into the lung while you're awake.
>
> They took a lot of specimens in the lung and sent them in for testing. When I went back to see the lung doctor, he said, "All the samples came back negative." I felt pretty good about that. But then he said, "I can't give you a clean bill of health with your history of smoking. I want you to go see the surgeon." (I had quit smoking only about two or three years before that.)
>
> I went next door to the surgeon. He looked at the x-rays and said, "Lung cancer." I argued that the tests had been clean. He said, "I know lung cancer when I see lung cancer." Then he explained what would happen and recommended surgery. He said, "If we get in and it's spread too far, then we'll just call off the operation and take a chemotherapy tack of treatment."
>
> They get you to the point where you're glad to have them cut it out. You hope that they don't find it's spread and they can still do something about it. I was so discouraged about the future, I just hoped they'd take it out. The decision seemed to be fairly easy to make.
>
> The surgeon took out the top part of my lung where the tumor was, and also took out the bottom lobe. I never knew why they did that. I overheard the doctor say later, "Well, if I'd known it wasn't malignant, I probably wouldn't have taken that much." I've never really forgiven him for that—taking out the bottom lobe. The doctors ended up saying that it was some kind of a tumor, although it was benign.
>
> While I was recovering, after the operation, I talked to another doctor in the hospital. I wanted to know how many times this kind of thing

> happens—where doctors operate and take out much of your lung and
> then the tumor isn't malignant. He hemmed and hawed and gave me
> some answers. By my calculations, the chances of that happening were
> about 1 in 15,000 of getting off the hook, with no cancer, if you were in
> my spot. The other 14,999 times, they would be right about it being lung
> cancer at that point.
>
> The doctors don't give you many outs—well it could be something else,
> but they don't hold that out very much. It was about six or eight weeks
> that I thought I had cancer before I found out I didn't.

You should consider traveling to an NCI-designated comprehensive cancer center for care, and perhaps enrolling in a clinical trial. Much of the best work done for lung cancer is performed at university medical schools. Chapter 20, *Clinical Trials*, describes how trials are structured. In Appendix A, *Resources*, the subcategories describing free treatment, drugs, travel, and lodging list charitable groups that might pay travel and lodging costs for you.

A word about managed care: your insurance provider may have restrictions regarding whom you may consult or where you may travel for care. Check your policy carefully for such restrictions and contact the provider before scheduling appointments that might not be covered. Some managed care providers charge only a modestly increased co-payment for out-of-plan doctors; others refuse to pay any of the doctor's fee; still others will pay most or all costs if medical necessity can be proved. If your HMO has a care coordinator, he may work with you to make special reinterpretations of the rules in your case. Many people don't challenge their HMO's rules, but those who do frequently win a full settlement or a compromise.

A lung cancer survivor diagnosed via surgery describes how he feels now:

> My advice to others? If you think something's wrong, keep pushing for
> answers. Looking back, I wish I could have been diagnosed eighteen
> months earlier when I first went in with symptoms; I wouldn't have had to
> go through everything.

Finding good specialists

If you have limited time to get recommendations, you can contact the nearest university medical school or the National Cancer Institute (NCI) at (800) 4-CANCER and ask for the names of several suitable surgeons and oncologists at their institution or in your area.

In addition to this technique, there are several more thorough ways to search for qualified surgeons and oncologists:

- The NCI designates both Comprehensive Cancer Centers and Clinical Cancer Centers. The former meet rigorous standards of excellence; the latter meet less rigorous, but still quite high, standards. If you phone NCI's Cancer Information Service at (800) 4-CANCER, they can provide you with a list of these centers. Be sure to tell them if you're willing to travel for care; otherwise, they are inclined to assume that you want only local references. Once you have these lists, you can phone the nearest center and ask for referrals. Note that any institution can simply include in its name the words "clinical cancer center" or "comprehensive cancer center." Be sure that the institution's title is NCI-designated. If you have a personal computer, you can access this information at the NCI's web site at *http://cancernet.nci.nih.gov.*

- The American Medical Association (AMA) maintains a list of all licensed doctors, AMA members or not, and can tell you if the doctor you're considering is board certified in a surgical specialty, such as lung surgery, or in medical or radiologic oncology. They can also furnish information, such as year of graduation from medical school and the location of residencies. The AMA Physician Select web site is *http://www.ama-assn.org/aps/amahg.html.*

- The American Board of Medical Specialties (ABMS) can refer you to board-certified specialists. Visit *http://www.certifieddoctor.org* or contact them at (800) 733-2267.

- *The American Medical Directory* and the *Directory of Medical Specialists,* available at your local library, both list doctors by specialty.

- The magazine *US News and World Report,* which can be found in your local library, annually designates hospitals as Centers of Excellence. Usually this "Best Hospitals" issue is published in July. You may be able to order a back issue of *US News and World Report's* "Best Hospitals" edition by calling (202) 955-2000 or by visiting the magazine's web site at *http://www.usnews.com.* Note that a hospital ranked best on some criteria does not ensure that it will be the best hospital for your circumstances, though.

- If your family doctor or primary care physician has recommended a surgeon or oncologist, ask him why he's recommending this person. Recommendations from another doctor can range from wonderful—"Because he gets such good results"—to lukewarm.

- Phone a reputable nearby hospital, ask for the oncology floor, then ask to speak with the head oncology nurse. Explain that you'd like a recommendation for a doctor who treats lung cancer, and that you'd value the nurse's opinion because he works extensively with so many oncologists.

- Phone a reputable nearby hospital, ask for the surgical floor, then ask to speak with the head surgical nurse. Explain that you'd like a recommendation for a surgeon who treats lung cancer.

- Use a personal computer to access the National Library of Medicine's Medline or have a friend or relative do so for you. Search the subjects "lung cancer surgery" or "lung cancer treatment." Scan the last two years' worth of papers and note the authors' names and institutional affiliations. The National Library of Medicine's free PubMed Medline search engine is at *http://www.ncbi.nlm.nih.gov/entrez/query.fcgi?db=PubMed*. Keep in mind, though, that many excellent oncologists are involved in research during their training years, then move into private practice and cease publishing. Lack of published material does not mean a doctor is inadequate, nor does the existence of many publications guarantee that he will be a good, caring practitioner or in clinical practice at all. Published papers are just one of many gauges of a doctor's ability. (For more information on using Medline, see Chapter 22, *Researching Your Illness*.)

- Your surgeon will almost certainly know medical and radiologic oncologists that are well regarded.

- The American Thoracic Society can refer you to good specialists; you can reach them at (212) 315-8700 or visit *http://www.thoracic.org*. Another good source of referrals is the Society of Thoracic Surgeons; you can reach them at (312) 644-6610 or visit *http://www.sts.org*.

Choosing treatment centers

Bear in mind that when you choose a doctor, you also choose by default a treatment center. Ask the doctors on your shortlist to which hospitals they have admitting privileges and with which, if any, NCI-designated treatment groups they are associated. Ask how many oncologic thoracic surgeries are done there annually and whether a surgical specialty team exists at the hospital. Studies have shown that oncologic surgical specialty teams in hospitals with specialty services have a better surgical success rate.

There are several different types of treatment centers: NCI-designated comprehensive cancer centers, university hospitals, cooperative lung cancer groups, community clinical oncology programs, research institutions, and community hospitals. A full explanation of each is beyond the scope of this chapter, but the point to be taken is that NCI-designated comprehensive cancer centers (the great majority of which are nonprofit university medical schools) are the best places to find cancer expertise.

University hospitals

In January 1999, the *New England Journal of Medicine* reported that although patients sometimes prefer the level of emotional support provided by community hospitals, teaching hospitals provide better medical care.

University hospitals or other research institutions funded by the NCI, such as Johns Hopkins in Baltimore or the Mayo Cancer Center in Rochester, Minnesota, are very likely places to find the latest advances in lung cancer treatment.

When regulatory agencies decide who will be allocated scarce resources or who will be given permission to provide rare services, such as PET scanning, the university hospital is a likely choice because the infrastructure, such as skill levels and staffing, is already in place. In addition, the cooperative and collaborative nature of the university hospital tends to attract the most talented medical researchers. In most cases, these same researchers are also expected to provide patient care. This means that the latest treatments are likely to be offered in this setting first, that the accumulated experience level among the staff is high, and that you'll be treated by some of the most talented and knowledgeable people in the country.

University-associated hospitals and cancer centers are the institutions most likely to be designated by the NCI as either Comprehensive Cancer Centers or Clinical Cancer Centers. All NCI-designated centers are nonprofit institutions.

Some people are afraid to receive health care at a university or teaching hospital because they fear they will be subjected to unproven or unnecessary treatment by newly graduated medical students who may not know what they're doing. It's true that a training mission incorporated into a hospital's charter means that you may be examined or cared for by more than one doctor, but this can be an advantage as well as a disadvantage. These advantages and disadvantages differ little from having a family doctor who is a member of a large practice: while it's true that you may not always see the same doctor, it's also true that you need not go without help if your doctor is not available. Newly graduated doctors, called interns (also called first-year residents, or postgraduate year-one students), are seldom charged with care or decision-making in the absence of your attending doctor or an oncology resident. You're always free to say that you prefer that a procedure or exam be done by someone with more experience.

In the US, unproven treatments are never performed without clear written informed consent if your hospital receives any federal funds or is governed by local laws regarding informed consent. If you are approached to take part in a study of an unproven treatment, called a clinical trial, you always have the right to refuse; if you do decide to enroll, you always have the right to withdraw later.

A most important fact of which all cancer survivors and their loved ones should be aware is that, for cancer treatment, a placebo is virtually never used. The new, unproven treatment is offered either in clinical trials that compare the new treatment to standard, approved treatment or that offer the new treatment only. For cancer, new treatments are never compared to an inactive sugar pill, as are drugs in other kinds of (noncancer) clinical trials. When there is no standard treatment to which the new treatment can be juxtaposed, such as the very first bone marrow purging procedures in the early days of bone marrow transplantation, this lack is clearly communicated by those attempting to ensure that consent is indeed informed consent.

Note that a community teaching hospital is not the same as a medical school training hospital, although the community hospital may have residency programs that accommodate certain university medical school training needs, such as emergency room rotations.

Cooperative groups

Cooperative groups comprise university hospitals and cancer treatment centers that take part in administering very large multicenter trials of new treatments. There are about thirteen clinical trial cooperative groups in the US. A current list of the centers in these groups can be obtained by phoning the NCI's Cancer Information Service at (800) 4-CANCER.

Community clinical oncology programs

This program links community doctors with the clinical trial cooperative groups described in the previous section. For a list of groups in your area, phone the NCI at (800) 4-CANCER.

Treatment at no charge

The NCI provides free cancer care to those who qualify, but only within clinical trials. A referral from your local oncologist is necessary for entry into a trial. Non-US citizens also may be admitted at the discretion of the principal investigator of the trial.

Some university and community hospitals have a policy guaranteeing that they will provide medical care for local residents who cannot pay.

Checking credentials of candidates

If a check on credentials wasn't part of the process you used to come up with a list of candidate surgeons and oncologists, you can check credentials now. Any doctors recommended by the NCI or from a clinical center have undoubtedly already had a thorough check of their backgrounds and qualifications; however, you might want to see them for yourself.

You can check doctors' professional qualifications in some of the same publications listed below as aids to locating qualified surgeons and oncologists:

- The *AMA Directory of Physicians* lists the doctor's name, medical school attended, year licensed, primary and secondary specialty, type of practice, board certification, and physician recognition awards. (Available in libraries or, if the doctor has agreed to be listed in the Internet directory, at *http://www.ama-assn.org*.)

- The official *ABMS Directory of Board Certified Medical Specialties* includes the specialty, when the doctor was certified, the doctor's medical school and year of degree, the place and dates of internship, place and dates of residency, fellowship training, academic and hospital appointments, professional association memberships, type of practice, and the doctor's current address, telephone number, and fax number. This service is available in libraries or by calling (800) 776-CERT or visiting *http://www.certifieddoctor.org*.

- To verify a surgical oncologist's credentials, contact the Society of Surgical Oncology at (847) 427-1400 or visit *http://www.surgonc.org*.

- Your state medical licensing board should be able to tell you the status of your doctor's license, when the doctor was first licensed by the state, and the status of any misconduct charges or disciplinary actions.

- An easy way to check on your doctor's credentials is to call Medi-Net, a consumer information service that provides healthcare consumers with a background check on any doctor licensed to practice in the United States, including credentials, degrees, training, and board certifications, as well as any disciplinary actions or sanctions taken against the doctor. Each complete Medi-Net physician profile costs $15.00 per doctor (less for subsequent profiles ordered at the same time). Preliminary information is provided on the telephone, with detailed reports usually mailed or faxed to callers the same day. To order a report, call toll-free (888) ASK-MEDI ((888) 275-6334) or (800) 972-MEDI ((800) 972-6334), or visit *http://www.searchpointe.com*.

Choosing the best from a shortlist

Once you have found one or more board-certified surgeons and oncologists who seem excellent, you can interview them to make sure they're good candidates. No matter how many recommendations you receive or sterling credentials you have uncovered, until you have a candid conversation with the human behind the stethoscope, you won't know if this is a person with whom you'll feel comfortable.

Schedule a meeting to ask any questions you have about the doctor's medical background, attitudes, and office policies, such as:

- How many surgeries for suspected lung cancer has the surgeon performed? If interviewing a medical or radiation oncologist, how many patients with your type of lung cancer has he treated?

- To what hospitals does he have admitting privileges?

- With which clinical trials is he familiar? It's important to have medical and radiation oncologists who are familiar with the latest research in lung cancer.

- With which institutions is he affiliated? For instance, does he have a faculty appointment at a medical school in addition to a private surgical or oncology practice?

- What surgery or treatment does he recommend? After the appointment, evaluate how this recommendation compares with what your reading has taught you.

- What is his policy for handling emergency calls during non-business hours?

- How will test results be communicated? Will ancillary doctors be given permission to communicate directly with you, the patient? Does the doctor object to leaving information on your answering or fax machines, if that's a method you prefer?

- Are family members welcome to call with questions? Some doctors prefer communicating only with the patient.

- Does the doctor's philosophy about health and life mesh well with your own? For example, does he espouse treatment at all costs over quality of life?

Use some of this interview time to describe yourself and your expectations, such as how much participation you would like to have in healthcare decisions.

Kathleen Houlihan describes what factors made her feel that her treatment center was best for her:

> I saw a jerk of an oncologist in my home city, who said we would do radiation and chemotherapy, but if it recurred, which it could do at any time, there would be nothing he could do. We went crazy over the weekend, trying to figure out how we could become experts on cancer treatments and alternatives to standard therapy in time to help me improve the 20 percent odds I was given for survival.
>
> I remembered having seen an ad for the Cancer Treatment Centers of America. I checked out their web site, and it was so uplifting and hopeful, in contrast to all the dreadful stuff I had been seeing about lung cancer. But I didn't think I could come here. I don't know why not, but I didn't think I could. On Sunday, we were still trying to figure out what to do. My husband Holt asked me what I wanted to do, and before I knew it I said, "I want to go the Cancer Treatment Centers of America." Boom! Holt was at their web site (http://www.cancercenter.com). He called their number. They had someone on call on Sunday. We started planning it. We felt it was urgent, since it had been going on for so long. So she called us back at 7:20 Monday morning, got my insurance information, made me an appointment with their pulmonologist for Tuesday morning, and got us plane tickets for Monday afternoon.
>
> Meanwhile, the jerk in my home city told Holt it would be a big mistake to go to CTCA. Boy, am I glad we didn't listen to him. We actually called back to cancel, but the counselor talked us into coming to see for ourselves.

Kathleen felt that the environment and philosophy of the center she chose matched what she was looking for in treatment:

> This CTCA center in Tulsa is housed in two towers. All the doctors' offices are in one tower, and everything else—regular hospital, radiation and MRI equipment, business offices, and "guest" rooms are in the other.

They used to be hospital rooms, but they took out the hospital beds and put in regular ones—we have a queen, and TV and phone, of course. Not luxurious, but plenty comfortable. And they cost $15 or $20 per night, depending on size. Meals cost $1.50 for breakfast and $3 for lunch and dinner. And it's mostly good, healthy food. (Call (800) 615-3055 or visit http://www.cancercenter.com for updated cost information)

It's pleasant here, not at all like a hospital. There are four floors with guest rooms, about 90 rooms in all, in the 30-story tower. The cafeteria is on 26, with an atrium open to 27. There's a big-screen TV and game tables on 28, with an atrium open to 29. So it's not claustrophobic at all, with two floors open to each other. We're on 29. The computer we use for email is just down the open-to-the-atrium hallway from our room. Each of the four guest room floors has a little kitchen with a fridge and freezer that we can put our own food in. And each has a laundry room with a washer and dryer that are not coin operated.

It's extremely convenient having everything in one place. And everyone knows your schedule, so they schedule appointments for you when you are free and call to tell you. If you are not in your room, there is voice mail. It's kind of like Club Med for cancer patients.

Then there are the weekly classes: nutrition, naturopathic medicine, mind-body, stress management, dance/movement, etc. And if you want an individual session with a counselor, physical therapist, or whatever, just call. No charge. They want you to do all this stuff. This is why I think I'm much better off here than at home. I've been going to classes—nutrition, naturopathic medicine, stress management, chemotherapy education, etc. And there are weekly appointments with my three or four doctors here. And meals—even though I haven't been that hungry, I've been trying to eat as much as I can. The naturopathic doctor said that, for my blood type, I should eat meat. Well, I tried a couple of days ago, but I think it's all still sitting in my stomach. I may add dairy back into my diet, but I don't think I can handle the meat. They do want us to have a lot of protein while we are in treatment, though.

So we are settling in. Holt keeps busy on the computer, taking walks, and whatever while I'm doing my thing. He will probably fly back home *and get a car in about a week or so. The transportation department has taken us around town some (movie, park, flea market, health food store, restaurants), but we could do a lot more if we had our own car here.*

Overall, you want to make sure that the surgeon and oncologists you choose have excellent medical credentials and extensive experience with lung cancer, and are affiliated with treatment centers that offer up-to-date resources. You'll also want to weigh in other considerations, such as communication skills, personal style, and office location.

Summary

Now that you have information regarding the differences among oncologists and surgeons, the wisdom of utilizing a board-certified specialist, and the advantages of care at a well-regarded cancer center or large cooperative lung cancer group, you are equipped to find a good doctor and turn your attention to such issues as the details of your treatment, communicating with medical personnel, and finding the emotional and instrumental support you will need.

CHAPTER 4

Interacting with Medical Personnel

How was it possible that he, a doctor, with his countless acquaintances, had never until this day come across anything so definite as this man's personality?

—Boris Pasternak
Doctor Zhivago

THE RELATIONSHIP YOU EXPERIENCE with your treatment team will play a critical part—indeed perhaps the most critical part—in your recovery from lung cancer. It's imperative that you and your treatment team communicate well with each other; that you, the patient, feel free to ask questions; that you become well-informed in order to make decisions; that there is enough mutual respect to disagree with each other amicably while adhering to a productive plan of treatment and care.

This chapter will assist you in learning how to communicate with medical personnel, improve communication, handle problems that arise, and move on to new and better patient/doctor relationships if improvements are not forthcoming. This chapter looks first at issues that may arise and when to address them. It then looks at the team members with whom you may communicate and discusses how their styles can influence your approach. Finally, the chapter describes a number of difficult situations and how you might handle them.

Issues that arise

Your doctor's staff phoned late on Friday to say that the doctor would like to meet with you to discuss your latest scan results. By the time you hear this cryptic message, it's too late to contact them for an appointment. On Monday, you're told that no appointments are available for two more days.

During your appointment on Wednesday, the doctor explains that the scan showed unusual shadows in the lung that may or may not be problematic, but additional tests are needed to clarify these results. She describes the purpose of the tests, but you don't hear much, because you're in shock. Your mind is tumbling with questions and doubts, and you find yourself losing track of what she's saying.

When you arrive home, you realize you forgot to set up the test appointments. You remember that you didn't write down the names of the tests—one of them sounded sort of like "pet"—nor did you ask what they'll entail nor how to prepare for them.

Parts of this scenario and others like it unfold every day for lung cancer survivors, and you may have other experiences that are equally hapless and frustrating. In contrast to receiving caring, intelligent, concerned, and respectful treatment from your doctor, instead you may experience condescension, paternalism, coldness, impatience, or black humor. You may experience indifference at the hands of certain medical personnel—in each case, a grotesque imbalance between some of society's most vulnerable and most privileged members.

Geri Capasso reinforces the importance of the relationship between doctor and patient from her experience:

> *I firmly believe that when a doctor isn't on "your team," it adversely affects the patient. It seems to me that there are doctors who have no hope for their patients—they just keep repeating the same treatments with dismal success rates—and there are doctors who are cutting-edge, who are at least reaching for the right treatment and treating this disease as the enemy that it is. There is no hope in surrender, and it is not an easy battle, seeing what my brother is going through, but I think that every cancer patient deserves doctors that are willing to reach out and fight this battle with them.*

Oncology personnel are human. Because they are human, they will at times be tired; they may be less successful listeners on busy days; thoughts of problems at home may interrupt their concentration; they have likes and dislikes that may be irrational; and they'll experience treatment failures that make them sad and depressed. They are busy people who need to keep abreast of advances in care for many different types of cancer, not just lung cancer. Often the stress of these demands emerges in their dealings with us. Doctors and nurses may develop techniques for dealing with patients that are in some measure a defense against their own pain.

Unfortunately, outright rudeness, ineptitude, or blatant lack of concern may also manifest; they must be dealt with promptly before your health is placed in jeopardy.

Larry Coffman says:

> *You have the right to demand a different treatment. You need to speak with your oncologist about YOUR wishes; involve your primary care physician and radiologist if necessary. Remind them that they are treating a person, not just a disease, and that "it ain't over till the pigs grow wings." I would inform them that you are a lung cancer survivor and not just a funding statistic.*

Only you can define what matters in your relationship with your doctor. You may prefer to have your doctor make all decisions for you, shielding you from uncomfortable details, or you may prefer to be privy to both the worst and most minute details concerning your care. You may find that you occupy a somewhat passive patient role initially, but at some point you may evolve into a more proactive patient. You may enjoy a joking, casual relationship, or it may make you feel belittled.

Keep in mind that, in the absence of your forthright requests for a certain quality of interaction, a doctor's assumptions about your needs are likely to shape how she interacts with you. The lung cancer experience, like most cancer experiences, can be a volatile one, and thus your needs may change from day to day. You're entitled to say, for instance, that, for today only, you want your doctor to do your thinking for you or that joking is not on the agenda.

Keep in mind, too, that the medical staff deserves the same respect you do. If your oncologist was the first person to give you the bad news about your having cancer, for example, you may unknowingly harbor resentment and anger toward her just because she was the bearer of bad news.

Larry Coffman describes his approach:

> *The patient and the caregiver have to take a proactive approach to treatment of this disease. After all, you can't separate the individual and the disease.*
>
> *I used my primary physician as my point guard in my battle. My primary physician had been with me for years, so he felt connected with me and insured that explanations were given and questions answered. He communicated with my oncologist, radiologist, and pathologist on a weekly basis, more if tests were being done or I was given chemotherapy*

that week. I believe the team approach is essential, be it at MD Anderson (an NCI center) or at your local hospital.

I have an unwavering belief that the disease can be beaten, while at the same time facing the realities square in the face. I feel strongly that my mental state has had as much to do with my survival as any doctor or drug. My life is mine. A doctor is kind of like an attorney: they can only recommend a treatment plan, the final decision will always be up to the patient. If the physician cannot accept that role, I personally would begin looking for one that will. My experience tells me that the physician that believes that their way is the way the patient must go is one that will not be completely honest regarding the positives and negatives of a certain treatment's outcome.

I think it's funny that my oncologist views me as one of his SCLC trophies. I accept that, as it seems to inspire him to keep a close eye on me.

The National Cancer Institute physicians at the NCI-designated cancer centers around the country have the right mental attitude, team approach, assets, and state of the art technology to work with.

When to voice concerns

Ideally, you have already developed the habit of clarifying your expectations at the beginning of a medical relationship. Few people do so, however—or need to—until serious illness entails complex long-term communication with the medical community.

If you're feeling disappointed with your care and haven't communicated your concerns to your oncologist, don't postpone doing so. Realign the relationship soon after you feel uncomfortable with it. Having an angry discussion regarding a long string of past disappointments is much less likely to succeed than realigning the relationship soon after you feel uncomfortable with it.

If you're the victim of blatant mistreatment or if you sense an unacceptable lack of concern for your well-being, it's best to address the problem immediately. The problem may be an honest mistake, and if so, the doctor and staff will be grateful to you for bringing it to their attention. Conversely, rudeness or indifference might be a bad habit that other patients have been too intimidated to challenge. Delay won't make these problems go away.

The team

This chapter assumes that the most common failure of good communication arises between you and your oncologist or your surgeon. Nonetheless, most strategies and tactics that may work in improving patient/doctor communication may also prove useful if problems arise with an oncology nurse, a radiotherapy technician, a member of the clerical staff, or your HMO gatekeeper.

Doctors have different styles of interacting with patients. The best among them may vary this style based on the perceived needs of the patient or by a patient's changing circumstances over time. A certain core style will generally emerge, though, and you may or may not be comfortable with it. The following sections discuss a few common styles found among doctors.

Paternalistic doctors

The paternalistic doctor is likely to be a fine, skilled practitioner who will provide you with excellent care. She views her responsibility to you as all-encompassing and is likely to err on the side of total, but accurate, control. If you're in need of a doctor who will make all decisions for you—and this is not at all a criticism, if this is what you want and need at any point—you'll be very happy with this doctor.

Your first clash with the paternalistic doctor may arise if you want to understand a great deal about your illness, ask many questions, and receive patient, detailed answers. Sooner or later, she's likely to ask you if you'd like to have your very own medical degree. She may even suggest that you ought not to read articles from medical journals, perhaps saying, "They'll just frighten you."

These replies hint that the accrual of medical knowledge is the province only of the doctor, never of the patient, and this behavior is the hallmark of the paternalistic style.

Given that you may not be able to change doctors because of certain constraints, such as geography or insurance requirements, here are a few ideas for dealing with the paternalistic doctor:

- Do your homework carefully. Find information from the NCI or from reputable medical journals. The doctor might never respect your efforts as much as you would like, but it will be harder (not impossible) for her to argue with pedigreed medical facts in print.

- Be matter-of-fact and forthright; don't slouch; use appropriate eye contact. Note that if you use humor with this kind of person, unless it's terribly urbane it's likely she'll decide you're someone that she doesn't need to take seriously.

- Be kind, but overt. Subtleties might waft right past this ego.

- If you're really annoyed by a particular exchange, you might try saying in a level tone, "Please don't say that. It sounds condescending, although I realize you didn't intend to sound that way."

The unethical doctor

If you have good reason to question your doctor's ethics, find another doctor. You might consider contacting your state regulatory agency to see what other actions might be appropriate, but don't endanger yourself by remaining in her care.

The impatient, insensitive doctor

Any doctor can have a bad day, perhaps seeming impatient or even cruelly insensitive, but if it happens consistently, you should consider finding another doctor.

If you are unable to change doctors, you should discuss with her your unhappiness about being offended or hurt as soon as possible. You may have some success in being very forthright and firm with this sort of doctor, because when humane factors cease being honored, what remains is a business relationship, and you're the paying customer.

Ironically, this doctor may be a very good and knowledgeable technician, but you're not likely to benefit fully from her expertise if you're upset each time you interact. Moreover, the stress of having to deal continually with a vexatious person might reduce the ability of your immune system to fight off infection, disincline you from adhering to a treatment regimen, or discourage you from phoning the doctor if you notice unusual symptoms.

The aloof, guarded doctor

Some doctors seem to want to distance themselves from patients. It's difficult to know if this person is cool by nature or is suffering the pain and burnout of being overexposed to the bittersweet results of practicing oncology. More often, they are genuinely concerned about you, as a patient and as a person, but momentarily lack the emotional wherewithal to express it.

You may find that this kind of doctor opens to you gradually, in response to certain aspects of your own attitude, your sense of humor, or things you have in common, such as parenthood. Many patients report finding a meeting ground with an aloof doctor gradually, as experiences are shared. To the extent that you warm to each other over time, you probably can expect expressions of compassion, support, and understanding from your doctor regarding your circumstances and the decisions you make.

The antismoking doctor

Often there are strong opinions against smoking in the medical community. Smoking is clearly a causative factor in many serious illnesses and should be avoided when at all possible.

Once you are diagnosed with lung cancer, however, no hint of prejudice against you or reduction in your care because of your having smoked is justifiable among medical personnel. They are doctors; you are ill. You are entitled to the best and most humane treatment, regardless of your medical history. The quality of mercy is paramount.

If you suspect your doctor is not treating you as well as she could because you do or did smoke, change doctors.

The equitable doctor

This is the doctor that most people probably prefer. She's able to sense whether you'd like a little information or a lot, and when; she seems to know when you need help making a decision or just more time to think; she doesn't react personally if you decide to learn as much as you can or if you decide to get a second opinion. If you're having an especially bad day, she seems to understand and doesn't hold a grudge.

You can tell clearly that she hurts when you hurt, and she's happy to be able to help you. She rejoices when she sees you evolve through the cancer experience into an informed patient, capable of making sound choices, and when she sees you succeed in finding a perspective that will give you some respite from worry.

The oncology nurse

The oncology nurse is the third most important person involved in your treatment, following only you and your doctor as key players.

Generally, oncology nurses are a uniquely loving breed. Not surprisingly, in some hospitals this specialty of nursing sees a high turnover of personnel because of feelings of vulnerability and burnout. They care deeply for their patients, often thinking of their charges long after returning to their own homes and lives.

If you take the time to befriend the nurse, you'll have an intelligent, well-informed, soothing ally to help you deal with treatment and its side effects.

The HMO case manager

Cancer survivors report disparate degrees of satisfaction with their health maintenance organizations (HMOs). Often the case manager is the pivotal factor.

The case manager's role is to streamline your treatment approval process, to keep costs down by eliminating redundant tests and treatments, to review your proposed care plan to ensure it meets certain standards, and to intercede for you to bend rules when your care must deviate from the standards of the HMO.

Some, but by no means all, HMOs use registered nurses or physician's assistants to oversee the approval of your care. When this is not the case, it means that decisions about your care might be made by someone with no medical training at all, who simply bases decisions on rules provided by her superiors.

It's to your advantage to get to know your case manager well and to communicate as thoroughly as possible. If you feel you are not being fairly treated, however, do not hesitate to ask to speak with a superior or to have the case reviewed by the HMO's medical doctor. HMOs often retain doctors for this purpose. At times, just the suggestion of a review by an MD is enough to cause the HMO to bend rules in your favor.

Family members

Family members and others intimately involved in the patient's care may find that they are in an awkward position when dealing with a loved one's doctor. Some oncologists cleave to the concept that their relationship is with the patient alone and, absent instructions to the contrary, all communications are considered the patient's privilege. If you sense this, while in the doctor's presence clarify your wishes regarding your doctor's sharing information with your loved ones.

Suggestions for successful interaction

Now that the players and the circumstances have been defined, specific ideas for improving communication are discussed.

Overinterpreting body language

Stress inclines people to react to visual cues more strongly than to the other senses. When we are terribly worried, we are inclined to scrutinize the faces and body language of those around us.

Take care not to overinterpret the actions and facial expressions of the doctors you communicate with. It's most likely they are not hiding anything from you—in the US, the days of lying to patients about cancer are over—and are relaying with their words the information you need. If you're intensely studying and interpreting facial cues, you might miss important verbal information.

Points of good communication

In general, the more you communicate, the better your chances of getting good care, even if the exchanges are not always smooth. Many patients make the mistake of not telling their doctors enough, perhaps because they feel intimidated or feel they'll be perceived as whining, or because they're afraid they're wasting the doctor's time. Here are a few tips to facilitate communication:

- Keep a journal between appointments of things that you notice and questions that arise.

- Before each visit, make a list of all your concerns, side effects, unusual happenings, and so on, and number them in order of priority—but be sure to relay all of them. What seems insignificant to you may be quite meaningful to your doctor.

- Allow the doctor to distract you only briefly. If she interrupts, be sure to get back to your list after answering her question. If she interrupts often, say calmly that you want to finish this thought before moving to another topic.

- Between appointments, do not hesitate to call your doctor about anything unusual that arises. At your next meeting, remind the doctor of these calls and reiterate your understanding of the content of her replies.

- Use a tape recorder to capture the doctor's wisdom. If she seems uncomfortable with this, you might offer a nonthreatening explanation, such as the well-documented fact that one's memory doesn't work well when under stress. After the meeting, review the recording with a friend or caregiver.

- If you don't have a recorder, ask your friend or caregiver to accompany you as an advocate. Lowell S. Levin, a professor at the Yale School of Public Health and Chairman of the People's Medical Society, says you should take along a family member or friend who is assertive, but diplomatic. You're likely to feel more relaxed and focused; you'll be perceived as wanting to be on top of your own issues; your friend may remember issues you'd discussed, but forgotten, or may think of things that neither you nor your doctor had considered. Make it clear that you want the medical staff to communicate as fully with your advocate as they do with you.

- As mentioned in Chapter 17, *Finances, Employment, and Record Keeping*, get copies of all your medical records and acquaint yourself with them.

- If you have many questions, offer to make an appointment just for this purpose. It's unfair to the doctor and other patients if your 15-minute follow-up exam turns into a 90-minute discussion.

- If your doctor is willing to have a phone consultation to answer many questions, offer to pay for her time.

- Tell your doctor's staff whether it's okay to phone you at the office. Clarify whether they may leave detailed messages on your answering machine without concern for violating your privacy. Make these arrangements in advance.

- If waiting over a weekend for clarification of disturbing news is unacceptable to you, tell your doctor, and find out her policy about being paged on weekends and holidays.

- Ask how you can reach the doctor or her staff during off hours.

- If you have a complaint, voice it first in a calm, objective way and suggest possible solutions. Explain that you understand the stress many oncologists face, but that this problem has caused you considerable distress. This leaves you with the option of being increasingly strident later if necessary, and reassures the medical staff that they're dealing with a reasonable, tactful person who understands compromise and human error.

- Keep written details of complaints you've expressed, including when and how often.

- Above all, strive to have good relations with all of the medical staff by remembering to say thanks, telling them if you're feeling especially stressed, giving them an idea of how much information you're comfortable hearing, and treating all people you contact with kindness, as if they're facing the same problems you're facing—because, in fact, they may be.

Larry Coffman describes his methods for communicating:

> *I always took a microcassette recorder to the oncologist's office and taped the conversation for later playback if I couldn't remember what the doc said, or I thought that I had misunderstood. I found that it worked so well that I began taking it to each appointment I had with other doctors.*
>
> *My motives were honest and I wasn't trying to trap the doctors, but have found that they are a bit more attentive and less likely to give me the "standard" answer to a question. Most physicians were very receptive to the idea; others were not, and those that were not I do not see anymore. If it makes them nervous, it just might make you wonder.*

Second and subsequent opinions

A second opinion is always in order if you have any concerns at all about the decisions made for your care. Although you may have to justify getting a second opinion to your insurance company and you certainly should tell your doctor that you want a second opinion, you do not have to apologize to your doctor for doing so. In fact, the Hippocratic Oath requires your doctor to seek outside advice when your well being is in question.

The NCI or the nearest medical school can supply you with the names of oncologists available for consultation. See Chapter 3, *Finding the Right Treatment Team*, for more information.

Other organizations, such as the American Medical Association and the Cancer Supportive Care Program, can also offer advice about subsequent opinions. See *http://www.ama-assn.org/insight/gen_hlth/doctor/second.htm* and *http://www.cancersupportivecare.com/second_opinions.html*.

Conflict resolution

Occasionally, problems arise between the patient and medical personnel that require more than tact and compromise.

Negotiation

If your concerns evolve around occasional mishaps and miscommunication rather than grossly inadequate care, trying to work through the problem with your doctor may be worthwhile. Schedule an appointment just for discussion, write down your main points and examples, and, unless you have had a great deal of experience negotiating, briefly rehearse beforehand what you'll say:

- Use "I" phrases, or neutral phrases, instead of accusations: "I felt belittled when you joked about my questions about sexual activity," or "That kind of answer about my questions strikes me as condescending," rather than "You like making your patients feel stupid, don't you?"

- Use a level, calm tone and appropriate eye contact. Getting angry will be a less useful tool in achieving good care than an honest attempt to communicate. Staring down the other party and avoiding eye contact entirely are both often interpreted as hostile, obstructive body language.

- Make it clear that your purpose is a permanent, workable solution, not revenge.

- Be specific. For example, don't say, "Whenever I ___, you always ___." Instead, say, "When I needed your help last week with understanding shortness of breath, you looked at your watch and told me that if I'd just stop worrying so much I'd breathe better."

- Don't repeat gossip heard from other patients, no matter what the volume or apparent accuracy of such third-hand information is.

- Recognize that anything perceived by the doctor as an insult is not likely to advance your chief goal of receiving good care. If, in order to satisfy your pain, you corner the doctor into admitting that she learned virtually no social skills in medical school or in life, plan to find a new doctor, because you'll almost certainly be punished later for humiliating the doctor if you continue in her care.

- Demonstrate calmly that you understand occasional mistakes or miscommunications may occur, but that you expect them to be fixed promptly and tactfully, and ask how you can help make this easier.

- Don't threaten to change doctors unless you mean it. If your doctor feels defensive, your care may suffer instead of improve.

Third-party intervention

The medical community is a rigid hierarchy. Use this to your advantage. If the doctor's staff continually disappoints you in spite of your tactful efforts to get satisfaction, tell the doctor. If a specialist to whom you were referred was unkind, tell the doctor. If the doctor repeatedly mishandles your concerns, say so. Unlike many relationships in life that require a great deal of subtlety and finesse, in this instance you can be quite overt as long as you're not cruel, incorrect, or unfair. Altruism and humanity aside, you are a paying customer. While tact is usually fruitful, superhuman efforts to be tactful, far exceeding those of the medical staff, for example, are not called for. It's your life at stake, not your reputation.

If you feel you have a problem with your current or previous doctor that you cannot resolve, you might contact your state health commission, the administrators or social workers at the hospital where the doctor treats you, or the local chapter of the Medical and Chirurgical (MEDCHI) Society, a group that acts as arbiters in disputes between doctors and patients.

Changing doctors

The decision to change oncologists is a wrenching one for many lung cancer survivors, but it need not be. If you believe you've done everything you can to resolve difficulties with your doctor or her staff, and if your medical insurance allows it, a clean break and a new start may be the best option.

It isn't absolutely necessary to tell your doctor you're leaving—the fact will become obvious soon enough when your new doctor requests information from your former doctor—but you might feel better if you handle this transition courteously, and certainly it will facilitate the pragmatic aspects of changing doctors, such as getting timely copies of medical records and doctor-to-doctor communication.

All states have laws providing for transfer of records, accomplished either by sending the records directly to the new doctor or to you. Expect to pay photocopy and shipment fees for this service.

Summary

Successful communication with medical personnel, especially with doctors, may require a variety of tactics. A combination of skills are required—language skills, listening skills, body language, assertiveness, diligent checking of facts, tenacity, compassion, and tact.

If a doctor is not inclined by nature or training to accord you kindness and respect, it will be up to you to attempt to level the playing field. If your needs for care, information, or emotional support from your doctor are continually unmet, however, or are met with hostility, do your best to discuss this with your doctor or consider finding a new oncologist or surgeon.

Key points to remember:

- Be respectful to all medical personnel. They're human, too, and some of them may be facing problems that are as serious as yours.

- Tell them if you're feeling stressed.

- Tell them how much information you want to hear today, and that your capacity to absorb information might change over time.

- Be assertive, but diplomatic. You have a right to good medical care, both by virtue of the doctor's Hippocratic oath and because you're a paying customer.

- Get the facts before communicating: keep good records and take your notes with you to appointments.

- Do not remain in the care of a doctor in whom you no longer have confidence or with whom you have a serious conflict regarding communication style. A second opinion or a change of doctors is neither selfish nor out of the ordinary.

- If you have a serious problem with a doctor or with HMO personnel, contact your state health department or state insurance commissioner for options open to you.

CHAPTER 5

What Is Lung Cancer?

It is not uncommon for individual lung cancers to manifest
biochemical features of both SCLC and NSCLC.

—Mabry, Nelkin, and Baylin
The Genetic Basis of Human Cancer

LUNG CANCER IS A TERM that describes a group of cancers, all of which affect the lung. Their treatments and outcomes differ.

In this chapter, we describe the characteristics of lung tissue and different lung cancers so that you can build a frame of reference for understanding your disease. First, we'll discuss briefly the structure and function of the lung. Next, lung cancers in the broader context of all cancers are described: types of lung cancer and variations in lung cancer by age, gender, race, geography, and other characteristics are discussed. Finally, we'll examine what is known about the possible and known causes of lung cancer.

What are the lungs?

The lungs are the body's means of exchanging oxygen for carbon dioxide and other gases. Oxygen is most critical, but other gases, such as nitrogen and water vapor, also are exchanged. Carbon dioxide is the main byproduct of these metabolic processes.

In normal circumstances, the expansion and contraction of the lungs called breathing occurs without conscious thought or effort. Normal breathing is the result of opposing but balanced forces that act like bellows.

Both the left and right lung absorb oxygen upon inhalation and expel carbon dioxide upon exhalation. The left lung is smaller than the right lung and consists of fewer lobes (see Figure 1-1 in Chapter 1, *Symptoms of Lung Cancer*), because it accommodates other left-side organs, such as the stomach and part of the heart.

Because of complex interactions between gravity, lung expansion, and blood circulation, when we are upright, most lung activity occurs in the lower lobes. When we rest in a horizontal position, though, the upper lobes of the lungs become more active in gas exchange.

The heart and the lungs work closely together; when disease exists in either, both often are affected.

What is lung cancer?

Lung cancer begins as the uncontrolled growth of cells that line the innermost surface of one lung or one airway leading to a lung. Lung tumors are known to progress gradually through stages of change from unusual overgrowths to cancerous tumors: hyperplasia, dysplasia, and neoplasia. As with other cancers, the wayward cells that characterize lung cancer do not always die as normal cells do (apoptosis), nor do they honor the cycles of orderly cell division as normal cells do: many have no resting phase, and instead divide continuously. What's worse, they divide without becoming fully mature, which makes them unable to function as the normal cells of the lung do. The body accumulates nonfunctional lung cells that crowd out other functioning lung cells and other nearby normal cells within affected organs, possibly blocking airways and causing pain in nearby bones or bleeding in lung tissue. For most solid tumors, an additional step must occur to cause serious illness and death: the abnormally proliferating cells must develop the ability to invade other organs. This invasiveness distinguishes benign tumors from malignant tumors; invasive strength distinguishes low-grade tumors from aggressive, high-grade tumors.

Differences from other cancers

The chief difference between lung cancer and other cancers is that a large percentage of lung cancers have one cause: exposure to tobacco smoke.

Lung cancer also differs from some other cancers in that there are no affordable, effective screening tests for which insurance companies are willing to pay. This means that most lung cancers are diagnosed at later stages when treatments are less likely to be successful.

Those diagnosed with one lung tumor are at high risk of developing a subsequent, but independent, lung cancer in remaining lung tissue. The genetic or environmental exposures that predispose one to developing lung cancer affect substantial amounts of lung tissue, creating multiple areas of abnormal cells with the potential for becoming cancerous—what is known as field cancerization or a cancerized field.

Unlike surgical approaches to breast cancer or colon cancer, for which removing all tissue might be a means of preventing recurrence of disease, removal of all lung tissue is not an option at this time.

Lung cancer differs from several other cancers in that individual cells of lung tumors demonstrate a great deal of damage to DNA, described below and in Appendix E, *Experimental Prognostic Markers*. In almost all lung cancers, the genetic damage includes the gain or loss of entire chromosomes, instability of short repeated gene segments (microsatellites), and a wide area of damage in the lung (field cancerization).

All persons with cancer are occasionally the target of some blame from the "healthy unaware" (See Chapter 16, *Getting Support*). People sometimes are blamed for having cancer because of their health habits, psychological type, negative thinking, "wishing" or "needing" to have cancer, and so on. Those with lung cancer are even more prone to be blamed, because of much-needed public health initiatives against smoking. Although smoking has been linked to the causation of at least eight other cancers, those diagnosed with other cancers seldom are asked by casual acquaintances whether they smoke.

Incidence and trends

According to 1996 Surveillance, Epidemiology and End Results (SEER) statistics from the National Cancer Institute, lung cancer is the second most commonly occurring cancer in the US, following breast and prostate cancers in incidence at 57 people affected per 100,000.[1] The American Cancer Society projects that new cases of lung cancer in 2000 will number 164,100.[2]

SEER statistics from 1973 through 1996 show an increase of 27.8 percent in lung cancer cases in that time span: a 2.5 percent decrease in incidence among males, and a 123.0 percent increase among females.

The American Cancer Society estimates that lung cancer will remain the most common cause of cancer death in the US, exceeding deaths from breast and prostate cancers. ACS estimates that about 156,900 Americans will die from lung cancer in 2000.

Detailed incidence rates for small cell and non-small cell lung cancers differ, though:

- SCLC incidence has increased 57.8 percent since 1973: an increase of 21 percent among males and 149.1 percent in females.

- NSCLC incidence has increased 23.6 percent since 1973: a decrease of 5.5 percent among males and an increase of 118.5 percent among females. Among NSCLC subtypes, adenocarcinoma has seen the largest increase.

Who gets lung cancer?

You'd be an unusual person if you didn't wonder why you developed lung cancer and where you are in the spectrum of others with the same disease. Much remains unknown about the causes of lung cancer, but several patterns emerge among those who are diagnosed. These are discussed below.

Geri Capasso discusses her brother's odds against getting lung cancer:

> My brother never smoked a day in his life and at age 46 he is diagnosed with NSCLC stage IV. I, on the other hand, smoked like a fiend for about 20 years and quit in 1991. By the way, I loved smoking and it was the hardest breakup I ever went through.
>
> My point is that getting cancer has no rhyme or reason. When I watched a certain HBO special, I thought it was very interesting to see that dinosaurs got cancer. It seems that just recently cancer research in general is finally headed in the right direction. And for anyone to point a finger at a smoker as being undeserving of the funds needed for a cure is simply not a nice person in my book. I pray every day for a cure.

Karen Parles, medical librarian and creator of Lung Cancer Online (*http://www.lungcanceronline.org*), describes why lung cancer deserves more study:

> I was diagnosed in 1998, at the age of 38, with advanced NSCLC. I had never smoked in my life, and I had not been exposed to second-hand smoke, radon, or asbestos. It was shocking to learn that I had lung cancer. I soon discovered, however, that I was not alone as a young, never-smoking female with lung cancer. In fact, I found that our numbers are increasing, and that more than 5,000 of us die each year from our disease. Many of us are mothers of young children.

*Our plight is unknown to the public at large and has been virtually
ignored by the medical profession. I have written countless letters to
medical researchers and the media trying to bring attention to this
epidemic of lung cancer among never-smokers. The general consensus is
that lung cancer research focuses on smokers and former smokers because
they represent the overwhelming majority of lung cancer cases. My view
happens to be that we never-smokers must be a highly susceptible group
and are therefore worth studying. Thankfully, because the absolute
number of never-smokers with lung cancer is substantial and on the rise,
researchers are beginning to take a harder look at this alarming
phenomenon.*

Smokers

Various inhaled toxins have been linked to the development of lung cancer and are
discussed in depth under "What causes lung cancer?" later in this chapter.[3] Chief
among these toxins is tobacco smoke, itself a mixture of thousands of chemical
agents. According to NCI statistics, the risk of developing lung cancer is 2,000 percent higher for smoking males than for nonsmoking males; for females, the risk is
1,200 percent higher for smokers versus nonsmokers.

Eighty to ninety percent of lung cancers develop in smokers or ex-smokers. About 10
to 15 percent of smokers develop lung cancer. Rates of lung cancer are lower among
cigar and pipe smokers than among cigarette smokers, but all tobacco smokers are at
increased risk of lung cancer and several other cancers, and risk increases with
increasing degree of exposure.

Kathleen Houlihan describes getting lung cancer in spite of significant lifestyle
changes recommended by many medical authorities:

*I quit smoking eight years before my lung cancer diagnosis, and since
then (even starting before then) became progressively more and more of a
health fanatic. I've been a virtual vegan (no meat, virtually no dairy, but
occasional eggs and fish) for several years, I take all kinds of vitamins,
minerals and herbs, drink green tea, eat lots of tofu and soy milk and
miso. Plus exercise—walking dogs twenty minutes in the morning and
usually over an hour in the evening. Plus no chemicals to speak of in the
house. Plus reverse osmosis water and almost all organic groceries. The
whole enchilada.*

Older studies suggested that about fifteen years after quitting smoking, lung cancer risk decreased to the risk faced by the never-smoking population. Newer studies show, however, that this statistic is too general:

- The earlier one starts smoking, the higher the risk remains throughout life.
- Fifty percent of lung cancers diagnosed today are in former smokers.
- Those who have smoked heavily for many years often have extensive and possibly irreversible precancerous changes and field cancerization in their lungs.

In addition to the greatly increased risks of cancer of the lung and bronchus among tobacco smokers, this group also faces a proven increased risk of cancers of the pancreas, urinary bladder, kidney, oral cavity, esophagus, uterine cervix, colon, rectum, pharynx, and larynx. Increased risks for cancers of the liver, stomach, and prostate are suspected.[4]

Passive smokers

Exposure to secondhand or sidestream smoke has been associated with lung cancer among those who have never smoked. Secondhand smoke also increases the risk of several serious or fatal illnesses, including such cancers as brain tumors, leukemias, and lymphomas, among the children of smokers of both genders.[5] Adult relatives who live with smokers are more likely to develop heart disease or benign respiratory diseases.

Gender

Although the rate of lung cancer is increasing drastically among females, it remains the case that more males are diagnosed with lung cancer than females. According to 1996 SEER statistics, the age-adjusted incidence among males is 70 per 100,000, whereas the age-adjusted incidence for females is 42.3 per 100,000. This incidence represents a rate decrease over the last decade among males and a pronounced and grim rate increase among females, as described earlier in "Incidence and trends." Smoking in women aged 15 to 25 is rising rapidly, with up to 40 percent of this population being current smokers. The US has the highest rate of female lung cancer deaths in the world. If the rate of increase in lung cancer among females continues unabated, incidence and prevalence of lung cancer among females will someday equal or surpass that of males.

Race

According to 1996 SEER statistics, African Americans are diagnosed with invasive lung cancer more often than Caucasian Americans: 73.9 per 100,000 versus 55.9 per 100,000.[6] African Americans with lung cancer are diagnosed in later stages and at an earlier age, and they survive for shorter periods of time.

This difference is thought by some to be an artifact of socioeconomic class rather than race: that is, attributable to differences in access to healthcare among socioeconomic classes in the US. One recent study has found, though, that even when socioeconomic factors are equal, African Americans with any cancer might be in receipt of less comprehensive care than Caucasian Americans. Other studies show that the higher incidence of and mortality from lung cancer in the African American population might be attributable to a reduced capacity to eliminate certain classes of carcinogens found in tobacco because of variations in the glutathione S-transferase M1 (GSTM1) gene.

The incidence of lung cancer diagnoses in all races per 100,000 US population is:

- 73.9 among African Americans

- 55.9 among Caucasian Americans

- 35.8 among Asians/Pacific Islanders

- 27.6 among Hispanics

- 18.6 among American Indians

Geographic distribution

The highest lung cancer incidence in both males and females is found in New Zealand among the Maori. The country with the highest male lung cancer death rate is Belgium; for females, Scotland.

Worldwide, more cases of lung cancer occur in urban areas than in rural areas. Air pollution in urban areas, especially industrial air pollution, is thought to be the cause of this difference.

China might emerge as the country with the highest incidence of lung cancer within ten to twenty years because of increased cigarette smoking and exceptionally high levels of indoor air pollution (coal, tobacco, and cooking oil). China is the world's largest producer and consumer of tobacco, with more than 1,900 cigarettes sold per adult per year, making China the world's largest market for cigarettes. Sixty-three percent of Chinese men smoke; 3.8 percent of Chinese women smoke. The average Chinese smoker spends 25 percent of his or her income on cigarettes. More than 72 percent of all Chinese are exposed to tobacco smoke. China is experiencing "an epidemic of diseases caused by tobacco."[7]

Age

The incidence of lung cancer rises with increasing age. The combined incidence for those under age 65 is 25.0 per 100,000 people; for those over age 65, however, the combined incidence is 348.6 per 100,000.

Socioeconomic class

One study of Americans has correlated an increased incidence of lung cancer to economic deprivation for most, but not all, ethnic groups, Hispanics being the exception.[8] Studies elsewhere also support a general tendency for lung cancer to occur more often among those of lower socioeconomic status.[9,10] Reasons offered for the correlation between lower socioeconomic class and increased lung cancer risk include:

- Increased rates of smoking among lower socioeconomic classes. Some studies have correlated increased tobacco smoking to lower socioeconomic status,[11] but other studies point out that tobacco smoking cannot be correlated to income in a meaningful way without consideration of other factors.[12]

- The tendency for lower-paid factory and production workers to be more frequently exposed to inhaled industrial toxins than are upper-level staff.

- The likelihood that the less wealthy will live closer to air-polluted areas.

- The inaccessibility of good health care to those with little money.

Family history

Those facing cancer often become concerned that family members might also be at risk. One recent study has shown that there is an inherited tendency to lung cancer, manifesting more often among younger people.[13] Another study has found a likelihood of increased lung cancer among nonsmokers in families with father, mother, or sibling having several other cancers, including breast, lung, airway, and digestive cancers.[14] Eleven studies discussed by Schwartz in *Lung Cancer: Principles and Practice* (Lippincott, 2000) describe a relative risk (risk compared to the general population, which is always assumed to be a risk of 1.0) for familial lung cancer ranging from 1.3 to 7.2.

A cancer survivor tells of how prevalent cancer is in his family:

> *Both my brothers and I were diagnosed with lung cancer. My younger brother passed away four years ago. My second brother was diagnosed last year, lung surgery. We had cancer on both sides of our family. My Mother passed away with cancer.*

The specific genetic variations that predispose one to lung cancer and that might be inherited are discussed more fully later under "What causes lung cancer?"

If you suspect that lung cancer in your family is inherited, contact the Genetic Epidemiology of Lung Cancer Consortium, listed in Appendix A.

Occupation

Those who work in environments containing certain inhaled toxins face an increased risk of lung cancer. Specific toxins are discussed under "Inhaled toxins." People whose occupations have these exposures are at increased risk.

It is important to note that studies done in other countries, although well conducted and meaningful in their context, might report on the effects of manufacturing techniques never used, or no longer used, in the US.

In the 1996 edition of *Cancer Rates and Risks*, the NCI lists the following occupations as high-risk occupations for lung cancer: miners, millers, textile workers, insulation handlers, shipyard workers (arc welders exposed to nickel or chromium fumes, for example, or those who handle asbestos), and cement handlers.

In Chapter 20 of the second edition of *Lung Cancer: Principles and Practice* (Lippincott, 2000), Schottenfeld describes these additional occupational risk factors:

- Roofers exposed to coal tar fumes

- Railroad workers exposed to diesel exhaust

- Smelters exposed to arsenic in mined copper, lead, zinc, or tin ore

- Producers and users of inorganic pesticides containing arsenic

- Plastic producers exposed to vinyl chloride, BCME, or CCME

- Early-stage refining of dust-heavy nickel ore for electroplating, steel manufacture, ceramics, battery manufacture, electric circuitry, and petroleum refining

- Coke oven workers in steel plants exposed to polycyclic aromatic hydrocarbons (PAHs)

- Any aluminum, nickel, or coal workers exposed to exhaust containing PAHs

- Workers exposed to PAHs in soot from combustion and diesel exhausts

- Retort coal gas plant workers

Other studies have found that those in the following occupations are at increased risk for lung cancer:[15,16,17]

- Plumbers, mechanics, and seamen exposed to asbestos

- Technical, chemical, physical, and biological workers exposed to asbestos

- Waiters and tobacco workers exposed to tobacco smoke

- Quarry workers

- Female construction workers

- Female barstaff

- Painters

These occupations appear to contribute to idiopathic pulmonary fibrosis, which often develops into lung cancer:[18]

- Farming

- Livestock handling

- Hairdressing

- Exposure to metal dust

- Raising birds

- Stone cutting or polishing

- Exposure to vegetable or animal dust

In China, females who do not smoke nonetheless experience high rates of lung cancer. This rate is attributed to indoor air pollution from coal stoves and from oil vapors generated during high-temperature frying.

Vietnam veterans

The US Department of Veterans Affairs (VA) recognizes exposure to dioxin (Agent Orange) as a risk factor for lung cancer and several other cancers. See Chapter 17, *Finances, Employment, and Record Keeping*, and Appendix A for more information. You can contact the VA at (800) 827-1000 or visit *http://www.va.gov*.

What causes cancer?

Before a clear discussion of the causes of lung cancer can ensue, you need to know a bit about what causes cancers in general.

Human DNA is stored on 46 paired chromosomes. With a couple of exceptions, each cell in the body has one copy of all 46 chromosomes, coiled tightly in a ball and stored in the cell nucleus. Each chromosome is composed of two long strings of genes held together like a ladder, with rungs consisting of electrochemical bonds.

All instances of cancer are accompanied by changes in the tumor cell's DNA. At times, one or more genes are entirely missing; have been altered by viruses that insert their own genes into the human genome; or have been half-spliced with another gene after DNA strands from two entirely different chromosomes accidentally overlap, break apart, and rejoin. In some cases, an entire chromosome may be missing. Often these mutations are harmless, but when a great many accumulate or a regulatory gene is affected, then uncontrolled growth, either benign or cancerous, may result. Regulatory genes that control cell growth, orderly cell death called apoptosis (the p53 gene, for instance), maturation of cell division, and cell reproduction are particularly important.

These changes become potentially harmful when genes are engaged to manufacture proteins. All of the body's work is accomplished using proteins. Our bodies build proteins from genes by reading the base pairs of DNA in groups of three, until special repeating sequences recognized as terminators are encountered. Each triplet encodes for one amino acid, and the complete string of amino acids comprises a protein. The string of amino acids that accumulates—that is, the protein built as the DNA is transcribed—is unique to that gene.

If the gene is damaged by the crossing-over of two chromosomes (translocation), for instance, a protein built from it will be based half on one gene and half on another and most likely will be completely nonfunctional, or even toxic. If one base pair is deleted from DNA, the transcription of the three base pairs into one amino acid is shifted off by one, almost exactly like placing one's fingers on a piano or computer keyboard in the wrong starting position. That is, every subsequent movement up and down the keyboard will produce wrong notes or wrong letters when the starting point is wrong. Thus, when one or more base pairs are missing, the resulting protein will be entirely different from that which the body is expecting to accomplish some metabolic task.

In most cases, cancerous growths are distinguished from benign growths by their ability to invade other tissues, although some leukemias can be fatal just by crowding out healthy blood cells from bone marrow without invading other organs.

Often, the higher the number of damaged genes, the more likely cancer is to result, as more and more cellular functions become affected by nonfunctioning proteins. Some cancers, though, such as acute promyelocytic leukemia, can result from damage to just two genes.[19]

What causes lung cancer?

Many people try to determine what gave cancer a foothold, sometimes from intellectual curiosity and sometimes from a determination not to suffer a recurrence.

Known causes

Asbestos, tobacco smoke, and ionizing radiation are proven causes of lung cancer.

Inhaled toxins

Many inhaled toxins have been linked to lung cancer. Chief among these are tobacco smoke and asbestos. It has been suggested that combined exposure to some agents along with tobacco smoke increases one's risk. Indoor radon is thought to contribute to about 14,000 lung cancer deaths in the US each year.

Other toxic inhaled substances that have been examined as possible causes of lung cancer include:[20] uranium ore dust; toluene;[21] vinyl chloride; cadmium; oil mists; acrylonitrile; beryllium; chromium fumes; nickel fumes; inorganic arsenic; silicon and ferrosilicon; mustard gas; chloromethyl esters BCME and CCME; hydrazine and other chemicals associated with rocket-engine testing;[22] fungal agents, such as microsporum canis;[23] byproducts of marijuana combustion (delta-9-tetrahydrocannabinol); polycyclic aromatic hydrocarbons (PAHs) from fossil fuel combustion; benzo(a)pyrene and possibly other airborne pyrenes; exhaust from soft smoky coal; wood smoke; and wood, metal, and stone dust.

Genetics

Many people diagnosed with lung cancer become concerned that their siblings or children also might face a risk of developing lung cancer. In fact, some families appear to be genetically predisposed to lung cancer. In these families, minimizing risks is especially important.

It might be difficult to understand any increased risk among family members if the way that many research studies use the word "genetic" is not understood. We who are not involved in research tend to use the word "genetic" interchangeably with "heritable" or "inherited," but the study of genetics encompasses a broader meaning, and researchers sometimes do not refer to genetics in the heritable sense when they use the word genetics. It is important to understand that genetic changes can be either inherited at conception or acquired via mutation throughout our lifetime. Many genetic changes occur within cancerous cells, but only genetic changes or errors that arise and persist in sperm or ova can be inherited.

If you have lung cancer, that by itself does not necessarily mean that your children will be more likely to get lung cancer. Many genetic changes accompany lung cancer, and knowledge is incomplete regarding which of these changes are heritable (that is, possibly predispose one's children to lung cancer) and which occur solely in the lung cancer patient as lungs become damaged and disease progresses. Even with the tools and methods available today, heritable changes are in some cases indistinguishable from environmentally induced genetic changes that initiate lung cancer or genetic changes that accumulate as disease progresses.

Research is in progress to determine which of these possibly inherited genetic variants or deletions is most meaningful: genes NAT1, NAT2, CYP1A1, CYP2D6, CYP2A6, CYP2E1, GSTM1, GSTT1, HRAS1, mEH, ERCC1, XPD, XPF, XRCC3, and XRCC1.

The following inherited sensitivities to substances that cause chromosome damage, thus predisposing one to lung cancer, are attributed to genetic variations that have not yet been mapped:

- Bleomycin mutagen sensitivity. This sensitivity is found most often in Mexican Americans and African Americans. This sensitivity can be further divided into chromosome 4 and chromosome 5 bleomycin sensitivity.

- Benzo(a)pyrene diol-epoxide (BPDE) mutagen sensitivity, found most often in Caucasians.

- Alfa-1 antitrypsin, controlled by Pi S or Z alleles.

Foods

The concept of avoiding lung cancer by making wise dietary choices is a tantalizing one, but variable results have been found.

Many studies have shown that a diet high in fruits and vegetables reduces the risk of lung cancer in smokers. This is consistent with findings for certain other cancers. A study of 88,000 women correlates a diet high in carrots (but not beta-carotene supplementation) to a reduced risk of lung cancer in female nurses.[24] Other fruits and vegetables noted in the medical literature for appearing to confer a protective effect include soybeans and tofu,[25] green vegetables, bananas, onions, and pumpkins.[26] One study notes that noncitrus fruits are more protective than citrus fruits,[27] but other studies have not found this. Several studies note that diet-based vegetable nutrients, but not supplements of vitamins A, C, or E, decrease the risk of lung cancer. Two large studies (CARET and ATBC) have revealed that beta-carotene vitamin supplementation increases the risk of lung cancer among male smokers.[28] Several studies have demonstrated a correlation between a diet high in fatty foods and an increased risk of lung cancer.[29] Other researchers believe this association is stronger for animal fats than for vegetable fats. Other studies have found that consuming cured foods raises risk, as is also true for certain other aerodigestive cancers. Several studies find high consumption of dairy products correlates to an increased risk of lung cancer. One study found a protective effect from consuming cheese, but an increased risk from consuming milk.[30] Other studies have found that consuming milk increases lung cancer risk for males more so than for females.

Medications, therapies

Those who have been exposed to ionizing radiation during treatment for other illnesses, such as breast cancer, face an increased risk of lung cancer.

Other illnesses

Some studies have found a correlation between benign respiratory illnesses and an increased risk of developing lung cancer: asbestosis, silicosis, idiopathic pulmonary fibrosis, emphysema (chronic obstructive pulmonary disease, COPD), chronic bronchitis, tuberculosis, and collagen vascular diseases, particularly progressive systemic scleroderma.

A recent study of both genders has found an increased risk of lung cancer among women with collagenous colitis, a form of chronic inflammatory bowel disease.[31]

Certain cancers, such as breast cancer or salivary gland cancer, appear to predispose one to lung cancer as a second primary cancer, especially in cases when radiotherapy was used as treatment for the initial cancer.

The aging immune system

Some researchers feel that the greatly increased rate not only of lung cancer, but also of most other cancers among those over age 65, hints at a general weakening of the immune system with age. Others feel that this increase in the rate of lung cancers with age more likely may be an artifact of the modern, industrialized world we live, in that genetic damage from substances in an industrialized environment accumulates over time and first becomes apparent among the oldest.

Summary

The preceding pages have attempted to categorize information about lung cancer so that you may begin to build a frame of reference for understanding this disease, to counsel family members and friends who might be at risk, and, if necessary, to consider lifestyle or occupational changes that might reduce the risk of lung disease.

CHAPTER 6

Prognosis

To lose one's health renders science null, art inglorious,
strength unavailing, wealth useless, and eloquence powerless.

—Herophilus, c. 300 B.C.

ALMOST EVERYONE WANTS TO KNOW how serious their cancer is and what their prospects are for survival. This concern is normal.

In this chapter, we first review factors that limit the ability of this book—or any printed resource—to predict outcomes for lung cancer. The last half of the chapter describes what risk factors have been studied and what factors matter the least and the most.

For any type of cancer, very few prognostic traits have meaning in the absence of a discussion about treatment. In other words, as new and better treatments emerge, they tend to dilute the effects of disease characteristics that once were considered deadly. For this reason, we do not discuss survival percentages in this chapter. When you've finished this chapter, you won't have an absolute, unchanging answer about your prognosis. However, you'll have an idea of factors that might influence your prognosis, a respect for the complexity of the topic, and an awareness of the dangers of predictions. Ask your oncologist for the most up-to-date information about your treatment and its success rate.

Limitations on accurate prognostics

The limitations on the ability to predict the course of lung cancer include the general limitations of all medical studies and statistics. There are still many unknowns, and not all unknowns can be predicted from what we do know. There are also limitations specific to lung cancer, such as the differences between various types of lung cancers and differences in patients. The following are factors to keep in mind when reading any discussion of the prognosis of lung cancer, no matter how recent.

Improving treatments

Because of intense research, information regarding prognoses stated unequivocally today might be obsolete tomorrow. Improvement in surgical techniques, the increasing use of adjuvant therapies, and the tremendous gains made in supportive care all contribute to improving survival. As always, your doctor, a well-trained and skilled person who you most likely chose carefully as outlined in Chapter 3, *Finding the Right Treatment Team*, is your best resource for the most current information. You might also choose to follow the progress of new treatments on your own. Ways to do this are discussed in Chapter 22, *Researching Your Illness*.

Difficult classifications

The various classifications and stages of lung cancer, which by some definitions overlap, make discussing research results complex. This means that multiple studies from different institutions, which yield conflicting results from the same treatment regimen, may not compare readily to one another and, most importantly, may not apply to you and your specific circumstances.

Limitations of statistics

Survival statistics are developed using groups of people, many of whom are not very much like you even if they appear to have the same disease. Your chances may be considerably better, for instance, than those of someone who has several chronic illnesses, such as heart disease, diabetes, or lupus, along with lung cancer. In addition, many of those whose cases find their way into medical journals and who become the basis for statistics regarding the success of one technique versus another are those who have had many different treatments. They might have one or more organ systems compromised because of repeated toxic treatments.

Those of you who studied statistics in school are aware that many different statistical methods exist to manipulate data, any two of which may in some cases give differing results. Statistical analysis is really just a method for making sense of large amounts of otherwise incomprehensible data. Consequently, sometimes the statistical model chosen represents only science's closest guess regarding how to analyze the outcome of treatment. Some statistical models chosen may not be a good fit for some collections of data. In spite of the best faith on the part of researchers and statisticians, these inconsistencies may creep into research papers. For more information on this topic, see Steven Jay Gould's essay, "The Median Isn't the Message." Steven Jay Gould is a popular evolutionary biologist and a survivor of a rare form of cancer called abdominal mesothelioma. His essay can be found at Cancerguide (*http://www.cancerguide.org/median_not_msg.html*) or in the June 1985 issue of *Discover* magazine.

Geri Capasso speaks eloquently on behalf of her brother Anthony regarding the limitations of statistics:

> *Statistics are created by the medical establishment, who sometimes play God. When people are told that there is no hope, they generally give up, and that is what helps to generate these dismal statistics.*
>
> *I believe that the mind is very important and can influence your fight and healing process. Just think about the moment before a car accident and how your blood pressure, heart, and adrenaline increase, and the hundred ways your body reacts to fright. I'm sure that if a coach told a football team not to bother trying, they had no chance of winning, a lot of players would just give up. But some players would work on a new strategy and fight and go on to win.*
>
> *My brother, age 46, was diagnosed with NSCLC IV metastases in the liver, behind his eye, spine, and pleural lining. When he stopped responding to the first line of chemo (cisplatin, Gemzar), he changed and is now on a second line of chemo (Taxol and thalidomide). He is in the hospital right now, having more fluid drained from his lung, and will undergo another talc procedure to stop the fluid accumulation.*
>
> *The road gets bumpy, but he is still positive, looks good, and feels strong, despite all the odds. My point is never give up hope, and if you believe in statistics, believe that you or your loved one will be in the surviving group! Have faith. My brother and family also believe in prayer.*

Larry Coffman, a five-year survivor of SCLC, has decided that statistics can't apply to him:

> *Statistics give some people a reference point and some people like me believe that it is a way of securing funding—nothing more, nothing less. There are so many variables when talking about lung cancer that no statistic can be used with any degree of accuracy. Problem is, we are bombarded with them so often that the first thing we look at is the statistic. There are only two "for sures" in this lifetime: birth and death.*

Five years ago, I was diagnosed with limited stage small-cell lung cancer located in the right upper lobe. The doctor making the initial diagnosis told me to "go home and get your affairs in order," and gave me a one in twelve chance for survival. That was a beautiful sunny December morning here in Texas. I walked outside and looked skyward, and the first thought I had was, "Man, I am going to miss this."

My oncologist said, "Let's get very aggressive," to which I replied, "We haven't started yet?" Treatment consisted of concurrent chemotherapy—five days a month for a year, using VP-16 (etoposide) and cisplatin in the beginning—and 25 course of radiation therapy. Treatment began a few weeks after diagnosis, and the last treatment with chemo was about twelve months after diagnosis.

So far, the "dragon" is dormant, and hopefully will stay that way. The treatment's extreme level of aggressiveness has pretty much changed my life, but I can still hug my kids, go to open house with them at school, and be here when they just need to talk to me. It's my belief that "I'll be okay either way, the Lord's will be done!"

I have felt all along that I would be my oncologist's "trophy," so to speak, and that I was a statistic, but I didn't and still don't care. I don't believe in statistics, as far as government and cancer go.

Each person has to do what he has to do, it is ultimately his decision, one he will have to make on his own. Consider another medical opinion (or a third or fourth)—whatever it takes to feel that the best-informed decision that can be made is being made.

Correlation is not causation

Just because a characteristic applies to people who have something in common does not mean that the characteristic causes that commonality. For example, say that everyone who has ever entered a college registration office has had a nose. You could say that there is a correlation between being able to walk into that office and having a nose, but you cannot say that having a nose causes a person to walk into that office, or that walking into the office causes a nose to grow. For example, a correlation between a particular occupation and a high lung cancer rate is not proof that this occupational exposure causes lung cancer, but is instead an indication that more study is warranted.

Complexity of the immune response

Humans and their capacity to withstand stressors are, thank goodness, always confounding medical theory. Everyone knows of someone who was told she had only three months to live, but was still alive long after. People can argue that these cases represent misdiagnoses, but this explanation is not likely to cover all such instances and gives no credit for variables, such as the many immune-system factors that are still unknown.

We have a great deal to learn about the immune system and are learning great amounts quickly because of well-financed cancer research and the sharing of knowledge across scientific disciplines.

Physical characteristics of patients in studies

Many lung cancer patients who enter clinical trials, especially phase I and II clinical trials, have had advanced disease and previous treatment that has failed. This means that the percentages of survival found in phase I and II studies of new substances or techniques might be lower than would be found if used on those with less advanced disease who had never been treated.

Staging of lung cancer is not an exact science. There can be significant differences among patients and the characteristics of their disease, even though their stage is nominally the same. See the discussion of staging controversies found later in this chapter.

Some lung cancer patients and survivors are genetically predisposed to lung cancer. It is possible that these patients will respond differently to chemotherapy or radiotherapy than will those who are not genetically predisposed. See the discussion of genetics later in this chapter and in Chapter 5, *What Is Lung Cancer?*, for details of genetic predisposition.

These variables mean that the same treatments used on any one person may produce better results than those recorded in trials; the same treatment used on the general population of lung cancer patients may produce better results than were seen in early clinical trials with pretreated patients.

Kathleen Houlihan describes her efforts to find sound information about her prognosis:

> *Last week my husband Holt and I flew to Houston to go to M. D.*
> *Anderson Cancer Center for a second opinion from an academic/research*
> *institution on whether surgery or any other kind of treatment would be*

appropriate for me at this point. We met with a doctor who went over my story, examined me, and asked us to leave my CT scans there so he could discuss my case with a group of medical, radiation, and surgical oncologists, all of whom specialize in lung cancer.

That discussion, which must have been "grand rounds," although he never called it that, took place this past Tuesday night, and Holt and I talked to the doctor via conference call on Wednesday morning. Their recommendation is exactly the same as the Cancer Treatment Centers of America: no surgery, follow with CT scans. In addition, the MDA doctor said that a "substantial percentage" of patients like me are cured (!) by the treatment I have had, so "that might be the end of it." Sounds good to me! He did also note, however, that a substantial percentage have recurrences. But he said the percentage of cures is not trivial. I had told him when we were in Houston that I didn't want to hear any grim statistics from him— I've already heard them. That's why he didn't go beyond "substantial" and "nontrivial." So the whole experience was quite reassuring, comforting, and encouraging. Well worth the exorbitant cost.

The progress of research

The pace of medical research can make the body of knowledge regarding prognostic factors for lung cancer outdated in just a few months.

At the time this book is being written, there are 105 trials of new treatments for non-small cell lung cancer and 40 trials for small cell lung cancer funded by the National Cancer Institute. This number does not include treatment trials funded solely by pharmaceutical companies and thus not included in the NCI's database. For a better understanding of what this progress might mean for those who are diagnosed today, consider that just ten years ago we didn't have:

- Intricate CT-guided or ultrasound-guided endoscopic procedures for removing all cancerous tissue in the least invasive way.

- Granulocyte colony stimulating factor, G-CSF (Neupogen) and Erythropoietin, Epoietin (Epogen, Procrit), for growing new blood cells when bone marrow has been suppressed by chemotherapy or radiation therapy.

- Stem-cell support for reconstituting bone marrow after high-dose therapy. Stem cell support following chemotherapy for lung cancer is now in clinical trials.

- Magnetic resonance imaging (MRI) for finding very small tumors that have spread to the brain and spine.

- Positron emission tomography (PET) for distinguishing benign lesions from cancerous lesions by detecting differences in glucose metabolism.

- Injected or inhaled imaging substances that permit the surgeon to detect and remove the smallest of cancerous lesions.

- Knowledge of growth factors that affect tumors and the blood vessels that feed them.

- Knowledge of the human genome that will permit custom-designed drugs to match and correct specific genetic aberrations.

- Stereotactic radiosurgery for treating brain metastases.

Thus, bear in mind that the not too distant future holds great promise.

The aging of printed material

Because of the amount of time it takes to enroll patients into trials, perform research, analyze results, write the research paper, peer review the research paper, print the results in a medical journal, and summarize many such papers in a textbook, there can be a lag of at least one year, and usually many more, between the completion of research and the results being disseminated among doctors and the concerned public. During this interval, research has continued and better information may have become available. For this reason, we encourage you to become familiar with clinical trials and medical journals that report progress in the treatment of lung cancer. Methods for finding and understanding the basics of research papers are discussed in Chapter 22.

Remember that what you read about survival and treatment success here, and in all but the newest texts, will never be as current as the information you can receive from a well-trained oncologist active in her specialty who has access to medical journals and to other researchers.

Which factors matter least and most

With all of the above in mind, please see the following summary of the features, both of lung cancer and of the patients who have lung cancer, that seem to affect or not affect outcome of treatment. This summary was prepared using the US National Cancer Institute's PDQ *State-of-the-Art Physicians' Treatment Statements* for small cell and non-small cell lung cancers and the second edition of *Lung Cancer: Principles and Practice* (Lippincott, 2000), edited by Harvey Pass. Many additional Medline and journal references from 1994 through 1999 were used to include the most recently discussed prognostic factors.

Even with the following list of risk factors, nobody is able to speak in absolute terms about your overall prognosis. You may have at least one risk factor for a poorer prognosis, and you will undoubtedly have several factors that point to a better prognosis.

The most important point to remember about your prognosis is that what are used today as reliable prognostic indicators may become meaningless when new treatments that surmount old difficulties are engaged. You might find it encouraging to read Chapter 23, *The Future of Therapy*, after you have read this chapter.

The order of the sections that follow does not imply a greater or lesser effect on outcome.

Stage (extent) of disease

Stage measures how far disease has spread. For some cancers, such as certain leukemias and lymphomas, stage is not strongly correlated to prognosis.

But for lung cancer, the US National Cancer Institute and every other authority on lung cancer state that stage is the most important prognostic factor. Other measures of tumor burden or tumor behavior have been sought and studied as means to predict outcome, but as of now, none is as important as stage of disease. Nonetheless, several exceptions and extensions to staging as a prognostic tool are discussed in the following sections.

SCLC exceptions to prognostic staging

In Chapter 34 of *Lung Cancer: Principles and Practice*, Ronald Feld and colleagues state that:

- SCLC patients with limited disease (LD) and no evidence of tumor activity in the mid-chest (mediastinum) have longer survival than those with mediastinal involvement.

- Those with extensive disease (ED) involving metastasis to the brain or other parts of the central nervous system have the worst prognosis.

- Patients with ED in the bone (not bone marrow) have longer survival than those with liver involvement.

- SCLC patients with LD and bone marrow involvement might have the equivalent prognosis of those with ED.

- Those with ED with metastasis to just one site have longer survival than those with metastases to multiple organs.

Larry Coffman defies the generalizations:

> I guess all of the negative aspects of small cell are evident. Most oncologists believe that, once it is large enough to show up on an x-ray, it's too late—at least that's what I have been told. I don't fret about the amount of time I might have left, nor do I want to be miserable.
>
> I have gone back to college and earned my Associates Degree in General Studies, and the wonderful part is, I have been able to do much of this from home, now that distant learning via computer has taken hold. My next challenge is a Bachelors Degree in Business Administration, majoring in Human Resources. As long as I am concentrating on positives I feel that my physical makeup will benefit as well. I get some of my best exercise walking to the classes that I have to attend on campus, which is even better now that I have the type of portable oxygen I can throw over my shoulder.
>
> My oncologist, pulmonary specialist, and primary physician gave me about an 8 percent chance to make it six months. Well, now I'm a long term, long-termer at five years! Hang in there, friends.

NSCLC exceptions to prognostic staging

When TNM stages are equal, the following traits appear to confer a better prognosis for those with NSCLC:

- No bone metastases
- For M1 disease, a single operable metastasis to only one distant organ when the lung tumor is also completely removed
- Single tumors in one adrenal gland (M1), which are more easily removed than single tumors at other distant metastatic sites
- No invasion of blood vessels by cancerous cells
- Tumors that cannot be visualized with a mediastinoscope
- No invasion of phrenic or vagus nerves in the aortic or supra-aortic region.

- No invasion of hilar lymph nodes

- No invasion of specific mid-chest (mediastinal) lymph nodes that drain areas beyond the immediate area of the tumor

- For bronchioloalveolar carcinoma (BAC), a solitary, nonmucinous tumor instead of a diffuse spread

- Two distinct operable lung tumors rather than one primary tumor and a metastatic secondary lung tumor

Tumor aggressiveness (tumor grade)

For many cancers, an aggressive tumor often (but not always) correlates to a bad prognosis. Almost without exception, SCLC tumors are very aggressive. For those with NSCLC, though, the findings are more heterogeneous because diagnosis does not occur at late stages as frequently as it does for SCLC, and because subtypes of NSCLC are more variable:

- The number of tumor cells actively dividing (known as the percentage of S phase content) is thought to contribute to recurrence of disease.

- An unusually high number of blood vessels in a tumor, a sign of robust tumor growth, is thought to predict recurrence. A tumor must grow beyond 2 millimeters in order to break apart and spread (metastasize). Tumors cannot grow beyond a few millimeters without an increased blood supply.[1]

- Invasion of lymph nodes, lymph vessels, or blood vessels indicates an aggressive tumor.

- Poorly differentiated tumor cells, an indicator of rapid cell division, are correlated to higher tumor grade and greater aggressiveness. Poorly differentiated tumors connote a worse prognosis than well-differentiated tumors diagnosed at the same stage.

- Tumors that can be grown readily and continuously in laboratory culture, a technique known as establishing a cell line, are thought to be more aggressive than tumors that cannot be established in a cell line.

Histology

Histology is the appearance of the tumor cell under the microscope. For all types of cancer, many studies have been done in an attempt to correlate a cancer cell's appearance with the patient's prognosis.

SCLCs with the characteristics of neuroendocrine tumors have a worse prognosis. Neuroendocrine differentiation is associated with advancing disease. One study has found that the mixed subtype of SCLC has longer survival time than the small or combined subtypes.[2]

The following considerations of histology apply to the prognosis of NSCLC:

- When the tumor is considered operable, histology might contribute to prognosis because squamous cell carcinomas tend to recur locally and adenocarcinomas tend to recur at distant sites. This means that the chances of removing all squamous cell disease with a first curative surgery are higher than the chances of removing all traces of adenocarcinoma.

- One study has found that large cell neuroendocrine carcinoma (LCNEC) has a worse prognosis than other NSCLCs.[3]

Blood values

Several blood tests that are commonly performed during routine health assessments can provide predictive information about the prognosis of lung cancer. These tests are meaningful only in concert with other findings, though. They cannot be used in isolation, for instance, as a screening tool, to confirm a recurrence of disease, or to determine prognosis.

For SCLC, these blood values, when assessed within a constellation of other prognostic findings, are indicative of a shorter survival time:

- High levels of lactate dehydrogenase (LDH)

- White blood cell counts greater than 10,000 (sometimes expressed as 10.0×10^9/liter)

- Elevated alkaline phosphatase (AP or AlkP) levels

- Low levels of albumin (Alb)

- Low levels of sodium (Na)

- High levels of uric acid

- Low levels of hemoglobin (Hgb)

- Low levels of blood cells called platelets (PLT)

- Abnormal levels of glutamic-oxaloacetic transaminase

- Abnormal levels of glutamate pyruvate transaminase

For NSCLC, these values in conjunction with other findings are indicative of poorer prognosis:

- High levels of lactate dehydrogenase (LDH)

- Low levels of albumin (Alb)

- Elevated alkaline phosphatase (AP or AlkP) levels, which might indicate bone metastasis

- Low levels of blood cells called platelets (PLT)

- High levels of calcium, which might indicate bone metastasis (Ca)

- Low levels of hemoglobin (Hgb)

- Raised white blood cell (lymphocyte and neutrophil) counts[4]

Tumor subtypes

There are two types of lung tumors that don't fit well into other categories, and this variance carries over into considerations of prognosis.

Neuroendocrine tumors

Small cell lung cancer often exhibits characteristics of neuroendocrine tissue; that is, tissue secreting substances normally secreted by glands, such as adrenal tissue. This type of small cell lung cancer usually is aggressive and has a poor prognosis.

Bronchial carcinoid tumors are another type of neuroendocrine tumor that can arise in the lung as well as other organs. Bronchial carcinoids have an excellent prognosis after surgery if isolated in the lung.

Well-differentiated neuroendocrine carcinomas of the lung are a type of NSCLC also called malignant carcinoid, metastasizing bronchial adenoma, pleomorphic carcinoid, nonbenign carcinoid tumor, and atypical carcinoid. These, like SCLC, occur mostly in cigarette smokers, but metastasize less frequently than SCLC. The five-year survival rate is greater than 50 percent in some studies, and surgical cure appears possible in most stage I patients.

Bronchioloalveolar carcinoma (BAC)

In general, BAC resembles other NSCLCs regarding prognosis in that the stage (degree of spread) is most important, but BAC tumors are more likely than other

NSCLCs to be diagnosed as a single lesion that hasn't spread. When early diagnosis of a single lesion of less than 3 centimeters is made, the patient's prognosis following surgical removal of the tumor is good.

Other factors that appear to contribute to improved survival time for BAC are presence of collagen; absence of mucin; absence of neutrophils (a type of young white blood cell) expressing interleukin-8; absence of invasion of deeper tissues, lymph nodes, and blood vessels; absence of sclerotic material; and absence of diffuse aerogenic spread—BAC can spread laterally across the interior surface of the lung, unlike many NSCLCs, which penetrate through the lung wall into non-lung chest tissues.

Patient characteristics

Many cancer survivors wonder if personal characteristics, such as their general health, ethnic background, diet, smoking, or gender, have a bearing on successfully fighting the disease. The following sections summarize the individual factors that appear to matter most for lung cancer.

Lifestyle choices

Continuing to smoke tobacco or continued exposure to inhaled particulate matter, including job-related exposures and fireplace smoke, can affect your prognosis by reducing the body's ability to withstand the pulmonary side effects of treatment, reducing blood flow, increasing the risk of infection, worsening infection during treatment that destroys white blood cells, and promoting the development of subsequent or simultaneous tumors.

Age

For both NSCLC and SCLC, some studies indicate that increasing age confers a worse prognosis, but other studies do not. When age is accompanied by other illnesses that reduce the patient's ability to withstand the side effects of anticancer therapy or surgery, resulting in delayed treatment or lowered doses of chemotherapy, age can be said to affect prognosis. For those with disease diagnosed at later stages, the effect of age on outcome diminishes.

Gender

Females with either SCLC or NSCLC have a better prognosis than males for reasons that are not well understood. This advantage holds even when stage and other factors are equal.

Weight loss

For those with SCLC and those with NSCLC level IIIA or higher, weight loss that is not deliberate indicates a worse prognosis.

Physical ability

Performance status (Karnovsky, Zubrod, or ECOG scales) measures the patient's ability to do everyday things, such as dress or bathe. For those with extensive SCLC or those with NSCLC staged as IIIA or higher, the lower the performance status at diagnosis, the poorer the outcome. This measure does not apply to temporary setbacks while coping with the side effects of treatment or recovering from surgery.

Tumor symptoms

NSCLC patients who have no pulmonary symptoms and no symptoms of distant metastasis have a better prognosis than those who have such symptoms.

SCLC patients are seldom diagnosed in early stages with no symptoms. Two clusters of symptoms in particular, those associated with Cushing's syndrome and with syndrome of inappropriate antidiuretic hormone (SIADH), are associated with shortened survival time. See Chapter 1, *Symptoms of Lung Cancer*, for a description of the symptoms associated with these syndromes.

Immune system response

For those with SCLC, a delayed hypersensitivity of skin to allergens is indicative of worse prognosis.

Emotional responses

Although there often are similarities in how people with lung cancer feel about the effect of their disease on the future and in how they choose to adapt to it, differences exist as well. Each person tends to find her own way along the path.

Denial

Some people prefer not to think about the possibility that lung cancer may shorten their lives. Denial about prognosis can be a very healthy way to live, as long as it doesn't cause you to miss doctor appointments or bypass valuable treatment.

Anger

Anger about the possibility of premature death is normal and expected. Moreover, because lung cancer is one of the cancers that some researchers have correlated to some lifestyle choices, some survivors who "followed all the rules" may feel angry that their prognosis is not good in spite of their having lived a healthy lifestyle.

Bargaining

When confronted with news about the possible outcome of your disease, it's possible that your first reaction will be to seek information about better treatments and better outcome. This can be a very fruitful reaction: many cancer survivors have found better treatment within a clinical trial because of this tenacious reaction.

For some survivors of lung cancer, bargaining takes other forms. Some diagnosed at a stage for which curative treatments might not succeed may bargain to live until their next birthday, or until Christmas, for instance. They may bargain with themselves and their caretakers for a pain-free death, and plan accordingly.

Depression

Depression about the uncertainty of the future after being diagnosed with lung cancer is entirely normal. In fact, depression is recognized as a major emotional consequence in those being treated for any cancer. The likelihood that one's prognosis might not be good will probably make depression worse.

Acceptance

Some survivors feel that they can face whatever the future holds. A conviction may develop that life is worth living and enjoying to its fullest, in spite of a possible decrease in the amount of time that remains.

Summary

This chapter has reviewed many of the known factors that might influence the outcome of lung cancer and its treatment. As stated at the beginning of this chapter, however, these factors are only relevant with respect to treatments in use at the time this book was written. Newer treatments may rise above current limitations, such as genetic damage or tumor burden. Your doctor is always your best source of up-to-date information.

CHAPTER 7

Types of Treatment

*The physician should look upon the patient as a besieged city
and try to rescue him with every means that art and science
place at his command.*

—Alexander of Tralles

LUNG CANCER IS TREATED in a variety of ways, including surgery, chemotherapy, radiotherapy, photodynamic therapy, inhalation therapy, and biological treatments (such as growth factor antagonists). This chapter outlines typical treatments used today.

The descriptions provided give you an overview of treatments and a starting point to find out more about the treatments your doctors recommend for you. This chapter will not outline which treatment is best for you, because such information changes continually. Nor will this chapter discuss rare treatments used outside the US and Canada, nor treatments classified as alternative.

Specific treatments for NSCLC and SCLC are found in Chapter 8, *Treating Non-Small Cell Lung Cancer*, and Chapter 9, *Treating Small Cell Lung Cancer*.

The information in this chapter is drawn from the National Cancer Institute's treatment statements, supplemented from various sources, such as the second edition of Harvey Pass's text, *Lung Cancer: Principles and Practice* (Lippincott, 2000); Jack Roth's 1998 edition of *Lung Cancer* (Blackwell Science); current research papers; pharmacological databases; and our medical reviewers.

A word of caution

Most medical writers approach a chapter such as this one with great caution, and so should the reader. The reason is this: no single publication of this type can possibly reflect the latest progress in lung cancer research. As you read this chapter, you must keep in mind that you will always get the latest information on the best way to treat your disease from the medical doctors and researchers in the trenches. Your surgeon and oncologists might recommend treatment options that are different from those you'll read here or elsewhere. You should always verify with your treatment team any treatment information that you find on your own.

Surgery

Surgical removal of a tumor, called surgical resection, is the chief means by which most early stage lung cancer patients are treated with the intention to cure (rather than simply to relieve symptoms). Surgery is the most accurate way to determine the spread of lung cancer, called staging the disease. A patient with clear presurgical evidence of widespread disease, however, is not likely to benefit from the additional staging information obtained from surgery. He might suffer unnecessary pain and discomfort from surgery that would damage the quality of his remaining life.

Clear margins

The goal of curative surgery for cancer is complete removal of all diseased tissue. If presurgical chemotherapy or radiotherapy—induction therapy—was used before surgery to shrink the tumor, tissue removal is targeted to the original tumor size, even if the tumor is smaller or gone.

One of the best determinants of complete removal is a finding called clear margins: a rim of healthy tissue, uninvaded by cancerous cells, on all perimeters of all tissue removed. Clear margins indicate a high likelihood that the entire tumor was removed, totally and intact, without being accidentally divided, punctured, left behind, or mechanically spread during removal.

The presence of clear margins in a given tumor sample can be determined only by microscopic examination and other testing in a pathology laboratory, not by a visual assessment during surgery. Clear margins might be difficult to assess if induction therapy was used.

Removing adjoining tissue

Removal of closely adjacent tissues is an essential part of curative lung cancer surgery for three reasons:

- Removing blood vessels, lymphatic vessels, and lymph nodes is necessary to eliminate all traces of disease by removing microscopic tumors that might be sequestered within nearby tissue.

- The removed tissue provides additional biopsy material for more accurate staging.

- Removal of blood and lymphatic vessels interrupts the outward path of any microscopic tumor or single cancerous cells that might remain.

For these reasons, it is extremely rare for a lumpectomy, often used for breast cancer, for example, to be used for lung cancer. Five-year survival of those who have had a lung wedge resection (roughly the equivalent of lumpectomy) for even small tumors tends to be lower than that of those who have had more tissue removed.

Access to the internal chest

An incision into the chest cavity is called thoracotomy. A small incision through which an endoscope is manipulated is called thoracoscopy or mediastinoscopy. An incision into the upper chest, near the collarbone, is called a cervicotomy.

Most lung tumors are removed in one of the following ways (in some cases, portions of one or more ribs are removed; which ribs are affected depends on the location of your tumor):

- With open surgery called posterolateral thoracotomy, involving an incision through all layers of chest wall into the lung through either the right or left side of the rib cage beneath the arm. Access is between two ribs, called the intercostal space.

- With open surgery called anterior thoracotomy into the front of the chest, involving separating the ribs from the breastbone (sternum) and penetrating the interior chest linings and wall into the lung.

- With open surgery called median sternotomy, involving opening the chest cavity by separating the ribs from the sternum or splitting the sternum down the middle, for accessing the space between the lungs called the mediastinum.

- With open surgery called posterior thoracotomy, utilizing entry through the patient's back and separation of one or more ribs from the spine.

- With thoracoscopy, involving several small incisions through all layers of the chest wall in either the front or side of the chest. Only very small, solitary lung tumors might be removed this way. This technique remains controversial because small incisions can limit visibility and the manipulation of instruments and tissue, possibly causing incomplete surgeries or contamination of healthy tissue with tumor cells.

Types of lung cancer surgeries

A considerable number of surgical options exist for treating lung cancer, so you must ask your surgeon for the details of the surgery he is planning.

Every effort is made to remove as little lung tissue as possible along with the cancerous tissue, so that adequate lung capacity remains for breathing. Surgeries for lung cancer are described below from least invasive to most invasive. Please refer to Figure 1-1 in Chapter 1, *Symptoms of Lung Cancer*, for information if you have questions about lung anatomy while reading the following descriptions.

For multiple tumors at different locations, two or more of these procedures might be adapted to suit the patient's specific circumstances.

Endoscopic procedures

The least invasive, most comfortable, and fastest healing surgery for lung cancer is removal of a single tumor, using either a bronchoscope inserted into the throat or an endoscope inserted through small incisions past the chest wall and linings into the lung, called thoracoscopy. A variation on this surgery is video-assisted thoracic surgery (VATS), which combines thoracoscopy with video viewing equipment. At times, ultrasound or CT scanning is used with bronchoscopy or thoracoscopy to locate tumors.

In practice, most lung cancer patients have a tumor that is too large, multiple tumors that have spread across too wide an area, or attachments to too many adjacent tissues to allow complete removal via thoracoscope. Moreover, endoscopic removal of tumor tissue can in some cases result in the microscopic spread of cancerous cells at the incision line that later develop into second tumors. This is thought to occur because the tumor is squeezed through the incision as it is removed.

Because of these risks and tumor characteristics, endoscopic procedures often can be used only to:

- Diagnose and treat fluid retention in the chest (a side effect of tumor growth called pleural effusion).

- Retrieve pieces of tissue for biopsy rather than effect a cure. Endoscopic procedures often are used to sample enlarged lymph nodes in the midchest to determine if cancer has spread to them.

- Remove a core of tumor, via scalpel or laser attachment, that is obstructing an airway, in order to relieve symptoms, not to effect a cure.

- Place braces known as stents in airways to hold them open.

- Stretch narrow airways.

- Place radioactive substances in or near the tumor.

Partial lung removal

To maximize the amount of healthy lung tissue remaining, several lung cancer surgeries remove just part of a lung or airway. The difference between these surgeries lies chiefly in the amount and location of lung tissue removed. At the time of this writing, though, removal of an entire lobe is considered more likely to provide long-term survival than do smaller, less invasive surgeries. The 1998 text *Lung Cancer*, edited by Jack Roth (Blackwell Science), describes several lung cancer surgeries, categorized as either lung-sparing or lobe-sparing:

- Lung-sparing surgeries leave part of the lung in place:

  - **Lobectomy.** An entire lobe—one of two lobes in the left lung or one of three in the right—and its blood supply are removed. Removal of many lymph nodes, called lymphadenectomy, is also performed.

  - **Bronchial-sleeve resection.** Part of one bronchial tube is removed, with reattachment (anastomosis) of the remaining ends. Removal of lymph nodes, called lymphadenectomy, is performed. Used against tumors high in a bronchial airway that would otherwise require removing an entire lung.

  - **Bronchial-sleeve lobectomy.** One lobe of a lung, its blood supply, and part of its bronchial tube are removed, with reconnection (anastomosis) of the two remaining ends of the bronchial tube. Removal of nearby lymph nodes, called lymphadenectomy, is performed.

- Lobe-sparing surgeries leave even more of the lung intact:

  - **Segmentectomy.** A segment of one lobe of one lung and its blood supply are removed. Removal of nearby lymph nodes and vessels, called lymphadenectomy, is performed.

  - **Sleeve segmentectomy.** A piece of the branched bronchial tube that enters one lobe segment is removed, along with that segment of the lobe and its blood supply. Reconnection of the two remaining ends of bronchial tube (anastomosis) and removal of lymph nodes, called lymphadenectomy, are performed. Used for tumors high in the airway that would otherwise require removing a lobe of one lung.

- **Wedge resection.** A wedge-shaped piece of a lobe segment is removed, usually from the outer (peripheral) edge. The location of the lobe segment affected by the tumor is a critical factor in the appropriateness of choosing this surgery. The success of this technique as curative surgery remains unclear. Lack of removal of lymph nodes and blood supply during wedge resection might contribute to a recurrence of disease. This technique is usually employed only when the patient is not a candidate for a larger, more effective surgery.

- **Precision dissection.** A very minimal "lumpectomy" of deep diseased lung tissue, using such sealing techniques as laser or cautery to close blood and lymphatic vessels after the tumor is removed. The success of this technique as curative surgery remains unclear. Lack of removal of lymph nodes and the tumor's blood supply during wedge resection might contribute to a recurrence of disease spread through either lymphatic ducts or blood vessels. This technique usually is employed only when the patient is not a candidate for a larger, more effective surgery.

Full lung removal

Removal of an entire lung and its blood supply, called pneumonectomy, is the oldest surgical technique for treating lung cancer. It remains an effective treatment for many patients who have disease involving more than one lobe of the lung. Removal of all lymph nodes and lymphatic vessels draining the lung, called lymphadenectomy, is performed as part of pneumonectomy.

Sleeve pneumonectomy involves removal of one lung, its blood supply, nearby lymph nodes, and part of its major bronchial tube, with reconnection (anastomosis) of the trachea and the other lung's bronchial tube. See also carinal surgery, described in the next section.

Extended surgeries

Often, lung tumors will grow through the lung into other chest organs, blood vessels, nerves, or supportive tissue. Several types of surgery address tumors that have grown beyond the lung.

En bloc surgery, mentioned several times in the descriptions that follow, is the removal in one joined piece of all adjacent organs invaded by the tumor. En bloc surgery is a means of removing all of a tumor without cutting into it, which might result in its spread.

- Chest wall tumors beyond the lung often can be removed during lobectomy for lung cancer, but in a separate step either before or after removal of the diseased portion of lung. If the tumor has invaded through the chest wall into bone, one or more ribs might need reconstruction using stiff mesh or other synthetic materials.

- Tumors of the superior sulcus, the area of the upper chest where the airways and blood supply pass through supportive chest tissue, are not always addressable with surgery. When surgery is used, superior sulcus tumors are removed using en bloc resection, a removal of the tumor and all organs to which it has attached, as a unit. This surgery usually is performed during lobectomy for the primary lung disease.

- Tumors of the carina, a ridgelike supportive structure wrapped outside the airway at the point where the trachea divides into the two bronchial tubes, are not always removable with surgery. When surgery is performed, the affected lung, all diseased airway tissue, and attached tissues outside the airway including blood vessels are removed. The end of the trachea and the remaining bronchus are joined to each other, as are the remaining ends of blood vessels. Some sources state that if rejoining is not possible because too much tissue has to be removed, a join should be reconstructed from other body tissue or synthetic materials.

- Invasion of the wide, thin-walled chest vein called the superior vena cava (SVC) by lung cancer is rarely addressed with surgery because involvement of the SVC usually indicates widespread disease not curable with surgery. When surgery is possible, a portion of the side of the superior vena cava might be removed, but often an entire cross-section must be removed and reconstructed. Engraftment using pieces of vein from elsewhere in the body might be attempted. Alternately, a surgical bypass of the SVC tumor might be done using veins grafted from other parts of the body. The latter surgery only relieves symptoms; it is not an attempt to cure the patient.

- Tumor involvement of arteries very near the heart—the aorta and main pulmonary trunk—usually cannot be addressed with surgery because surgical risks, postoperative complications, and the risk of spreading the tumor throughout the bloodstream are too dangerous. When in carefully selected patients it is possible to remove these structures surgically, tumors are removed using en bloc resection, a removal of the tumor and all organs to which it has attached. Sections of the tumor-affected artery that must be removed often are replaced using bypass methods similar to those used for heart disease.

- Tumors that have invaded the spine near the lungs might be addressed via en bloc surgery of all affected organs, including part or all of a vertebra, if penetration into the bone is not too deep. Tumors invading the spine far from the lungs or invading bones that are not spine or ribs are not treated with surgery.

- Tumors that have invaded the lining of the inner chest (mediastinal pleura), the lining of the heart (pericardium), or the diaphragm might be addressed with surgery if no lymph node involvement is found.

Distant sites

In addition to surgeries of the lung and adjacent organs, surgeries that address lung cancer that has spread to other parts of the body are in some cases possible:

- Removal of brain metastasis using traditional surgery or a radiation technique called stereotactic radiosurgery (once called the gamma knife) might be recommended if a solitary brain lesion or just a few lesions are found, and if all tumors elsewhere have been completely eliminated.

- If one of the two adrenal glands has been invaded by lung cancer, surgical removal might be suggested if no other metastases exist and if all tumors in the lung have been completely eliminated.

- If one small liver tumor exists, or a few small tumors in just one liver lobe with no encroachment on major blood vessels, surgery might be considered by some researchers who are testing new techniques that are now in clinical trials for other cancers, such as colorectal cancer metastases. Contact your doctor and the National Cancer Institute at (800) 4-CANCER for more information.

Other surgical considerations

There are many considerations your surgeon will weigh when planning your surgery. Most concern the finer details of surgery; you can and should entrust these decisions entirely to your surgeon. The following general surgical issues and techniques, however, might affect your outcome and should be evaluated by both you and your surgeon:

- The training, skill, experience, and board certification of your surgeon.

- The medical center to which your surgeon has admitting privileges.

- Any lung impairment caused by smoking, cancer, or other diseases that affect the amount of pulmonary function you have. These constraints will determine the kind of surgery chosen—or whether surgery is even an option.

- The location of cancer in either the left or right lung. The left lung is smaller and of different structure from the right lung, because other organs (such as the heart) occupy space in the left chest. This means loss of the right lung reduces breathing capacity more significantly than loss of the left lung. Moreover, the entry into the body and the surgical techniques chosen by your surgeon for left-lung disease differ from those for right-lung disease to avoid damage to the heart and its major blood vessels.

- Mechanical staplers might in some cases compress healthy lung tissue, into which staples are placed to a greater degree than sutures would be. Although this is not likely to cause a recurrence of cancer, it might compromise pulmonary function in remaining lung tissue.

- If tumors are removed through the small incisions that are made during thoracoscopic or video-assisted surgery, great care must be taken not to contaminate the incision with cancer cells as the tumor is being removed, called seeding the cancer. Cases of metastasis along incision lines following thoracoscopic surgery have been reported, a disturbing phenomenon that is the subject of much discussion among thoracic surgeons.

Draining chest fluids

The chest contains sacs and layers of tissue that surround the lungs and heart. These structures normally contain a small amount of fluid that acts as a cushion and lubricant, reducing friction as the heart pumps and as the lungs expand and compress during breathing.

Lung cancer patients sometimes develop fluid in the chest related to tumor activity, such as blockage of lymphatic channels or overproduction of fluid. Stress on organs, such as the kidney, also can cause fluid to accumulate around the heart and lungs.

Draining chest fluid is necessary if:

- It is needed for diagnosis.
- The patient is losing too much blood into the fluid.
- It interferes with the patient's heart function or ability to breathe.

Draining lung fluid (pleural effusion)

Excess fluids surrounding the lungs, known as pleural effusion, may or may not contain cancer cells; the fluid can be drained using the following procedures:

- Thoracentesis, involving inserting a narrow needle with a large reservoir through the chest wall for one-time drainage via suction aspiration.

- Tube thoracostomy, involving the temporary implantation of a chest tube to drain away fluid continuously.

- Pleurodesis (sclerotherapy), involving injecting a substance that will cause scarring in the tissue layers between which fluid has been collecting. Scarring causes the two layers to adhere, which discourages the collection of fluid. All fluid must be drained away first.

- Pleuroperitoneal shunt, involving the insertion, under anesthesia, of tubing that transferred fluid from the pleural space into the abdominal space called the peritoneal cavity, where it is absorbed and processed by the body. Fluid is transferred to the peritoneal cavity via a pump. A pleuroperitoneal shunt can be left in place indefinitely.

- Pleurectomy, a surgery that removes the sacs and layers encompassing the lung. This technique is not often used in lung cancer patients because it is a risky surgery for those whose pulmonary function and other body systems are compromised by lung cancer.

Draining pericardial fluid

The heart is contained in a protective sac known as the pericardium. Excess fluids surrounding the heart, known as pericardial effusion, occur in 5 to 10 percent of lung cancer patients, and can be drained using the following procedures:

- **Pericardiocentesis.** With local anesthesia and EKG monitoring, the insertion of a narrow needle with a large reservoir through the chest wall for one-time drainage via suction aspiration.

- **Pericardiotomy (pericardial window).** The opening and partial removal of the sac containing the heart to release, drain, and sample accumulated fluid while the patient is under general or local anesthesia. A central incision near the breastbone is used, and temporary drains are installed to remove any remaining fluid over the following days or weeks.

- **Sclerotherapy.** The injection of substances to cause scarring in the tissue layers between which fluid has been collecting. Scarring causes the two layers to adhere, which discourages the collection of fluid. All fluid must be drained away first.

Chemotherapy

Chemotherapy, or cytotoxic therapy, as it is used for lung cancer is a whole-body (systemic) treatment using drugs that have been proven to kill cancerous cells. Chemotherapy can be done:

- Preoperatively, to reduce tumor size and to kill microscopic cancer cells before surgery

- Postoperatively, to kill any tumors or microscopic cancer cells that remain after surgery

- Alone or with radiotherapy when the patient is not a good candidate for surgery

When chemotherapy is used with surgery, it is called adjuvant chemotherapy, because it is intended only to boost the chance of success of surgery as cure. When used before surgery, it is called neoadjuvant chemotherapy. When combined with radiotherapy, it is called chemoradiotherapy or combined-modality therapy. When multiple drugs are used in a chemotherapy regimen, it is called combination chemotherapy.

Geri Capasso describes her brother Anthony's diagnosis and treatment:

> My brother, age 46, was diagnosed with Stage IV NSCLC, metastases to eye, bones, and possibly liver. My brother is determined to win this awful battle, and my hope is for all to win, and a cure to finally be found. He is currently taking cisplatin/gemcitabine and he is in a protocol double-blinded phase III trial taking AG3340. So far he is tolerating the chemo well; he has less pain in his legs, and he is not coughing as much. He never was a smoker, and he just had chest x-rays six months prior to diagnosis that were included in a physical. The x-rays didn't spot the tumor. The first symptom was when he noticed that his vision was off in one eye. From there they found a tumor behind his eye, and diagnosed it as a secondary tumor.

Several weeks later Geri is encouraged by treatments:

> My brother has just completed two rounds of cisplatin/Gemzar and has been in a double-blinded trial study of AG3340. He had CT scans this week and his doctor said there is a 20 percent improvement in the lung tumor. My family is so grateful.

For access to the newest drugs being considered for any type of lung cancer, contact the NCI at their web site *http://cancernet.nci.nih.gov/trialsrch.shtml* or by calling (800) 4-CANCER.

How anticancer drugs are given

Many patients tend to focus on which drugs they are receiving, but the route and schedule of administration of chemotherapy can greatly affect outcome. Chemotherapy can be administered in several ways and on different schedules:

- Into a vein or into a central or peripheral venous catheter (see Appendix B, *Tests and Procedures*) by a doctor or nurse, repeated once a week or several times a week for several months. This is called bolus infusion.

- Orally, as pills.

- Through a semipermanent catheter that empties into a vein, once a day or throughout the day for several days, using a portable continuous infusion pump that is either implanted inside or carried on the outside of your body.

- Directly into the chest cavity for disease that is causing pleural effusion, a buildup of fluid in the chest.

- Into the central nervous system and brain via spinal puncture or an Ommaya reservoir.

- Inhalation therapy for bronchioloalveolar carcinoma (BAC) is in clinical trials.

See Chapter 11, *Experiencing Chemotherapy*, for the practical aspects of this treatment.

How anticancer drugs kill tumors

Drugs that are used or have been used against lung cancer fall into several categories of action:

- **Alkylating agents**. Form new bonds within double-twisted DNA strands that resemble ladder rungs. This disrupts many normal functions of DNA, including its ability to divide. Alkylating agents are able to affect a cancer cell's DNA even when the DNA is not uncoiled and separated—in other words, they are not cell-cycle specific, which may explain their relatively high activity against many cancers.

  Cyclophosphamide, ifosfamide, procarbazine, and lomustine are alkylating agents. Mitomycin, derived from the fungus Streptomyces caespitosus, is an atypical alkylating agent. Mitomycin is also capable of creating oxygen-free radicals, which damage DNA.

Cisplatin and carboplatin are similar, but not identical, to alkylating agents in their mode of action against cancer. Like alkylating agents, cisplatin and carboplatin are able to affect a cancer cell's DNA even when the DNA is not uncoiled and separated.

- **Antiangiogenic agents.** Most tumors trigger growth of many new blood vessels to support the increased metabolic needs of the tumor. This growth of new blood vessels is called angiogenesis. Antiangiogenic agents interrupt the ability of the body to grow new blood vessels, causing tumors to shrink. Low molecular weight heparin (dalteparin), marimastat, carboxyamidotriazole, thalidomide, BMS-275291, AE-941 (shark cartilage extract), and prinomastat (AG3340) are antiangiogenic agents in clinical trials for lung cancer. See also "Biological therapies."

- **Antimetabolites.** As the word antimetabolite implies, these substances in some way impede the cell's metabolism—its building up and breaking down of cell parts.

  Methotrexate is a folate antagonist recommended by the NCI for use against SCLC. Folate or folic acid, a B vitamin found in many green vegetables, is needed to make the building blocks of DNA, purines and pyrimidines. Absent these, new copies of DNA cannot be made. Methotrexate blocks the action of an enzyme called dihydrofolate reductase, which is necessary for the metabolism of folate.

  Gemcitabine is an analog of deoxycytidine triphosphate (dCTP), a natural body substance that lengthens a DNA strand as it's being copied. Gemcitabine substitutes in deoxycytidine's place, and, because gemcitabine differs from deoxycytidine in critical ways, the DNA cannot be copied.

- **DNA intercalators.** Insert themselves between DNA base pairs and change the shape of the DNA helix, thus interfering with the copying of DNA. The DNA strand cannot be lengthened after its shape no longer matches the configuration of other agents responsible for copying DNA. Doxorubicin is a DNA intercalator used against lung cancer.

- **Matrix metalloproteinase inhibitors.** These drugs inhibit the ability of cancer cells to anchor in a new location. Marimastat and AG3340 are matrix metalloproteinase inhibitors in clinical trials for lung cancer.

- **Radiosensitizing drugs.** Research has shown that some drugs that can kill cancer cells on their own also appear to heighten the cancer cell's vulnerability to radiotherapy. Paclitaxel and cisplatin have this effect, and fluorouracil (5-FU) is being studied for this purpose.

- **Rescue drugs.** Some drugs are effective in offsetting certain dangerous effects of chemotherapy. Colony stimulating factors, described under "Biological therapies" later in this chapter, help bone marrow produce more red and white blood cells and platelets after they have been suppressed during chemotherapy. Mesna is used along with cyclophosphamide or ifosfamide to prevent bladder damage.

- **Topoisomerase inhibitors.** Topoisomerases are enzymes that our cells use to untwist DNA before copying, and to repair breaks in DNA after copying. Topoisomerase inhibitors interfere with DNA replication, causing the cancer cell to die because damaged DNA cannot be translated into the proteins, such as transport and digestive proteins, that each cell needs to breathe or eat.

  Doxorubicin, etoposide, and topotecan are topoisomerase inhibitors used against lung cancer. Irinotecan is in clinical trials. (Doxorubicin also acts as a DNA intercalator, described above.)

- **Tubulin binding agents.** When a cell has made a copy of all of its chromosomes and is ready to divide, spindles made of tubulin form to pull the two copies of each chromosome apart into two identical clusters of 46 chromosomes apiece. Tubulin binding agents stop spindles from forming, thus stopping the cell from dividing.

  Some tubulin binding agents currently used against lung cancer are vincristine, vinblastine, vinorelbine, docetaxel, and paclitaxel.

Radiotherapy

For lung cancer, radiotherapy on its own, radiotherapy combined with chemotherapy, or adjuvant radiotherapy before, during, or after surgery might be recommended to combat the spread of disease or to control symptoms. For tumors that are inoperable or borderline operable, reducing tumor bulk prior to surgery might permit safer, more complete surgeries that increase the chance for cure.

When radiotherapy is used with surgery, it is called preoperative or neoadjuvant, intraoperative, or postoperative radiotherapy. When combined with chemotherapy, it is called chemoradiotherapy or combined-modality therapy.

How radiotherapy is given

Radiation therapy can be administered in several forms, broadly grouped into two categories, external radiotherapy and internal radiotherapy.

External radiotherapy

External radiotherapy techniques are the most common forms of radiation therapy used against lung cancer:

- **Traditional external-beam radiotherapy.** Administered from outside the patient's body, either before surgery to reduce tumor bulk, increasing the chance of clear resection, or after surgery to kill microscopic remains of diseases.

- **Whole-brain irradiation (WBI) and prophylactic cranial irradiation (PCI).** Forms of external radiotherapy used to prevent or destroy metastatic tumors in the brain.

- **Stereotactic radiosurgery.** Once called the gamma knife, this is a finely targeted one-time dose of radiation matched exactly to the tumor's size, shape, and location. It is most often used for brain metastases. Often a CT scan or MRI is used on the spot to visualize the tumor (instead of beforehand in a simulation session) for very accurate targeting. When it is a one-time treatment, the dose delivered is higher than the dose used for conventional fractionated external beam radiotherapy. When the dose is fractionated, smaller doses, but more of them, are administered over several sessions.

- **Fractionated stereotactic radiosurgery.** Resembles stereotactic radiosurgery, described in the previous item, but is administered over several sessions (as is traditional two-dimensional external-beam radiotherapy).

- **3D conformal radiotherapy.** Treatment using external beams specifically matching the tumor's shape, directed from many more angles than used in conventional external-beam radiotherapy. Lead shields or leaflets are designed by a computer to match the beam exactly to the tumor from all angles, thus sparing nearby healthy tissue. While the shields or leaflets might be designed in a pretreatment simulation session, they are easy to change dynamically with the computer's software as the tumor shrinks with treatment. The additional angles allow more radiation to be delivered to the tumor very precisely, while affecting a smaller amount of healthy tissue. The treatment usually uses a fractionated dose of radiation; that is, small doses delivered over several sessions.

- **Cyberknife.** The cyberknife and the Peacock system, a variant of the cyberknife, use miniature radiation equipment and robotics to move around the patient, delivering hundreds of small doses of radiation from many angles.

Internal radiotherapy

Some lung cancer patients benefit from radiotherapy designed to deliver a dose from within the body:

- **Brachytherapy.** The positioning of a source of radiation, such as iridium-192, in a container contiguous to the tumor to enhance the radiobiologic effect of the radioisotope.

- **Endobronchial brachytherapy.** Sometimes used for lung cancer to deliver a dose of radiation to a tumor that is blocking the airway.

- **Interstitial brachytherapy.** Involves implants of radioactive material, such as iodine-125 or palladium-103, within a tumor, stored in capsules, wires, foam, or similar sealed delivery vehicles, often as permanent implants at the time of surgery.

- **Intraoperative electron beam irradiation (IOERT).** Directed against specific sites of disease while the patient's body is open during surgery after the tumor has been removed. This is rarely used for lung cancer.

- **Radioimmunotherapy.** Injecting a radioisotope into a vein; is in clinical trials for lung cancer. When combined with a monoclonal antibody as a homing device, radioimmunotherapy might also be classified as a biological therapy, about which more is said below.

See Chapter 12, *Experiencing Radiotherapy*, for the practical aspects of these treatments.

How radiotherapy kills tumors

Radiation therapy interferes with the growth and replication of cancer cells by changing the structure of molecules that make up the cell's DNA, after which the DNA strand can no longer be copied, lengthened, paired, and twined correctly.

Similar damage is possible in healthy cells that happen to be in the path of the radiation beam, especially if they are in the process of dividing.

Much research over many years has revealed that fractionating, or dividing, the dose over many days for several weeks has a higher kill rate for tumor cells but protects healthy tissue. More recent research has shown that hyperfractionating the dose to several times per day and accelerating the dose into a shorter schedule might offer even better tumor kill.

Radiotherapy dosage

Dosage of radiation therapy always is tailored to the patient's specific circumstances, depending on the kind of lung cancer treated, where the tumors are located, whether cure is possible or only pain control is being attempted, and how much radiation a given organ can withstand. The liver, spine, heart, and healthy lung tissue, for instance, are very sensitive to radiation and must be shielded or avoided by careful targeting.

Doses for control of symptoms are lower than those used for cure. They are delivered the same way curative doses are delivered, but for fewer sessions.

If higher dosage is required for certain sites, more sessions are added, but the dose per exposure is not raised. Because external beam radiation often must pass through healthy tissue to reach the site of the tumor, a moderate dose per exposure has been determined to be the best means for killing lung cancer cells while allowing healthy cells to recover.

Some patients question why lower doses over a longer period of time aren't used to reduce the side effects of treatment. Doses lower than those currently recommended might allow a surge of cancer growth to go unchecked; some researchers have noted accelerated growth in head and neck cancers that were apparently stimulated by radiotherapy. Although this finding is not directly applicable to lung cancers, the risk of cancer regrowth after reducing the single fractionated dose is considered too great in the absence of more solid information.

Biological therapies

There are a number of biological therapies. Each one works differently, but in general the therapies are manmade copies of natural body substances and enhance the action of these substances.

- **Anti-growth factor therapies.** Therapies that target any one of many growth factor receptors identified for SCLC or NSCLC, such as angiogenic or epidermal growth factor receptors. An antiepidermal growth factor (EGF) substance known as Iressa (ZD 1839) is in Phase III clinical trials. The manufacturer, AstraZeneca (*http://www.astrazeneca-us.com/default.asp*), is making the drug available to those in and outside clinical trials in accordance with the FDA's Investigation New Drug program.

- **Monoclonal antibodies.** Manmade copies of proteins—antibodies—that our white blood cells secrete. Because a particular cell surface protein, or antigen, attracts a particular antibody, natural antibodies are responsible for attaching to foreign substances in the body and for initiating an attack against invaders, such as viruses and bacteria.

  When mass-produced in the laboratory, antibodies can be made all of one type (monoclonal) to target preferentially a certain kind of invader. Because cancer cells are different in some ways from healthy cells, such as in the number or combination of proteins that extend from their surface, manmade monoclonal antibodies (abbreviated moabs, or mabs) can be made to aim preferentially for cancer cells by targeting these surface proteins. They are capable of attaching to healthy cells as well, but the aforementioned differences in expression of surface proteins between healthy and cancerous cells result in a higher likelihood of attachment to cancerous cells.

  A monoclonal antibody may be naked or it may be coupled, or conjugated, with another substance called a payload: a toxic substance, such as ricin; or a radioactive substance (radioisotope), such as iodine-131 or yttrium-90. When the conjugated monoclonal antibody attaches to a cell's surface protein, the proximity of the toxic substance damages or kills the cell. There are no data that prove the benefit of monoclonal antibodies for the treatment of lung cancer, but several are being tested for use against lung cancers.

- **Cytokines.** Substances the body uses to trigger other immunologic events. Interferon-alfa-2B, for instance, is a cytokine that can halt growth of some tumors, force cells to mature, and interrupt cell motility.

- **Colony stimulating factors.** Substances causing growth of new blood cells in marrow:

  - **G-CSF.** Granulocyte colony stimulating factor (Filgrastim, Neupogen) is a man-made copy of a protein that causes bone marrow to grow new white blood cells called neutrophils.

  - **GM-CSF.** Granulocyte-macrophage colony stimulating factor (Sargramostim, Leukine), like G-CSF, is a manmade copy of a protein that causes bone marrow to grow both new white blood cells called neutrophils and new monocytes. Macrophages, which develop from monocytes, are cells that surround and digest foreign material and microorganisms in the body.

  - **EPO.** Erythropoietin (Epoetin alfa, Epogen, Procrit), like the colony stimulating factors, is a manmade copy of a substance made by the kidney (and in lesser quantities by other organs, such as the liver and adrenal glands) that causes bone marrow to produce new red blood cells.

– **TPO.** Thrombopoietin, like G-CSF and EPO, is a man-made copy of a body product that causes bone marrow to grow new platelets. Man-made thrombopoietin is not yet approved by the FDA.

– **Interleukin-11.** IL-11 (Neumega, oprelvekin), approved by the FDA in 1997 for certain cancers, stimulates growth of new platelets to aid recovery from marrow-suppressing chemotherapy.

• **Tumor vaccines.** Tumor vaccines, now in clinical trials for lung cancer, are an attempt to re-educate the body to attack tumor cells. For reasons still unknown, at some point the body stops attacking cancer cells, even though evidence suggests that it does mount an immune attack against cancer cells when they are still small and few in number.

• **Stem cell support.** Use of stem cell support in conjunction with high-dose chemotherapy for SCLC is being tested in clinical trials. Stem cells are very young blood cells that can repopulate depleted bone marrow. Reintroducing stem cells to the body after high-dose treatment permits very high doses of chemotherapy or radiotherapy to be used—that is, doses high enough to kill all cancer, and also to destroy bone marrow.

For more information on many other treatments still in the experimental stage, see Chapter 23, *The Future of Therapy*.

Photodynamic therapy

Early-stage lung cancers that have not penetrated very far into the lung wall might be treated with photodynamic therapy. Squamous cell carcinomas of the lung are sometimes treated using this method.

Photodynamic therapy uses three components: a drug that sensitizes cells to light, a light source (usually a laser), and oxygen:

• A light-sensitizing drug that is absorbed more readily by tumor tissue than by normal cells, usually Photofrin or HpD, is administered into a vein two to five days before treatment.

• While the patient is sedated, the laser light source is introduced, via bronchoscope, into the airway near the tumor.

- The tumor is exposed to highly focused laser light in the presence of oxygen for 10 to 40 minutes.

- Several electrochemical events involving transfers of energy take place that transform oxygen into a toxic form called a singlet oxygen species. The singlet oxygen destroys cell walls and internal cell membranes.

These changes occur both within cancerous cells and within the blood vessels that feed the tumor. Cell division halts and the cell disintegrates. Although it appears that DNA is not directly damaged by this treatment, as it is by most anticancer treatment, damage does occur both to the nuclear membrane that contains DNA and to the main cellular membrane and mitochondrial membrane. (Mitochondria, a subcomponent of all cells, use oxygen to fuel all cellular activities.)

Watch and wait

Certain slow-growing types of lung cancer, such as some nondiffuse bronchioloalveolar carcinoma, might not warrant treatment until a period of growth or regrowth. This approach is known to medical professionals as watch-and-wait, or watchful waiting, but patients usually call it "watch and worry."

Summary

A variety of lung cancers exist, and their presentations differ. Many treatments have been developed to address these differences. It's not unusual to meet someone with lung cancer who is being treated with a different surgical, chemotherapeutic, or radiotherapeutic regimen than you've had. It's also not unusual to have patients with the same type of lung cancer receive the same treatment, but show a different response—both in therapeutic outcome and possible side effects. The histologic type of lung cancer and the treatment regimen may be the same, but each patient is unique.

If you have questions about the appropriateness of treatment information you've found here or elsewhere, please rely on your doctor for clarification and updates.

CHAPTER 8

Treating Non-Small Cell Lung Cancer

There are no such things as incurable, there are only things
for which man has not found a cure.

—Bernard Baruch

HOW NON-SMALL CELL LUNG CANCER (NSCLC) is treated depends on what subtype is found, the number and spread of tumors, the general health of the patient, how much lung function exists, and the patient's willingness to undergo certain therapies.

This chapter will discuss treatment of NSCLC by stage of disease. The information in this chapter is drawn from the National Cancer Institute's treatment statements, supplemented from various sources, such as Harvey Pass's 2000 text, *Lung Cancer: Principles and Practice* (Lippincott); Jack Roth's 1998 edition of *Lung Cancer* (Blackwell Science); current research papers; pharmacological databases; and our medical reviewers.

Before you agree to any treatment for NSCLC, you should consider newer treatments that are still being tested under the auspices of the FDA and the National Cancer Institute. The NCI recommends that all lung cancer patients at any stage consider clinical trials to gain access to potentially better treatments.

Treatment options for NSCLC

There are several ways to treat NSCLC, depending on its subtype, location, and spread. All are described in detail in Chapter 7, *Types of Treatment*:

- Surgery to remove all cancerous tissue. Surgical removal, called surgical resection, is the chief means by which most early-stage NSCLC patients are treated with the intention to cure (as opposed to relieving symptoms or extending life). Surgery also can cure some NSCLC patients who have minimal tumor spread outside, but very near the lung, or who have single tumors in the brain, liver, or adrenal gland—but only if these tumors meet very strict criteria of size, number, and degree of invasiveness.

- Many patients treated with surgery develop tumors in other organs, however. If you have any stage of NSCLC, you should consider clinical trials to gain access to possibly better treatments.

- Stage I and some stage II patients who are not good candidates for surgery might be cured with radiotherapy, but for some patients radiotherapy is less effective than surgery.

- A review of nine studies showed decreased survival when radiotherapy was used *after* curative surgery for stage I or II,[1] so radiation therapy following surgery should be discussed carefully with your treatment team if it is suggested for stage I or II disease.

- Tumors spread outside the lung but confined to the superior sulcus (a groove in the upper lung and its sac through which runs a major artery) can in some cases be cured with surgery, radiotherapy, or both. In some cases, surgery after radiotherapy is done to verify the success of treatment and to remove dying tumor tissue.

- Solitary tumors that have traveled to just one other organ or second solitary tumors in the lung can sometimes be treated with surgery, radiotherapy, or tools that mimic surgery:
  - Tumors that have invaded a limited section of the chest wall might be treated with surgery, for example.
  - Solitary brain tumors might be treated with surgery followed by whole-brain irradiation or with stereotactic radiosurgery, a form of radiation therapy once called the gamma knife.
  - Radiofrequency ablation, heat waves that are capable of killing tumors, is being tested against certain isolated tumors or a few small tumors.
  - A solitary tumor in an adrenal gland can in some cases be removed successfully with surgery.

- Photodynamic therapy can be effective for cure of very early lung lesions of certain subtypes of NSCLC amenable to laser illumination, such as squamous cell carcinoma.

- Treatment with chemotherapy and chest radiotherapy, or chemotherapy before surgery, improves survival odds in some instances for some stage IIIA patients.

- Treatment with chemotherapy and radiation therapy might extend survival in some stage IIIB and stage IV patients.

- Widespread stage IV disease often is treated with body-wide (systemic) chemotherapy to extend life and improve the quality of life, usually not to cure disease.

- Biological therapies work in a variety of ways, usually by mimicking or augmenting a natural body process, such as immunity. Some biological therapies for attacking the tumor are being tested in clinical trials; other biological therapies are for supportive care, not cure.

- For certain kinds of NSCLC confined to the lung, inhalation therapy might be recommended.

- Treatments aimed at eliminating the collection of fluid in the chest are common for NSCLC.

Treatment of NSCLC by stage

The treatment guidelines listed below were adapted from the National Cancer Institute's state-of-the-art treatment statement for physicians as of November 2000, and in some cases were amended by our medical reviewers. You should discuss your specific treatment options thoroughly with your own oncology treatment team. You should consider calling the NCI periodically at (800) 4-CANCER or visiting the NCI PDQ web site at *http://cancernet.nci.nih.gov/pdq/pdq_treatment.shtml* to obtain updated standards of care.

Chemotherapy drugs are not mentioned by name in the NCI's treatment statement for any stage of NSCLC except stage IV. Nonetheless, some drugs in use today for NSCLC, often in combinations of two or three, are:

- Carboplatin
- Cisplatin
- CPT-11 (irinotecan)
- Docetaxel
- Gemzar (gemcitabine)
- Mitomycin
- Paclitaxel
- Vinblastine

- Vinorelbine

- VP-16 (etoposide)

See Appendix D, *Chemotherapy Drugs and Regimens*, for other drugs that might be used for NSCLC.

Occult NSCLC

An occult tumor is a tumor that is not readily detectable. Tests are used to find the primary tumor and to best determine its type and stage. Treatment is geared to the stage found.

Stage 0 NSCLC

Stage 0 lung cancer is the most superficial of tumors, contained within just a few layers of the lung's internal surface cells, not usually visible on radiographic studies, and usually curable with surgery.

Treatment options recommended by the NCI and our medical reviewers include:

- **Standard treatment.** Consists of surgical removal, using the least invasive method possible (segmentectomy or wedge resection) to best preserve lung function, because patients with stage 0 NSCLC face a high risk of second lung cancers.

- **Endoscopic photodynamic therapy.** An alternate form of treatment that might be recommended for central tumors that do not extend more than 1 centimeter within the bronchus.

- **Radiation therapy intended to cure.** Might be recommended for those who have a tumor that could be cured with surgery, but are unable to withstand surgery because of other health problems.

Stage I NSCLC

This stage delineates T1 and T2 tumors with no lymph node involvement and no metastasis. (For TNM status, see Chapter 2, *Diagnosis and Staging*.)

Treatment options recommended by the NCI and our medical reviewers include:

- **Standard treatment.** Consists of surgical removal of a wedge, segment, or lobe of one lung, possibly with removal of part of a bronchial tube (sleeve resection), as well. Removal of an entire lobe appears to reduce recurrence.

- **Radiation therapy intended to cure**. Might be recommended for those who have a tumor that could be cured with surgery, but are unable to withstand surgery because of other health problems.

- **Experimental approaches**. Include:
  - New chemotherapy regimens that are still in clinical trials.
  - New drugs used for preventing second tumors; that is, drugs that are still in clinical trials.
  - Endoscopic photodynamic therapy; being evaluated only for carefully selected patients with T1, N0, M0 tumors.

Stage II NSCLC

This stage describes a tumor with:

- T1 or T2 tumor size/location status and N1 lymph node status
- T3 tumor with N0 node status

For TNM definitions, see Chapter 2, *Diagnosis and Staging*.

Treatment options recommended by the NCI and our medical reviewers include:

- **Standard therapy**. Includes surgical removal of the whole lung, one lobe of the lung, a segment of a lobe, a wedge of a segment, or part of a bronchial tube.

- **Radiotherapy intended to cure**. Might be recommended for those who have a tumor that could be cured with surgery, but who are unable to withstand surgery because of other health problems.

- **Experimental approaches**. Being evaluated. Note that adjuvant therapy is not yet conclusively proven to be of value for this stage of lung cancer:
  - Enrollment in a clinical trial of a new chemotherapy regimen after curative surgery
  - Enrollment in a clinical trial of a new radiation therapy regimen after curative surgery

Stage IIIA NSCLC

This stage describes a tumor with:

- T1 or T2 tumor size/location status and with N2 lymph node status
- T3 tumor size/location status with N1 or N2 node status

For TNM definitions, see Chapter 2.

One of our medical reviewers pointed out that, in spite of the three NCI recommendations for stage IIIA listed below, neoadjuvant chemotherapy followed by surgery has become the standard of care for stage IIIA patients who have a tumor that could be removed entirely by surgery. Regarding neoadjuvant therapy, the NCI says, "…results are encouraging, and combined-modality therapy with neoadjuvant chemotherapy with surgery and/or chest radiation therapy should be considered for patients with good performance status who have stage IIIA NSCLC." It is likely that the NCI recommendations for treating stage IIIA will remain the subject of controversy among medical professionals—and thus a source of some confusion for patients—until more conclusive information is gained from studies.

Treatment options recommended by the NCI include:

- In patients with no large tumors in nearby lymph nodes, surgery alone with no chemotherapy or radiotherapy
- Radiation therapy alone
- Chemotherapy combined with surgery or radiotherapy; recommended by the NCI and strongly recommended by one of our medical reviewers

Superior sulcus tumor (T3, N0 or N1, M0)

Superior sulcus tumors are tumors in a narrow area of the upper chest where the airways, nerves, and blood supply pass through supportive chest tissue.

Treatment options recommended by the NCI include:

- Radiation therapy and surgery
- Radiation therapy alone
- Surgery alone in carefully selected patients
- Chemotherapy combined with surgery or radiotherapy
- Enrollment in clinical trials of a new drug regimen or radiation therapy regimen

Chest wall tumor (T3, N0 or N1, M0)

Tumors that have breached the lung and invaded the chest wall might require a special approach.

Treatment options recommended by the NCISurgery include:

- Surgery and radiation therapy
- Radiation therapy alone
- Chemotherapy combined with surgery or radiotherapy

Stage IIIB NSCLC

Stage IIIB NSCLC is characterized by:

- A tumor of any T size/location status, node status N3, no metastasis to other organs
- A tumor of T4 size/location status, any nodal status, no metastasis to other organs

For TNM status, see Chapter 2.

Treatment options recommended by the NCI include:

- Radiation therapy alone.
- Chemotherapy combined with radiation therapy.
- Chemotherapy and concurrent radiation therapy followed by surgery.
- Chemotherapy alone. One of our medical reviewers emphasized this option for patients with pleural effusion.

Stage IV NSCLC

Stage IV disease is disease that has spread to any distant organ, such as bone, the adrenal gland, or brain. Stage IV is designated as:

- Any T tumor size/location status
- Any N nodal status
- Any metastasis

For TNM status definitions, see Chapter 2.

Treatment options recommended by the NCI and our medical reviewers include:

- Chemotherapy:
    - Cisplatin, vinblastine, and mitomycin
    - Cisplatin and vinorelbine

- Cisplatin and paclitaxel
- Cisplatin and gemcitabine
- Carboplatin and paclitaxel

- External-beam radiation therapy for relief of symptoms, not for cure.

- Endobronchial laser therapy and/or brachytherapy for removing obstructing airway lesions.

- Experimental treatments still being evaluated, including new chemotherapy regimens still in clinical trials.

Our medical reviewers note that topotecan is now approved for lung cancer and that docetaxel and gemcitabine are now widely used.

Summary

This chapter summarizes the latest information regarding treatment for NSCLC. New treatments evolve continuously, however, and it's in your best interest to keep abreast of these changes. Your surgeon, medical oncologist, radiation oncologist, the NCI, and cancer research journals are your best sources of information for current treatment choices.

CHAPTER 9

Treating Small Cell Lung Cancer

Diseases come of their own accord,
but cures come difficult and hard.

—Samuel Butler

TREATMENT FOR SMALL CELL LUNG CANCER (SCLC) is selected based on the spread of tumors, the general health of the patient, and his willingness to undergo certain therapies, including promising experimental therapies in clinical trials. At this time, chemotherapy is considered the keystone of treatment for SCLC.

This chapter discusses treatment of SCLC based on extent of disease. The information in this chapter is modeled on that provided by the National Cancer Institute, supplemented from various sources, such as Harvey Pass's 2000 text, *Lung Cancer: Principles and Practice* (Lippincott); Jack Roth's 1998 edition of *Lung Cancer* (Blackwell Science); current research papers; pharmacological databases; and our medical reviewers.

Before you agree to any treatment, you should consider newer treatments that are still being tested by the National Cancer Institute. NCI recommends that all lung cancer patients at any stage consider clinical trials to gain access to potentially better treatments.

Treatment options for SCLC

There are several ways to treat SCLC. All are described in detail in Chapter 7, *Types of Treatment*:

- Surgery is appropriate for certain carefully screened patients with early-stage (limited) disease. Surgery for SCLC is rare because at diagnosis, disease often is too widespread to be cured by removing tumors surgically.

- Combining chemotherapy with other types of treatment can cure some patients with limited disease and may lengthen survival and improve the quality of life for other patients.

- Radiation therapy, alone or combined with surgery or chemotherapy, can cure some patients with limited disease and may lengthen survival and improve the quality of life for other patients.

- Biological therapies work in a variety of ways, usually by mimicking or augmenting a natural body process, such as immunity.

- Treatments aimed at eliminating the collection of fluid in the chest are common for SCLC.

Larry Coffman, five-year survivor of SCLC, describes his chemo protocol:

> I can't speak for current chemotherapy protocol, but mine was 5 days on, 21 days off. The infusions started about 9 AM and I was done and home usually by 12:30. Just in time to watch my cooking shows. And please consider getting a port (central venous catheter) before starting treatment. They didn't have me get one, as they were sure that I wouldn't make it 90 days into chemotherapy. Now my veins are a mess.
>
> Would I do it again if I had to? You bet! In a heartbeat!!

Treatment of SCLC

The treatment guidelines listed below were adapted from the National Cancer Institute's state-of-the-art treatment statement for physicians as of November 2000. You should discuss your specific treatment options with your own oncology treatment team, and you should consider calling the NCI periodically at (800) 4-CANCER or visiting the NCI PDQ web site at *http://cancernet.nci.nih.gov/pdq/pdq_treatment.shtml* to obtain updated standards of care.

The NCI mentions specific drugs and drug regimens for both limited-stage and extensive-stage SCLC. Other drugs being used are:

- Vinorelbine
- Docetaxel
- Gemcitabine

See Appendix D, *Chemotherapy Drugs and Regimens*, for other drugs that might be recommended for SCLC.

Limited-stage SCLC

Limited-stage small cell lung cancer describes a tumor or tumors still entirely within the chest, confined to areas that can be irradiated "tolerably," that is, areas small enough to produce only side effects that the patient can tolerate.

Treatment options recommended by the NCI for limited-stage SCLC include:

- Chemotherapy with one of the following regimens, plus chest irradiation, with or without preventive prophylactic cranial irradiation (PCI) for patients who respond completely to chemoradiation:

    - EC: etoposide and cisplatin plus chest irradiation

    - ECV: etoposide, cisplatin, and vincristine plus chest irradiation

- A multidrug chemotherapy regimen, with or without preventive cranial irradiation (PCI), in patients who have a complete response to chemotherapy. This option is used for patients who cannot have chest irradiation because of impaired pulmonary function or other health problems.

- In carefully chosen patients with stage I tumors, surgery to remove the tumor(s) followed either by chemotherapy or chemotherapy plus chest irradiation, with or without preventive cranial irradiation (PCI) in patients who have a complete response to chemoradiotherapy.

- Experimental use of new drugs, new drug doses or schedules, and new combinations of chemotherapy and radiotherapy.

Larry Coffman, five-year survivor of limited-stage SCLC, describes a part of his treatment intended to prevent brain metastases:

> Keep one thing in mind as you go forward: according to my oncologist, chances of metastases to the brain with recurrence run about 30 percent. Whole-brain radiation (WBR) reduces that possibility to about 5 percent with various side effects, which are different for each person. I chose intrathecal chemotherapy that reduced the possibility to about 5 percent, as well, with little or no side effects. But it was a little more uncomfortable to get.
>
> One other thing to keep in mind, according to my primary physician, pulmonologist, and oncologist: if you make it 24 months from the time you are diagnosed with SCLC, chances are pretty slim that it will recur at all. My primary physician said, "If you outlive the disease, you are on easy street." Managing the side effects has been my major battle.

Extensive-stage SCLC

Extensive-stage small cell lung cancer describes disease that is too widely spread to fit the definition of limited-stage disease. For this reason, your treatment team might greatly individualize your treatment regimen.

Treatment options for extensive-stage SCLC recommended by the NCI include:

- Chemotherapy with one of the following regimens, with or without preventive (prophylactic) cranial irradiation (PCI) given to patients with complete responses to chemotherapy:
    - CAV: cyclophosphamide, doxorubicin, and vincristine
    - CAE: cyclophosphamide, doxorubicin, and etoposide
    - EP: etoposide and cisplatin
    - EC: etoposide and carboplatin
    - ICE: ifosfamide, carboplatin, and etoposide
- Other regimens that are less well studied, but appear to produce similar outcomes, include:
    - Cyclophosphamide, methotrexate, and lomustine
    - Cyclophosphamide, methotrexate, lomustine, and vincristine
    - Cyclophosphamide, doxorubicin, etoposide, and vincristine
    - CEV: cyclophosphamide, etoposide, and vincristine
    - Single-agent etoposide
    - PET: cisplatin, etoposide, and paclitaxel
- Radiation therapy to relieve symptoms from tumors that are unlikely to be relieved immediately by chemotherapy, especially brain, spine, and bone tumors
- Experimental treatment using new agents being tested in clinical trials, with the understanding that the patient can switch to standard therapies described above if there is no response to the new agent

Summary

The cornerstone of treatment for SCLC is chemotherapy. For some patients, radiation therapy to the chest might be recommended. In rare cases, the disease is diagnosed early enough to cure with surgery.

CHAPTER 10

Experiencing Hospitalization

There shall be no card playing or dicing and such patients
as are able shall assist in nursing others, washing and
ironing linen and cleaning the rooms and such other services
as the matron may require.

—Regulations of the Philadelphia General Hospital, 1790

TREATMENT OF LUNG CANCER often involves hospitalization for chest surgery. Additional hospital stays might be necessary to administer chemotherapy or radiation therapy, to drain chest fluid, to treat a collapsed lung or a blocked airway, or to address a side effect of treatment, such as infections that develop when white blood cell counts drop during chemotherapy.

Some people are frightened by the idea of being admitted to the hospital, even while realizing that the best care for a particular problem can be delivered only with the round-the-clock medical scrutiny available in a good hospital. This chapter will attempt to help you view the experience in a positive light and will highlight the precautions you can follow to make your stay brief and fruitful. We will examine the experience chronologically, beginning with preparation and admitting procedures and finishing with discharge and home care. Separate sections on radiotherapy, chemotherapy, and infection are included.

General concerns

In the US, generally you are limited to using hospitals at which your doctors have admitting privileges. It's best to consider this limitation in advance, as discussed in Chapter 3, *Finding the Right Treatment Team*. Ideally, the hospital should be an NCI-designated comprehensive cancer center, as discussed in Chapter 3, or affiliated with a medical school. At the very least, it should be accredited by the Joint Commission on Accreditation of Healthcare Organizations (JCAHO). Call JCAHO at (630) 792-5000 and also ask the hospital's administrators about the outcome of their latest evaluation by JCAHO. For more detailed information on selecting a hospital, see *A Cancer Survivor's Almanac*, published by the National Coalition for Cancer Survivorship.

Preparation

If you know in advance that you'll be admitted to the hospital, you can plan to make your stay brief and successful. If your admission is for surgery, for example, copious helpful information, including what to take, will be given to you in advance by the staff. Preoperative tests, such as a chest x-ray, lung capacity tests, electrocardiogram, and blood testing will be conducted.

On the other hand, you might be admitted via the emergency room if symptoms are unusual, have a rapid onset, or are associated with immediate danger, such as copious bleeding from the lungs or pronounced difficulty breathing. You might be taken directly into surgery from the emergency room if a collapsed lung or a blocked or perforated airway is suspected. If you have symptoms of an infection following chemotherapy, your doctor might insist that you proceed directly to an isolation room in the oncology wing while your loved ones deal with the admitting paperwork in the germ-filled front lobby.

You might have little control over some of these happenings, but it's best to avoid the emergency room during treatment, if possible, by careful tracking of symptoms and timely communication with your doctor. Emergency-room care can be greatly delayed or can vary in quality, based on several factors beyond your control, such as the seriousness of the illnesses of others waiting or the experience of the medical staff on duty. If you must use an emergency room, be sure to call your treatment team and let them know what's happened.

Arrangements

Here are a few general tips for preparing in advance against a hospital stay:

- You can smooth the path of abrupt admissions by having an overnight bag ready that contains much of what you'll need. See the next section, "What to take."

- If you're being admitted for surgery or any other procedure, call your insurance company to see if the procedure must be precertified. Keep a written log of whom you spoke with and when.

- If you're being admitted for surgery, verify that the surgeon is board certified in thoracic surgery or general surgery, with a second specialty in oncology. The Official ABMS Directory of Board Certified Medical Specialists is a publication that can be found in a local library, and the American Medical Association also can verify board certification: see Appendix A, *Resources*. Your state licensing board or state medical society can verify how many years of experience your surgeon has had.

- If you're being admitted for surgery, obtain and review all consent documents. Strike any clauses that connote that staff other than your surgeon might be participating in your procedure, unless you and your surgeon already have discussed who else might be participating and you're comfortable with these additional personnel. There are varying risks associated with surgery done under general anesthesia, including excessive bleeding from the incision site and a very small risk from the anesthesia itself. Your doctor and the hospital staff will explain fully the risks that apply most closely to your surgery.

- Hospitals that receive federal funding or are governed by certain local laws must adhere to federal or local laws regarding informed consent prior to use of human subjects for research. Government-funded hospitals include most university, state, and nonprofit hospitals. Verify whether your hospital receives any federal funding, and phone your state health department to determine if your state has its own laws regarding consent issues. If your hospital is a private for-profit hospital that receives no federal funding and is not governed by similar local laws, closely question any treatment suggested for you. Ask your doctor if your proposed treatment represents state-of-the-art treatment as defined by the NCI or if you'll be treated in an investigational study.

- Ask if you can donate your own blood (autologous donation) in advance of surgery. Receiving your own blood is safer than receiving donor blood.

- Read as much as you can about the procedure you'll be having.

- Arrange to have any biopsied material kept forever so that it will be available in the future if tumor-based treatments such as tumor vaccines are planned.

- Make notes about all health problems you have, related to lung cancer and otherwise. Make several photocopies of these notes, because each group of medical caretakers you meet will ask the same questions again.

- Arrange for child care, if needed. Most likely, this care will be provided by a well-informed relative; but if not, prepare abundant information well in advance, in writing, including phone numbers of relatives and pediatricians.

- Contact a pet-sitter, if necessary. Provide clear written instructions regarding feeding and any health problems. Provide your veterinarian's address and phone number and those of an emergency all-night veterinary service. Leave all supplies, including carrier and medications, in a prominent place.

- Have the mail and newspapers held if nobody will remain at home. Make arrangements for a plant-waterer, if needed.

- Pay any upcoming bills in advance.

- Plan transportation to and from the hospital, allowing plenty of time in everyone's schedules for check-in and check-out procedures. Hospitals are not very good at checking patients out quickly, especially if you need special instructions about home aftercare.

- Call the hospital and ask about parking arrangements, such as less expensive long-term passes for those who will be visiting you during an extended stay, special parking for outpatient units, or discounted or waived fees for those accompanying you during a surgery.

- If you'd like to take a laptop computer, first verify if the hospital has digital phone lines. If so, borrow or buy an adapter so your modem won't be ruined if it's not capable of handling digital input. Tell email friends if you'd love to receive email during your stay, but point out that you might not be able to respond. Ask them not to be offended, but instead to keep on writing.

- Contact your employer, not only to arrange for use of sick time or disability pay, but also to ensure their emotional and professional support when you return to work. Ask for a copy of company leave policies and the federal Family and Medical Leave Act in order to become acquainted with all employment-related options.

- Check your calendar and cancel any commitments that conflict with your hospital schedule.

- Arrange for a visiting or live-in home nurse if you think you or your caretaker will need extra help after your hospital stay. Many insurance companies will pay part of this service if your doctor says you meet certain conditions, such as being temporarily unable to bathe.

- If you're having radiation therapy for lung cancer that involves placing radioactive material into your airway, let your family and friends know that children and pregnant women might not be able to visit you at all and that others should plan for brief visits only, until the hospital staff say it's okay. During the time the radioactive substance is very active, you and your body wastes will constitute a radiation exposure risk to others.

- Discuss with your family and other loved ones what aftercare or special considerations you might need when you arrive home. Many types of surgery require that you avoid driving for some number of weeks, for instance, or internal radiation therapy may require that you dispose carefully of body wastes for a few days. A supplemental oxygen supply might be needed for a period of time after surgery. A tube to drain lung fluid might be left in place for a few days or weeks after discharge and might require daily care.

What to take

Some people take too many, or inappropriate, things, to the hospital; others pack too little, assuming that the hospital will provide everything. Here are a few suggestions:

- Ask the hospital staff for a list of things that will be useful. Remind them of your treatment plan so they can give you detailed suggestions.

- Prepare several copies of lists of your medications, both prescription and over-the-counter: never assume that the hospital has spoken with all of your doctors.

- Take your health insurance card and your certificate showing you donated your own blood for use during surgery, if applicable.

- Take your own over-the-counter medications if you suffer from athlete's foot, tooth sensitivity, or other conditions not related to lung cancer. You must remember to inform the staff first, though, if you need to use these supplies: they are medications, and they might interact unfavorably with medications your doctor has ordered.

- You might feel better in your own clothing if you have someone who can launder it for you. Leave behind any clothing with metal zippers or snaps because you might need diagnostic tests, such as CT scans or MRI, and metal in clothing could interfere with these tests. Choose clothing that won't press on your incision or cause you undue strain as you dress. Choose shirts with easy sleeves that can accommodate IV lines. Add something dashing or seductive to the overnight bag if you think an ego boost will help.

- If you pack a razor, avoid the plug-in electric variety, as the local fire code or the proximity of hospital oxygen supplies may regulate against them. Battery-operated razors generally are most acceptable; however, a disposable razor may do, provided you're able to manipulate it while feeling less than your usual self.

- Take eye and ear coverings for sleep. Hospitals can be noisy places at odd hours.

- If music will help you relax and sleep, take a personal player with a headset to avoid disturbing your roommate.

- If you anticipate a long stay, take pictures of home, family, pets, and loving experiences.

- Remember warm socks. (The nursing staff love wild socks.)

- If this is a return trip, take the phone that they might have sold you during your prior stay.

- An old sock full of quarters will help you and your family make postsurgical phone calls, pay for parking, buy newspapers, or buy those sometimes unavoidable vending-machine meals. Unlike a purse or a wallet, a ratty old sock doesn't look worth stealing.

- Take a laptop computer if you enjoy Internet email support from other friends with lung cancer. Take a bike lock to anchor your PC to the bed if the hospital has experienced theft.

- Pack a list of phone numbers of friends and family.

- Most hospitals provide some toiletries such as soap, washcloths, and a toothbrush, but you might prefer your own. Avoid heavily scented products, though, as they might make you or your roommate ill, or might make breathing more difficult.

- Prepare several copies of your advance directives (living will, durable power of attorney) to inform the staff of your wishes for or against extreme life-support measures.

- Take books that are lightweight. You might be groggy and achy for a spell. Don't plan to read and analyze the Hardy-Weinberg equilibrium or to hold open a seven-pound tax code manual during your hospital stay.

- For females, pack a long, loose shirt or tunic top for the times when you're told to "take everything off, and put on this gown with the opening in the front." Sooner or later you will indeed have to open these in the front, but you'll feel less the victim of someone else's poor sartorial taste.

- For both males and females, pack a pair of baggy boxer shorts for the times when you're told to "take everything off, and put on this gown with the opening in the back." A wild, glow-in-the-dark pair, for instance, can give your sense of individuality a boost and might give others a smile.

What not to take

Taking certain items to the hospital can turn into a hindrance:

- Leave all jewelry at home. If you want to wear your wedding band, ask the staff about this first. They can secure it with tape during surgery, for example.

- Don't take scented toiletries. You might feel nausea after certain procedures, and scents might take you (or your poor, captive roommate) beyond the edge of gastric comfort. Moreover, you might come to associate your once-favorite scent with a hospital stay, or you might find it more difficult to breathe if heavy scents surround you.

- Leave your purse, wallet, credit cards, and money, beyond incidental change for newspapers and the like, at home or in a safe-deposit box.

- Leave your worries and your work behind. Let your family and the hospital staff coddle you. When you're allowed to eat, order everything on the hospital menu and share it with your pals.

Admission

Admission will start with paperwork, phone calls, questions about next of kin, phone and TV service preferences, attachment of a plastic ID bracelet, and directions to the correct room and floor. Have copies of all insurance paperwork and medical records ready.

After admission, a volunteer might be assigned to stay with you briefly until you've arrived in your room and become oriented, especially if you're having surgery.

Once you have arrived in your room, the nursing staff will take control and prepare you for whatever care you will need. They'll check vital signs, such as pulse and temperature, and might start an intravenous line (IV) for administering drugs. You'll probably find that nurses will return a hundredfold any small effort you make to be friendly and kind.

Ask now about the meal menus, as there is usually a delay in getting meal preferences to newly admitted patients.

If you're being admitted for most procedures, you might be sharing a room with someone else. If you're scheduled to be treated with a radioactive substance introduced into your airway via a bronchoscope, you might be given a private room immediately or very soon.

The staff

The nursing staff is the first group you're likely to encounter in your hospital stay, but they're just one group of a confusing array of medical personnel you'll meet.

Note that you may refuse care administered by any staff member with whom you don't feel comfortable and can ask for a more experienced person to attend to you.

Nurses

Hospital nurses will provide most of your care:

- Nurses' aides and licensed practical nurses (LPNs) will help to wash you, help you in and out of bed, make your bed, and perform simple nursing tasks, such as checking your pulse and temperature. LPNs, but not nurses' aides, have completed vocational training and may provide medication.

- Registered nurses (RNs) have earned a college degree in nursing and passed a licensing examination. RNs are able to provide more complex and critical medical care than LPNs, such as changing wound dressings, communicating with doctors, starting IVs, and administering IV medications.

- Nurse practitioners or clinical nurse specialists are RNs who have undertaken extensive additional training and are licensed to provide many of the same services that doctors provide. In some states, they are able to prescribe drugs under the auspices of a physician. In some hospitals or clinical settings, they can perform simple surgeries and procedures, such as lancing abscesses.

- Head nurses and nurse managers are in charge of other nurses, entire floors, or patient centers. Although all nurses now face the additional burden of administrative work that deprives them of time they prefer to spend with their patients, head nurses and nurse managers usually handle administrative issues exclusively and seldom provide patient care unless staffing is inadequate.

Doctors

In teaching hospitals, you'll encounter the full spectrum of doctors in various stages of training. In some community hospitals, you'll encounter just residents and attending physicians. In other community hospitals that have training agreements with nearby medical schools, you might find an amalgam of the two systems. Doctors in various stages of training include:

- Medical students, who have completed four years of college and are undertaking four additional years of medical school. Medical students do not treat patients, although often they accompany an attending physician on rounds, and the physician may elicit their opinions.

- Interns, also called first-year residents or postgraduate year-one students, who have completed four years of medical school and are in the first year of three to six years of primary specialty training. They will not give you care unless supervised by much more experienced personnel, such as the attending physician or a more experienced resident, but that supervision can be distant. If you prefer not to be treated by an intern, say so.

- House officers (once called residents), who might be postgraduate year-two students, postgraduate year-three students, etc. These physicians are still receiving primary training that can last from three to six years, depending on the field.

- Fellows, or teaching fellows, who have completed their six years' primary training and have undertaken three years of additional training in a subspecialty.

- The attending physician, who is in charge of all fellows, residents, and interns. In university hospitals, she is likely to be a faculty member. In community hospitals, she is hired to oversee patient care in her area of specialty based upon her reputation in the medical community.

Surgery

The different surgeries used for lung cancer are discussed in Chapter 7, *Types of Treatment*, as well as in the 1998 text *Lung Cancer*, edited by Roth and colleagues (Blackwell Science), and the 2000 text *Lung Cancer: Principles and Practice*, edited by Harvey Pass et al (Lippincott).

You'll meet with your surgeon to discuss in detail what will be done during surgery. You'll receive extensive instructions, will meet with the anesthesiologist, and will be monitored to ensure that no food is taken before surgery requiring general anesthesia.

You'll be asked to sign a lengthy consent document that describes all risks associated with your surgery. Certain tests, such as x-rays, bronchoscopy, CT scanning, ultrasound, or MRI, might be repeated before, during, or after surgery to target tumors that need to be removed or to track progress after surgery.

If you do not have a central catheter, an IV will be placed in your arm or hand—upon admission, one day before surgery, or directly before surgery.

Just before surgery

The risks associated with this surgery will be explained to you, and you might be asked to re-sign additional copies of the consent forms.

The site of the incision will be cleaned, shaved, and possibly marked for proposed incision lines. If you're especially hairy, ask that a large area be shaved, including the IV site on your arm. Sticky bandaging can hurt terribly when it's removed if it pulls against hairs that have not been shaved.

If you're feeling nervous, ask for a sedative. The hour or two directly before surgery are likely to be the most tense.

If you have had nausea associated with anesthesia in the past, tell the anesthesiologist. Experiencing nausea after anesthesia is essentially nonexistent if premedication with such drugs as Zofran is done.

You will either be asked to walk into the surgical suite or be taken in on a rolling bed and shifted to the table. Your arms might be positioned on armrests that facilitate giving medications by IV. After you're asleep, a breathing tube might be inserted from your mouth into one or both of your lungs, as might drains for the bladder (urinary catheter) be inserted into the urethra, or a drain to empty fluid from the lung or chest cavity through the chest wall. Coating your eyelids with a lubricant while you're asleep to keep them from drying might also be done, because pre-surgical medication might include drugs to dry body fluids and reduce bleeding.

And now, the good part: you'll fall asleep, and you won't care what they do.

Surgical recovery

When you reawaken slowly, you'll be in the recovery room. You might notice that you've acquired rubber pump-up support stockings or a series of tubes attached to various body parts—but you won't care too much, because you'll be groggy for several more hours. You might also notice that your hearing returns first, well before sight does, and that you can remember odd or humorous things the staff said as the surgery was ending. If a ventilator or respirator is used to help you breathe, it's likely that sedation will also be used, because some patients fight the ventilator.

You might feel pain upon waking. Be sure to make clear your need for pain medication as soon as you are awake and are experiencing pain because excessive pain can interfere with healing. The nursing staff will not administer painkiller, though, until you're clearly awake, in order to avoid overdosing a patient possibly still affected by anesthesia. This means that, if you're feeling pain, you must tell them distinctly as soon as you are able. Groaning, for example, is not considered a clear indicator that you're awake. The nurses will attempt to get you to speak to be sure you're awakening normally.

Eventually, you'll be returned to your room, but the first few hours are likely to be a hazy memory if you've received general anesthesia. If you received a sedative instead of general anesthesia, you'll be groggy, too, but it will resolve more quickly than the aftereffects of general anesthesia.

Some patients require assisted breathing with a respirator after surgery. Often, sedation is used to make this experience easier on the patient. Recent research has shown that shallow respiration provided by a respirator can, in some cases, promote better recovery, but shallow respiration can make patients feel short of breath, and perhaps anxious in spite of its benefits.

Additional pain medication from day one will be given freely if you ask. Most patients find they need a minimum of three days of strong pain medication after chest surgery, particularly if ribs were partially removed. Many hospitals now use patient-controlled infusion (PCI) pumps, because they yield a more even dose— about twenty microdoses per hour— than pain medication given by tablet or IV. PCI pumps also yield a limited amount of additional medication if the patient pushes a button on the pump for this purpose. Don't worry about overdose. The pump won't allow it. The minicomputer within the pump counts the number of patient pushes so that the staff will have a good idea of your need for pain medication. Kathy describes her husband's experience with pain:

> A nurse let us know in a roundabout way that they would not
> proactively give Marty drugs at the four-hour mark (he could only get a
> shot every four to six hours), we had to ask for the shot. So we learned to
> ask as soon as the four hours were up. Most of the time, the pain would
> return in two to three hours.

If you feel any nausea at all, even transient nausea, tell the nursing staff immediately. Vomiting with a fresh incision is a very painful experience, and inhaling (aspirating) vomitus into the lung can cause life-threatening pneumonia, or even suffocation.

Use of anesthesia and painkillers slows the activity of various organs, including the kidneys, urinary bladder, and intestinal tract. Your liquid and solid waste will be monitored after surgery until the staff note that your body systems are once again functioning as they should. A surgical patient recalls:

> *The surgeon went in through the back, removed all those ribs. I was in*
> *no shape when I was in the hospital to have any therapy. I also had a*
> *heart condition. I was in the hospital for ten days. I would describe it as*
> *hell on earth.*

Do the physical therapy, walking, coughing, or breathing exercises you're given as soon as possible and as often as possible. Exercise will help you heal more quickly, and will reduce the chance of developing such complications as blood clots or the type of pneumonia that's associated with lying flat for long periods. If possible, ask a caretaker to bend your arm and leg joints. Oddly, having someone else move your limbs will increase your respiratory rate, because nerve endings in our joints respond in this way. This should be done along with real exercise, of course—not as a replacement for it.

Getting in and out of bed can be painful if you have a chest incision, especially if many bones were separated to gain access to the tumor. Raising the head of the bed before getting out or in might reduce pulling on trunk muscles and drains. You might find that timing your exercise to five or ten minutes after the painkiller is used gives you enough relief from pain to allow you to exercise before sleepiness sets in.

After surgery to remove a tumor and most of one lung, one man recalls the pace of his recovery:

> *After the operation, in intensive care, the nurses kept wanting me to get*
> *out of ICU. One nurse started pulling on my arm, my bad arm. I was*
> *about ready to hit her and yelled at her not to pull my arm.*
>
> *In the hospital, I didn't feel a lot like doing much. Getting out of bed*
> *and walking, taking a shower, took about three or four days. I didn't want*
> *to do any activity that would pull on anything. I was in the hospital for*
> *eleven days.*
>
> *I didn't have a great deal of activity. But I did have a lot of breathing*
> *therapy—lung capacity, how much could you breathe, inhale antibiotics,*
> *respiratory therapy—trying to increase capacity.*

Hospitalization for infection

If you're being treated with chemotherapy for lung cancer, or if you've recently had bronchoscopy, you might also be hospitalized to treat infection.

About seven to ten days after certain chemotherapies are given, it's common for one's white blood cell counts to drop to dangerously low levels, called neutropenia. Without adequate numbers of white blood cells, the body cannot fight infection.

If you're hospitalized for infection, most likely you'll be placed alone in a hospital room, a procedure called isolation. The air might be scrubbed with a high-energy particulate air (HEPA) filter or controlled via laminar airflow.

Although some studies have shown that infection during neutropenia most often arises from pathogens already within the patient's body, restriction of visitors, gifts, and certain foods will be enforced. For example:

- All who enter will be expected to adhere to safety measures, such as vigorous handwashing and, perhaps, covering the mouth with a mask.

- Gift plants with pollen-bearing stamens or potting soil or silk plants with mossy, fungus-bearing camouflage at their base might be returned or held outside your room.

- Certain foods, such as fresh fruit or yeast breads, might be denied to you.

Isolation procedures might seem odd—after all, you're already infected—but the goal is to prevent your coming in contact with additional, and potentially very serious, infectious agents.

You'll be given oral or IV antibiotics, antivirals, or antifungals, depending on your symptoms and the results of various cultures. You might also be given drugs to help you grow new white or red blood cells. If you have pneumonia, you might need oxygen or a respirator to help you breathe or a heart pump to assist your heart.

You'll stay in isolation until your white blood cell counts rise and the infection is bested, either by the antibiotics you're given or by the infection-fighting ability of your own increasing white blood cells.

Chemotherapy

Some chemotherapies are given in the hospital in order to simultaneously administer additional agents that offset the damage to healthy organs, or to monitor the state of affected organs.

The procedures used will vary, of course, depending on the agents given; but you can most likely expect an IV line to be inserted if you don't have a permanent venous catheter. Also, you'll receive frequent and perhaps somewhat embarrassing attention from nurses regarding normally routine and personal phenomena, such as blood pressure, how much urine or feces you've passed, whether bowel movements are painful, and so on.

If copious oral or IV hydration accompanies your treatment, unless a urinary catheter is in place, you'll be compelled to rise frequently to urinate, and you might become quite tired because of lack of a full night's sleep.

Internal radiotherapy

For those with lung cancer, two types of internal radiation therapy might require a hospital stay. In addition to the more common treatment of lung cancer with external beam radiotherapy, radioactive substances also can be used by:

- Permanently implanting a radioactive material embedded in wires, seeds, capsules, foam, or needles into a tumor and surrounding tissue during the surgery that removed a primary tumor or, less frequently, in a second surgery (interstitial brachytherapy)

- Briefly placing a radioactive substance into tubes in the throat that are inserted just beforehand with a bronchoscope (brachytherapy) while you are sedated

If your implants are not permanent, a stay in a lead-shielded isolation room or surgical suite might be necessary while radioactive material is inserted under sedation, left in place for a few minutes, then removed. Containment measures will be used while the radioactive substance is being handled and while it is in place. Visitors will be limited, kept at a distance of six feet, or forbidden altogether. Although hospital staff will provide you with all the care you need, for their safety during this time they must minimize their contact with you—by wearing protective clothing, for instance.

To avoid having tubes or implants shift, you might be asked to stay in bed while they are in place.

Once the radioactive substance is removed, you are no longer a risk to others.

When treatment has ended, implants might be either left in place or removed. Often, tubes that are temporary can be removed with little or no pain at the end of treatment, but you should tell the hospital staff if you are experiencing pain or discomfort during or after removal.

Your throat and nose might be sore or might bleed following radiation therapy.

Thriving versus surviving

Very few people look forward to being hospitalized. Ultimately, it's your life, and, in spite of perhaps temporarily diminished capacities, you're still very much in charge.

Here are several key points:

- Read your medical chart. Ask questions if anything is unclear. Ask for definitions of terms the staff uses, such as NPO (*noli para os*, or nothing by mouth). If you're not well enough to do this, have a friend or relative do so.

- Verify all drugs and treatments given to you. Ask about oral medications before swallowing, and read the contents of the IV bags on your pole. If you're not well enough to do this, have a friend or relative do so.

- Tell the nursing staff right away if something seems wrong. Don't let seemingly simple things, such as a nosebleed, shortness of breath, or feeling constipated, become major problems. Severe constipation can cause sweating and panting breath, for example, which is uncomfortable and frightening after lung surgery.

- Move about your room and the corridors as much as possible, especially if you've had surgery. You'll heal faster, improve your remaining lung capacity, and diminish the likelihood of serious complications if you move about. If you feel too bad to get out of bed, flex your arms and legs a good deal. Studies have shown that just manipulating joints, even if done by a second person, increases respiration. If your white blood counts are low (neutropenia), ask if you and your IV pole can cruise the corridors while you wear a mask and surgical slippers. If you feel conspicuous wearing a mask, you might make a prank of it by adding a toothy grin with waterproof ink.

Additional ideas for dealing with your hospitalization include:

- If you're not on a restricted diet, ask friends and loved ones to bring you your favorite foods. This will make you feel better and will help those friends who would otherwise not know what to do feel useful and loving. Most hospitals now permit outside food to be brought into the patient's room, a change more in keeping with the European model of families caring for patients. Bringing food will help family members feel a part of your care if they are not permitted to do much else—for instance, if their time with you is restricted during certain radiation therapy treatments.

- At first, take pain medication on schedule if it is prescribed, even if you think you won't need it, because you'll heal better and can be more mobile if pain is adequately controlled. As time passes, you'll be a better judge of how much painkiller you really need.

- Befriend the staff. They'll repay you tenfold for your kindness. It's surprising how much can be asked of others if it's done in a nice way.

- If you're a caretaker, pitch in and do what you can to help the nurses help your loved one. Stay overnight, if at all possible; if the staff decline, insist. A wife recalls how she was able to help during her husband's recovery:

    When my husband was hospitalized after his abdominal surgery, he was on morphine, which slowed his ability to urinate. Often during the night he needed to use the john, and he and his IV pole would stand there in front of the toilet doing not much of anything for ten or fifteen minutes. Because I stayed with him overnight, I was able to help him in and out of bed repeatedly without his calling a nurse.

Discharge and departure

Discharge might be an anticlimax after your hospital stay, but you should use this time to have the staff answer all your questions about aftercare. Make sure you understand:

- First, whether you're really going to be able to handle being at home. Hospitalization times vary based on the patient's condition and the type of insurance in effect. If you feel you need to stay longer in the hospital but your insurance policy limits your stay unless the doctor requests otherwise, be sure to make your needs known to your doctor and the nursing staff.

- How to operate the pump to drain fluid from your chest and lungs if a pump and drain have been left in place. Although some drains rely on gravity, some drain into the abdomen using a manual pump that the patient engages several times a day.

- How to obtain and use oxygen supplies, including a cart or pouch to transport the oxygen canister, and how the oxygen is replaced or regenerated.

- What medications you'll be taking. When you are discharged, you probably will be given a prescription for oral pain medicine, for example. If you've had a bronchoscopy, ask about an antibiotic to prevent infection.

- Whether the hospital pharmacy can fill your prescriptions before you leave. If not, get the doctor to phone your pharmacy or get a family member to fill them beforehand.

- How to care for your incision if you've had surgery.

- What side effects or aftereffects you should watch for that might signal a problem.

- What follow-up appointments should be scheduled.

- Any diet restrictions.

- Your bill. Always ask for an itemized bill.

The person helping you with your trip home should take the car to the exit in advance and should make as many preliminary trips as necessary to remove your personal effects and gifts from your room, perhaps warming or cooling the car in advance as well. Most important, though, is that by leaving you for last, your escort can devote attention to you alone as you're exiting. This is a useful arrangement because you might need help getting into the car, for example, but most hospitals' assistance and liability end at the door.

Use the restroom before you leave, even if you think you don't need to. Even a small amount of stress on the trip home or cold temperatures, for example, can cause the brain to signal the bladder or bowel to empty. A full stomach or bowel can press upward on the diaphragm and temporarily decrease lung function by decreasing breathing space.

Most hospitals have a regulation stating that you must be escorted to the door in a wheelchair. This reduces the chance that patients, possibly weakened by extended bed rest, will pass out or suffer a misstep while exiting. Although many people leaving the hospital find using a wheelchair embarrassing, it safeguards both you and the hospital. Fortunately or unfortunately, you'll have plenty of chances to prove you're mobile again once you're out the door.

After many surgeries, one is restricted from driving for several weeks. Certain other activities, such as climbing stairs, might also be restricted. Full recovery can take as long as six weeks and might include pronounced fatigue. As one man recalls:

I looked like warmed-over death for quite a while after I got out of
there. My weight went down under 140. I lost a lot of weight before went
in for the operation; I guess it was the infection that did that.

After radiation therapy, you might be surprised to feel more tired over time instead of less tired. This is normal and will reverse eventually. The areas irradiated might feel sore or burnt for days or weeks after therapy.

Summary

Current treatment for lung cancer often includes hospitalization and chest surgery. The lung cancer survivor also might face hospitalization for infection or for radiotherapy, chemotherapy, or photodynamic therapy. This chapter offers insights and several checklists to help make your stay brief and successful.

For several good books that deal exclusively and in depth with being hospitalized, see the Appendix A, *Resources*. For many excellent ideas on dealing with surgery and recovering afterward, see *Surgery and Recovery* by Kaye Olson, RN.

If you want detailed knowledge about the surgery that will be performed, see Chapter 7. Other good sources of information include the 1998 text *Lung Cancer*, edited by Roth and colleagues (Blackwell Science), or the 2000 text *Lung Cancer: Principles and Practice*, edited by Harvey Pass et al (Lippincott).

CHAPTER 11

Experiencing Chemotherapy

*Surely every medicine is an innovation, and he that will not
apply new remedies, must expect new evils.*

—Francis Bacon

NOT SURPRISINGLY, MANY PEOPLE have concerns about what chemotherapy will be like and how they'll make it through treatment. This chapter, along with Chapter 13, *Adverse Effects of Treatment*, will describe what you're likely to experience.

Most chemotherapy for lung cancer is administered in the outpatient setting. Accordingly, we will walk you through an outpatient chemotherapy treatment, beginning with your preparations and scheduling, entering the treatment office, encountering certain medical personnel and other patients, advancing through the treatment itself, and finishing with what you can expect afterward. Keep in mind, though, that what you experience may differ from what is described in this chapter.

Use of continuous infusion pumps and certain standard and experimental treatments categorized as biological therapies and biological response modifiers—monoclonal antibodies, interferons, colony stimulating factors, anticancer vaccines, and the like—also are discussed in this chapter. Biological response modifiers often are injected, as are other chemotherapies, and pose some of the same risks.

The theories behind lung cancer treatment and the side effects of treatment are discussed separately in other chapters.

The information this chapter provides is not a substitute for your doctor's knowledge. Always ask your doctor when an aspect of your treatment is unclear, and report immediately to your doctor any adverse reactions that arise during or after treatment.

Preparation

Improvements in supportive care, such as excellent new antinausea drugs, have made chemotherapy a much easier experience than it once was. Nonetheless, people can have a wide range of responses to chemotherapy, even if they're receiving the same drug and dose. You won't know for certain how you'll respond, so it would be best to make sure you have certain supplies and assistance if you need them. Some of the drugs given for chemotherapy or to prevent side effects can cause drowsiness or affect concentration, for instance, or you might be sitting for many hours in a room that is overly warm or too cool.

For these and other reasons, it would be wise to have a friend or loved one along, not only for emotional support during your first treatment visit, but to handle issues such as safely tucking away written instructions for diet and aftercare; helping carry an oxygen supply; understanding and remembering verbal instructions; relaying information to the medical staff for you if you're hoarse; communicating insurance information; handling the co-pay, if any; and assisting with the drive home. As you adapt to treatment, you may need someone to drive if you take medication for nausea before leaving home because many of these drugs cause drowsiness.

Comfort should be high on the list of priorities for anyone having chemotherapy. Come prepared for a few hours' testing or treatment by wearing comfortable, layered clothing; bringing along relaxing friends or music cassettes; and asking in advance what to expect. Don't arrive with an empty stomach. Eat light food up to two hours before treatment.

Although the antinausea drugs in use today are excellent, store a bucket in your car because of the possibility of nausea during the ride home. Call the doctor a day or two in advance to get nausea medications and take them beforehand if instructed to do so.

Before your initial treatment, ask about wearing cosmetics, jewelry, or nail polish, because skin and nail bed color are useful ways for the medical staff to assess your well-being and response to drugs. Ask about using lotions or aftershave; these products may cause skin irritation, depending on the treatment given, especially if radiotherapy has been administered. If you feel strongly about wearing cosmetics and nail polish to treatment to improve your frame of mind, ask them about a compromise, such as leaving one fingernail bare for visibility or for using the thimble-like oxygen sensor that slides over your finger.

Ask if your chemotherapy will be administered into an arm vein. If so, plan to wear a short-sleeved top, and bring a cardigan for the parts that needn't be uncovered and might get chilled.

Ask about the advantages of having a central or peripheral venous access device, commonly called a catheter, put in place.

Tell the staff about dental appliances, contact lenses, surgical staples, pacemakers, and other synthetic materials that may interfere with treatment.

Certain drugs used for chemotherapy may react badly with certain foods or food supplements. Ask your doctor if you should avoid certain foods (such as grapefruit, cured meat, or cheese) for a week or two before or after treatment; some of these foods interfere with metabolism of some drugs by the liver. Vitamins, antioxidants, or any kind of supplements should also be approved by your doctor before use. For example, potassium supplements may trigger a dangerous metabolic imbalance, tumor lysis syndrome, that imperils the kidneys if you have a large tumor that is killed rapidly by treatment.

You may also receive instructions about avoiding other possibly dangerous circumstances, such as excessive sunlight or crowds. Some of the drugs used for lung cancer cause skin to become overly sensitive to sunlight. Protective clothing, sunglasses, and sunscreen lotions may be recommended. Some chemotherapies cause white blood cell counts to drop, which leaves you more susceptible to infections. In some circumstances, you may be advised to avoid crowded places, such as shopping malls.

Kathy describes Marty's chemotherapy and the supportive care he received:

> We met the oncologist, whom I am so impressed with. He is so kind and gentle. Marty was sent home from the hospital with lots of pain prescriptions. It took at least a week to get him used to taking the pills instead of getting shots.
>
> He started chemo (Taxol/carboplatin) the Monday after he was discharged. We chose carboplatin instead of cisplatin because it was easier on the kidneys—we had learned Marty only had one kidney.
>
> Marty was starting to get back to normal within a week or two of starting chemo and getting used to the MS Contin (60 milligrams three times a day) and constipation. He had to figure out just the right combination of Senokot S and lactulose prescribed by the doctor. Chemo went along fine; on the third day after treatment he would get exhausted, he lost taste and lost his hair. He had a lot of anxiety, so he took lorazepam to help his nerves.

Scheduling

The schedule on which chemotherapy is administered is based on years of research that determine a drug's effectiveness at a certain dose and interval. Some chemotherapies are given daily; some are given weekly for several months; some are given once a month for many months. Those delivered via portable pumps may enter the body throughout the day for many days. Oral medications taken at home may be taken once a day or several times a day.

If you can't afford or don't want to miss time from work, you might prefer scheduling weekly treatments to occur just before a weekend break so you'll have several days to adjust and recover without the additional stress of meeting work responsibilities.

Don't be surprised if the schedule on which your chemotherapy is administered differs from the schedules you hear others discussing because your schedule will very likely be tailored to your particular circumstances. You may, for instance, be receiving a drug that might be toxic to the heart, but on a less condensed schedule that is intended to lessen toxicity to the heart.

Depending on what drugs are being used, the timing of subsequent therapy may be influenced by the quantity of blood cells remaining in your bloodstream after your last treatment. Thus, for certain regimens, your blood will be tested when you arrive, or perhaps a few days in advance, if your doctor recommends or if you prefer. A standard measurement known as a complete blood count (CBC) is used to assess the status of your immune system (white blood cells), blood clotting ability (platelets), and oxygen transport capacity (red blood cells). If your blood counts are too low, treatment may be delayed for a few days or a week.

A delay of a few days or one week is not likely to affect the success of treatment, but a great many delays, or a delay of long duration, may. For this reason, oncologists sometimes prescribe either blood transfusions or injections of colony stimulating factors to bring your blood counts up to safe levels to undergo treatment. Colony stimulating factors are synthetic copies of natural body products that cause bone marrow to produce more new blood cells than it otherwise would.

For therapy administered from an IV bag or syringe rather than by infusion pump, it's not unusual for one chemotherapy session to last for several hours. High-dose therapies that must be administered over several days (with or without stem cell rescue) may require a hospital admission, but the trend is toward outpatient treatment for all but the most rigorous procedures or the sickest patients.

Arrival

Often, your treatment is not started until a doctor, nurse, or medical technician has weighed you, taken your blood pressure and temperature, done a brief physical, asked you about symptoms and side effects, and drawn blood to check blood counts. If you have a portable pump, however, you might be briefly examined, refilled, given replacement batteries, and discharged fairly quickly.

Your first visit is a good chance to begin to make friends with the nursing staff. Oncology nurses are a unique breed, generally cheerful and unusually kind. Often they'll have great ideas for helping you that might not occur to your doctor to mention, such as where to buy satin pillow covers to reduce hair loss and how to ease breathing difficulties. Interaction with a good nurse may well be one of the finest and most rewarding experiences in life, exemplifying the best humans can offer one another. Many oncology nurses say that they get much more from their patients than they give.

You may also find that your fellow patients in the waiting or treatment areas have good insights to share about experiencing chemotherapy. Often, those waiting in an oncologist's office are reluctant to start a conversation with others because the people nearby seem worried or withdrawn or because they themselves have so much mental and emotional processing underway. You might find, though, that deep, instructive, nurturing friendships are formed among cancer survivors in this setting.

After you're settled in the treatment area, waiting or being treated, consider having your companion visit the pharmacy to buy ice bags or a pill organizer, to fill any prescriptions or buy any over-the-counter drugs, including stool softeners and antidiarrheals, that you'll need later. With this arrangement, if you feel bad or fatigued after treatment, your medications and supplies will be available immediately.

The setting

Chemotherapy may be administered in a doctor's office, in a hospital outpatient setting, or, if given in the form of tablets or a portable pump, actively or passively in your home. If it is administered in a doctor's office or outpatient department, it may be administered by a chemotherapy nurse or by the doctor. It may be administered in a large room with other cancer patients who are seated in reclining chairs in partitions divided by curtains, or it may be administered on a bed or chair in a private room.

Sometimes the setting in which chemotherapy is given is dictated by what insurance companies will pay for. Injections of colony stimulating factors, for example, which may be necessary to stimulate bone marrow growth of new blood cells, may be administered safely and easily by the patient or another at home. Some insurance companies, however, will pay for these injections only if they are administered by a doctor.

Kathleen Houlihan describes how well her first chemotherapy session went:

> On Tuesday night I had my first weekly dose of chemotherapy. In my home city it would have been administered in one hour, but here they drip it in over five hours, preceded by one hour of antinausea, anti-allergy medication. It's supposed to be more effective, as well as better tolerated. The preliminary medication made me a little woozy, but I didn't feel anything with the chemo itself.
>
> It was done at the infusion center here (Cancer Treatment Centers of America), where they have small, private hospital rooms with TV, phone, bed, bathroom, chairs—all the modern conveniences. I just lounged on the bed, ate the dinner I had brought with me, watched TV, and dozed a little, for six hours. My husband Holt was with me most of the time. I did it from 5:00 to 11:00 PM. Some people do it overnight. They go in around 9:00 or 10:00 PM and just sleep through it. But because of one of the chemicals they are giving me, Taxol, they put an automatic blood pressure cuff on me that pumps up every fifteen minutes. I don't think I could sleep too well through that.
>
> So far so good on my first week of chemo. The hardest part of the week was just spending an extra six hours a day in bed. It's okay to lounge around and watch TV for six hours for a day or two, but after that it gets old. I felt like my muscles were wasting away. I didn't have to stay in bed, but after the Benadryl and other pre-meds, I didn't feel like getting up or doing anything except vegetating. Oh, well. It's a small price to pay.
>
> All my checkups continue to be very encouraging. The tumor has shrunk a little more since May. And the tumor marker we are watching (CEA) is way down, from 66 in March to 8.4 last week. Normal is under three (author's note: under three for never-smokers, under five for smokers and some ex-smokers; norms vary by lab), and I'm getting close.

Some chemotherapies and tumor types are known to be associated with risks that are best handled in a hospital setting. Cyclophosphamide (Cytoxan), for example, is known to damage the bladder at very high doses, and in this instance is administered simultaneously with heavy bladder irrigation, such as that provided by intravenous fluids. Large tumor masses of the chest or abdomen that die quickly when treatment is started may require IV fluids to protect the kidneys only at the start of treatment. For this reason, you may be admitted to the hospital to receive these treatments. See Chapter 10, *Experiencing Hospitalization*, for what to expect.

How chemotherapy is administered

There are several different forms of chemotherapy for lung cancer and different ways to administer it:

- Intravenous therapy
- Oral therapy
- Skin (subcutaneous) injections
- Portable pumps
- Monoclonal antibody injected therapy
- Intrathecal chemotherapy into the spine or via an Ommaya reservoir

Intravenous therapy

Chemotherapy for lung cancer often is administered into a vein using a temporary or semipermanent IV line in the forearm, or by any one of a number of venous access devices (VADs), such as a central catheter that has been implanted into a large vein in your chest.

If you have difficulty finding a usable vein, see Appendix B, *Tests and Procedures*, for suggestions that may make this process easier. If you continue to experience trouble with inaccessible veins or if they worsen during treatment, discuss with your doctor the advantages and disadvantages of venous access devices, such as central catheters.

Some of the drugs used will be in plastic bags that are hung from your IV pole. They may be mixed with a saline drip to dilute them as they enter your vein. Others may be injected directly into your IV line from a large syringe. This method is called a bolus push.

Some drugs used for intravenous chemotherapy are damaging if they come in contact with skin. Notify the medical staff immediately if you experience any pain, swelling, redness, or burning near the injection site.

You may feel a warm flush or sweating when certain drugs are administered. Verify with the medical staff that this is normal for your drug regimen.

Oral therapy

Your chemotherapy regimen may include oral medication along with, or in place of, intravenous injections; or you may be given oral medication to offset nausea or reduce coughing. You might be given tablets to take at home, perhaps several times a day or perhaps every other day. You may be given prescriptions for antidiarrheal or antinausea medications to take with your chemotherapy.

Although taking pills may seem easy, you should be aware of several potential issues.

Chemotherapy drugs and radiation therapy targeted to the high chest can cause some problems in swallowing pills. After several days or weeks of treatment, you may notice your mouth becoming increasingly dry as the rapidly dividing cells in your mouth die. A good habit to cultivate is wetting your mouth before attempting to swallow a tablet.

It's easy to forget what medications you've taken when you have quite a few and when some of them are making you drowsy. Each day, keep a new list of what you must take and check them off as you take them. Consider buying a plastic pill organizer to assure that all doses are taken.

Subcutaneous injections

Colony stimulating factors, such as granulocyte colony stimulating factor (G-CSF), thrombopoietin, or erythropoietin (EPO), frequently are injected under the skin or, less often, into muscle.

If your insurance company will pay for the drug, you may be able to give yourself these injections at home. The medical staff will teach you the quick, painless poke-in-the-thigh method, using pinching, stretching, or slapping to anesthetize the area first. Small syringes of the type used for insulin usually will do. The staff will give you a "red bag" for needle disposal, which should be returned to the doctor's office when full, not put into the trash.

If your insurance company will only pay for these injections if they are administered in a doctor's office, you may have to make twice- or thrice-weekly trips to the doctor.

Portable (ambulatory) pumps

Some studies have shown that, for certain patients, a continuous infusion of one or more anticancer drugs for lung cancer is more effective than a single daily or weekly administration. By using a portable infusion pump, it's possible to have certain anti-cancer drugs administered throughout the day for many days or to have multiple drugs delivered at the same time. These pumps can be programmed to deliver, or not deliver, a steady or varying dose of drugs for hours, days, or weeks.

If you have a venous access device such as a central (chest or neck) catheter or a peripheral (arm) catheter, most likely it can be used for delivering drugs via portable pump. If you don't have a venous access device, almost certainly one will be put in place before treatment starts. A very small battery-powered pump—about the size of a paperback book—is connected to this line. The pump can be implanted under the skin or carried in a satchel that you can wear around your waist or over your shoulder.

The advantages of a portable continuous infusion pump are:

- The possibility of a better anticancer response to chemotherapy
- Fewer and shorter doctor visits, yielding less disruption of your schedule

Disadvantages are:

- The possibility of greater side effects with continuous infusion, entailing a temporarily reduced quality of life.
- The inconvenience of having to adjust to and carry an attached pump all day long.
- The need to have a venous access device put in place. See Appendix B for a description of this experience.
- If an implanted pump is used instead of an external pump connected to a catheter, it might need to be put in place while you are under general anesthesia.

Implanted and portable pumps have advantages and disadvantages, as well. Implanted infusion pumps might be more expensive and might require a surgery to implant, but they are less likely to clot or become infected as a central venous catheter might when it is attached to an external pump.

The reservoir in your pump can be refilled on a schedule determined by your oncologist. Implanted pumps might be accessed through the skin; external pumps and balloon reservoirs might just be replaced.

There are several kinds of portable infusion pumps and many different regimens for delivering drugs at optimal levels. You should keep in mind that there is a variety of approaches. Have no concern if you hear of someone whose treatment schedule or pump type is different from yours.

Monoclonal antibody therapy

Monoclonal antibodies are a manmade version of a natural body product, a protein secreted by our white blood cells. They are injected into a vein via an IV line or catheter.

It's possible to have an allergic reaction to monoclonal antibodies because often they are formed from combined human and mouse antibodies, and over time, the patient can develop an intolerance for the mouse antibody. This reaction is easily controlled, but it must be addressed immediately to keep it from becoming serious. To avoid this allergic reaction, antibodies usually are injected very slowly over several hours.

Intrathecal therapy

Some chemotherapies are aimed at preventing the spread of disease into the central nervous system, including the brain. These chemotherapies are injected directly into the spinal column with a syringe or via a temporary device implanted beneath the scalp, called an Ommaya reservoir.

Some doctors combine intrathecal therapy with a spinal tap, if one is considered necessary: spinal fluid is removed for analysis and replaced by the chemotherapeutic agent. See Appendix B for a description of a spinal tap, also called a lumbar puncture.

Larry Coffman describes his intrathecal therapy:

> Some possible side effects of whole-brain radiation (WBR) were explained to me by my medical oncologist: memory might start to fail, ability to drive might be impaired, ability to walk might be impaired. I chose not to do WBR as a preventive measure. (My radiation oncologist, on the other hand, didn't feel the need to explain the worst and best case scenarios, but only the best case.)
>
> My medical oncologist chose to inject the chemo directly into the spinal cavity in order to increase the amount of the drug reaching the target and to reduce the possibility of metastases to the brain. The brain filters its

supply of blood in order to protect itself. The long-term effects are much less for the kind of treatment that I experienced versus radiation therapy—that is, according to my oncologist.

Departure

Before you leave the doctor's office, be sure you have received written instructions regarding necessary dietary or behavioral changes, information about possible side effects, prescriptions, and phone numbers for emergencies.

Do not leave feeling unwell. If you are feeling unwell, tell the medical staff.

Use the restroom before leaving if you received your treatments via IV line. Often, IV drugs are accompanied by a saline drip. The volume of fluid that your kidneys have processed from this treatment may surprise you halfway home. If you have received doxorubicin by IV, you might note that your urine has an orange or reddish tint. This tint is harmless and temporary.

Most chemotherapy treatments do not result in infection or side effects that require hospitalization. However, occasionally such problems do occur. Carefully note all symptoms and communicate immediately with your doctor if problems arise.

Kathleen Houlihan tells of her comfort with and adaptation to chemo as it progresses:

> *After I finished this round of treatment, my friend LH went to the airport with me on Tuesday and saw me to my plane. I just took it easy, conserving energy; not even doing my usual morning or evening walks starting Monday night, and made it back just fine without crashing like I did last month. Not having to change planes on the return helped quite a bit. I also tried those motion sickness wristbands this time and didn't have any queasiness on the flight. My husband Holt met me at the gate and ushered me home, where he's been doing all the chores. He even assembled the new airbed he had picked up earlier in the day. It's pretty nice: air bladders inside a foam mattress that can be adjusted from firm to soft at the touch of a button.*
>
> *I'll return to the treatment center in a month, when I'll be scanned "from head to toe"—brain MRI, bone scan, CT scans. If there is no evidence of cancer anywhere other than the original tumor site, next month will be my last round of chemo and I'll go on a three-month checkup schedule for the next three years. I'll become a former cancer patient. Sounds good to me!*

Dosages

If you feel inclined to do so, you can verify your chemotherapy dosage. See "How to verify your chemotherapy dose" in Chapter 22, *Researching Your Illness*.

Summary

This chapter, in combination with Chapter 13, aims to make the chemotherapy experience a less frightening one.

Many of the topics we touch on in these chapters are well described in other books. See Appendix A, *Resources*, for several excellent books that can offer you much more information.

Key points to remember:

- Plan in advance for side effects by purchasing prescriptions in advance and taking nausea medications as prescribed.

- If your insurance plan provides a liberal allowance for prescriptions, ask your doctor to prescribe the most effective antinausea medication (antiemetic), regardless of cost.

- Consider scheduling your first few treatment appointments near a day off so you can recover before attempting to return to work or other responsibilities.

- Take along an advocate who can speak for you and take notes.

- Dress for comfort, avoiding clothing that will interfere with access to veins, ports, or pumps.

- Talk to the other survivors in the waiting and treatment rooms.

- Report any unusual feelings or discomfort immediately to the medical staff.

- After treatment or during continuous infusion via pump, report any illness, fever, or unusual side effects to your doctor immediately.

- If you note blood in the line leading from a vein to a portable infusion pump or in your catheter, notify your oncologist.

CHAPTER 12

Experiencing Radiotherapy

*Poisons and medicine are oftentimes the same substance
given with different intents.*

—Peter Mere Latham

BY NOW YOU HAVE CONSULTED with several types of oncologists and decided that radiation therapy is a good choice for treating your lung cancer. Perhaps it will be used
before surgery to shrink a tumor, perhaps one of several sites will be irradiated to
alleviate unpleasant symptoms, or perhaps irradiation of the brain will be chosen to
prevent the spread of cancer or to remove a single tumor. Often radiation is used in
conjunction with other therapies, such as chemotherapy or surgery.

We are justifiably afraid of radiation. We know that sunlight can burn us, that x-ray
technicians leave the room and wear lead aprons when they treat us. We know we
should be wary of too many diagnostic x-rays and that large amounts of radiation
caused tremendous damage at Hiroshima, Nagasaki, and Chernobyl. In spite of fears
about radiation, though, many lung cancer patients are pleasantly surprised to find
that radiation therapy is a smooth, quick, silent, painless treatment.

External radiotherapy is the most common form of radiation therapy used for lung
cancer. As with the chapter for chemotherapy, this chapter will acquaint you with a
typical radiotherapy experience. Most radiotherapy used for lung cancer is administered in the outpatient setting, so we will walk you through an outpatient treatment.
We will begin with your preparation, including treatment simulation and the cre-
ation of braces and shields; scheduling; arriving at the treatment office; encountering
certain medical personnel and other patients; advancing through the treatment itself;
and we'll finish with what you can expect afterward.

Brachytherapy and radioimmunotherapy are discussed briefly in this chapter.

The theories behind radiotherapy as treatment for lung cancer and the side effects of
treatment are discussed separately in Chapter 7, *Types of Treatment,* and Chapter 13,
Adverse Effects of Treatment.

Although there are different kinds of radiation, including x-rays and electron, proton, or neutron beams, for the sake of readability we will not distinguish among them. We will use only the term radiation.

The information this chapter provides is not a substitute for your doctor's knowledge. Always ask your doctor when an aspect of your treatment is unclear, and report immediately to your doctor any adverse reactions that arise during or after treatment.

If you would like greater detail on radiation therapy, *The Chemotherapy and Radiation Therapy Survival Guide* by Judith McKay and Nancee Hirano (New Harbinger, 1998); *Making the Radiation Therapy Decision* by David Brenner and Eric Hall (Lowell House, 1998); and *Coping with Radiation Therapy: A Ray of Hope* by Daniel Cukier, MD, and Virginia McCullough (Contemporary Books, 1996) are books that focus on radiation therapy from the patient's perspective.

Where radiotherapy is targeted

For most types of lung cancer, radiation therapy is targeted to the chest. For small cell lung cancer, the brain also might be irradiated to prevent or control metastases. Occasionally, lung cancer tumors that have traveled to organs other than the chest or brain are irradiated to reduce or eliminate painful symptoms.

External radiation therapy

External radiation therapy might be used before surgery to shrink tumors or after surgery to kill any remaining microscopic tumor cells or to control metastases. The following sections will walk you through preparation and treatment simulation, scheduling, receiving therapy, departure, and the days that follow treatment.

Preparation

Your responsibilities when preparing for treatment include planning for accompaniment to treatment and learning what products or clothing to avoid at the time of treatment.

Radiation therapy is a brand new experience for most people. It often makes patients increasingly tired as it progresses. Some patients receiving radiation to the brain can become confused. For these reasons, it would be wise to have a friend or loved one along, not only for emotional support, but to handle such issues as saving written instructions for diet and aftercare; understanding and remembering verbal instructions; communicating insurance information; handling the co-pay, if any; and assisting with the drive home.

Make a point of discussing nausea and pain medications with your doctor before treatment starts. Excellent painkillers and antiemetics are available; you shouldn't have to endure these side effects.

Ask about skin care, too. External beam radiation must pass through your skin to reach tumor sites, and irritation may result. Newer, higher voltage equipment used today causes less damage to skin because the damaging rays concentrate in deeper layers, but some skin reaction still is possible. See Chapter 13 for a discussion of radiation therapy's effects on skin and other tissue. In general, you should ask for instructions about using your favorite lotions, deodorant, talc, and topical medications; about how to shave, bathe, and dry your skin; and about avoiding sticky bandages, extremes of heat and cold, and sunlight. These factors might interfere with treatment, or they might cause your skin to become hypersensitive when exposed to radiation.

Ask as well about clothing with metal zippers, pacemakers, and surgical staples. Most surgical staples do not react with radiation, MRI, or CT scanners, but they might appear as unknown entities on a simulation scan.

Simulation

If you are receiving fractionated radiation therapy spread out over several weeks, your first one or two treatment visits to the radiation oncology treatment offices will be spent determining the precise details of how best to treat you. This process of fine-tuning radiation treatments to your individual circumstances is called simulation. Simulation allows very precise delivery of radiation to be calculated and delivered only to the tumor; irradiation of healthy tissue and side effects can be minimized.

You'll be positioned on the treatment bed and perhaps marked with small dots of temporary or permanent ink or tattoos. If you have a brain tumor, you might be fitted with a head frame marked for targeting accuracy. Shields for sensitive organs might be constructed. A CT scanner might be used to plan your treatment if either fractionated stereotactic radiosurgery or 3D conformal radiotherapy (3D-CRT) is planned. All of these preparations are called simulation; they might take several hours spread over one or more visits.

Several medical specialists are involved in this stage of your treatment: your radiation oncologist; the radiation therapy technician who will administer the treatment; a dosimetrist, who calculates the correct dose; a radiation physicist, who calibrates the machine; and perhaps a CT technician. Some of these staff members might work behind the scenes.

For these initial visits, which might be lengthy, make yourself as comfortable as possible by wearing clothing that doesn't bind, goes on and off easily, and has no metal zippers. Take a cassette player if you like, and use the restroom before the simulation starts.

None of these preparations are painful, but you might feel claustrophobic if a face shield is made for whole brain irradiation. To make a face shield, a soft plastic compound is shaped to your face and left there to harden. While it is hardening, you must hold very still. Some people find this experience unsettling.

If you will be having fractionated stereotactic radiosurgery or 3D conformal radiotherapy to the brain, an immobilization frame might be fitted against your scalp to restrain your head. This frame is considered uncomfortable by some, but it is not surgically attached to the skull with pins as is done for non-fractionated stereotactic radiosurgery.

Depending on the location of your tumor and the type of radiotherapy used, shields or blocks might be made to shape the radiation beam to match your tumor's shape exactly, allowing the treatment to avoid sensitive healthy organs. Beams of invisible radiation generated by some older machines are emitted shaped like rectangles, from two to fifteen inches in any dimension. If these beams were trained against your tumor, nearby healthy tissue within the two- to fifteen-inch rectangle would be irradiated, too, suffering damage. To avoid this effect, shields or blocks with cutaways in the silhouette of your tumor are created using your x-ray or CT films as guides. The shields made for you are used only by you. You might see the same kinds of devices belonging to other patients hanging nearby or in other treatment areas.

Some of the machinery used during simulation looks and moves just as the genuine radiation equipment does, but instead it generates only a plain light beam to verify positioning, ink markings, and the fit of shields.

After all shields, frames, and blocks are made and your skin is marked, the entire simulation will be repeated with all pieces in place—exactly like a dress rehearsal.

If you will be receiving 3D conformal radiotherapy, simulation might be done on a computer without the patient.

As your treatment progresses and your tumor shrinks, or if you lose a substantial amount of weight, new ink markings or shields might be remade to match the new shape of your tumor, and simulations might be repeated.

Scheduling

Years of research have shown that a large amount of radiation can be delivered to a tumor safely if the dosage is spread out over several weeks. This kind of delivery is called fractionating the dose, or simply fractionation. It spares healthy tissue from unnecessary damage and gives it time to recover. Hyperfractionated doses are delivered several times a day for several weeks instead of once daily for several weeks. Accelerated hyperfractionated doses are delivered several times a day for fewer weeks than hyperfractionated doses.

Kathleen Houlihan talks about the beginning of her treatments:

> I started my twice-daily radiation treatments. In the first treatment center I visited, they would have been given once a day, but here they break it up into two lower doses. It's supposed to be easier on the patient, as well as more effective. Each round takes about five minutes, including getting on and off the table.

Most people receiving radiotherapy for lung cancer receive traditional external beam radiotherapy, 3D conformal radiotherapy, or fractionated stereotactic radiosurgery in an outpatient setting. If you will receive non-fractionated stereotactic radiosurgery, also called a gamma knife, the treatment usually is done in one sitting or in the hospital, not spread out over several weeks.

Dosage fractionation means that you will have to visit the treatment center several times a week, or perhaps once or more times per day, for several weeks, depending on your treatment plan. It also means that each dose of radiation lasts only two to four minutes. If your tumor is irradiated from several different angles (and most are), each angle might take two to four minutes after the machine is repositioned. After the lengthy time spent in simulation, you might feel that ten to thirty minutes of treatment time is an anticlimax.

At the halfway point, Kathleen continues to do well:

> This past Monday marked the halfway point of my radiation treatments, fifteen days down and fifteen to go. May 17 is my expected last day, after which I'll return for the monthly chemo treatments for five more months. I'm still hanging in there, one day at a time. My joints are

better, thank goodness. I get a little queasy on occasion, but drinking club
soda takes care of it (thank you, Mrs. F in my support group!). I just
started getting a "radiation burn," but it's not too bad, and I have a cream
that helps a lot (thanks to JM's suggestion). I'm tired most of the time,
even first thing in the morning, but that's just the way it goes. My days
are punctuated by naps now, even though I have never been a napper.

This month's chest x-ray showed the tumor has shrunk a little more
since last month. In its long dimension, it's "only" about 4.5 centimeters
now, down from about 8 centimeters in March. And the CEA tumor
marker, which was 66 in March, is down from 8.5 last month to 6.5 now,
heading toward the normal level of three or below. So all those indications
continue to be encouraging.

Don't be surprised if the schedule on which your radiotherapy is administered differs from the schedules you hear others discussing. Your radiation schedule always is
tailored to your particular circumstances, based on the size, number, and location of
tumors; your overall health; your body size; and the type of lung cancer you have.

For each treatment, you might want to call the treatment center before leaving home
or work. Radiation therapy machines sustain heavy use and must be taken offline
periodically for recalibration or repair. You can save your valuable time by calling
first to see whether appointments are running on time.

After a few treatments, you might begin to feel that most of your time is spent traveling or chatting in the waiting room, because treatment itself is so brief.

Arrival

Upon arrival, you might be asked to change into a hospital gown. Depending on what
treatments are being used, the timing of your radiation therapy might be influenced
by the quantity of white blood cells remaining in your blood after your last chemotherapy or radiotherapy treatment. Your blood might be tested when you arrive, using
a standard measurement known as a complete blood count, or CBC. If your white
blood counts are too low, treatment might be delayed a few days or a week.

If you become nauseous after treatment, though, request a change in medication.
Although the new antinausea drugs (antiemetics) are excellent, ask for suppositories
in case oral medications won't stay in your stomach. If nausea becomes a problem,
subsequent treatments might be preceded by an injection of one of the new antinausea drugs, such as Zofran.

If you develop mouth or throat pain (esophagitis), call your doctor promptly. In some cases, strong painkillers (even morphine, temporarily) are needed to control this pain and enable you to eat because adequate nutrition is supremely important. A brief stay in the hospital to receive intravenous feeding might be necessary while your mouth and throat heal.

The setting

The source of radiation will be a machine that either safely contains a radioactive substance, such as Cobalt 60, or generates its own radiation as needed. Like a CT scanner or a gamma camera, some radiation machines are designed to move around you and your bed as you hold still, but others do not move and are repositioned as needed by the staff. Many models are almost silent, but some make a sound like a vacuum cleaner, and they might click and whir if they reposition automatically. They tend to be large machines, and some patients find their size and movement unnerving.

The room in which treatment is given has thick walls and is lead-clad to prevent the very small amount of radiation that rebounds from its target, known as scatter, from affecting the medical staff, those in the waiting room, and random passers-by. For the safety of the staff, the treatment room will contain only you when the machine is engaged. (The small dose of radiation they would sustain if they stayed with you would probably not harm them, but if they stayed with all patients, all day, every day, the dose from scatter would indeed accumulate to dangerous levels.)

The staff can see and hear you at all times because there are microphones and cameras connecting you and them. If you feel at all bad, just let them know. Music and wall art sometimes are available in the treatment room to lower your boredom and stress levels.

Delivery of external radiation therapy

Although simulation can take hours, treatment takes just a few minutes.

External radiotherapy is administered using the blocks and shields that might have been made expressly for you, perhaps with sandbags or a head frame to hold you very still and blankets to keep you warm.

You should feel no pain, no heat, no sensation at all during treatment, although some survivors say that they feel a sensation of energizing—not quite a tingling—in the area of the tumor during treatment. It might indeed be that some people can sense a highly active biological entity, such as a tumor, reacting to the disruption of its DNA.

Some find the absence of sensation eerie, but most people are grateful that the treatment is comfortable and brief.

During delivery, it is most important to hold very still, but you can breathe normally. If newer technologies, such as the cyberknife or the Peacock system, are used, continuous CT scanning will track any small movements you make and adjust the machine accordingly.

Departure

After each of your first few treatment sessions, make sure before leaving the doctor's office that you have received written instructions regarding any necessary dietary or behavioral changes; information about possible side effects, such as possible inflammation of throat tissue; prescriptions; and phone numbers for emergencies. Often, side effects of radiation therapy do not emerge until you've had two or more weeks of treatment. If you have prepared for these possibilities by asking questions during the treatment visits when you feel well, side effects might be easier to deal with.

You are not likely to feel unwell after your treatments, but if you do, do not leave without telling the medical staff of your problem.

Kathleen Houlihan tells of her happiness as the end of her radiation therapy sessions approaches and she prepares to leave the center where she has been receiving treatment:

> We're getting ready to go home! I had my last chemotherapy session, for this go-round, this past Monday, and next Monday will be my last day of radiation. I'll have a chest x-ray and see all my doctors on Monday before we leave. The chest x-ray I had after three weeks of treatment showed the tumor had shrunk some. We're expecting to see it quite a bit smaller on this next x-ray. A generalized tumor marker they are using to track my tumor is down. Normal is under 5, but I'm getting there. And finally, the shoulder pain I've had since last July, which apparently was the first symptom of the cancer, disappeared completely after a couple of weeks of treatment. So all indications are good.
>
> We'll be home for a month and then start a routine of coming back here one week a month for five months for additional chemo. I probably will lose my hair then, according to my doctor. Oh well, it will grow back.
>
> Things are going well. I'm feeling better and better. Must be time to go home.

Internal radiotherapy

Although various types of external beam radiation therapy are the most common forms of radiotherapy used for lung cancer, for some lung tumors, a radioactive substance placed very close to or within the tumor might offer the best chance for cure. This treatment, known as brachytherapy, might be combined with surgical removal of as much tumor as possible.

Endobronchial brachytherapy

During endobronchial brachytherapy, a bronchoscope is used in conjunction with an external imaging tool, such as a CT scanner, to position an empty tube through the nose down into the airway alongside the tumor. You will be sedated during this timed exposure, and a topical anesthetic will be used to numb your nose and throat. Once the tube is in place, a team specially trained to handle radioactive material manipulates the radioactive substance (such as iridium-192), perhaps remotely, into the tube. It might be left in place for only a few minutes or for a few hours, depending on the dose required and the isotope used.

All of the above might be done first without a radioactive substance as a simulation.

Typically, brachytherapy delivers a high dose of radiotherapy for a short period of time. This means that while your body contains the radioactive substance, the radiation will pass through your tissues and will continue to travel beyond your body. Your bodily wastes might contain radioactive byproducts. Consequently, during this time and for a short time afterward, you and your bodily wastes will represent a radiation hazard to others. Visits from family and friends during treatment will be discouraged or denied, and nursing staff will wear protective gear and limit their contact with you. They will provide you with all the care you need, but they might, for example, speak to you from about six feet away instead of from the bedside.

After the designated amount of time has passed, the team will return to remove and dispose of the radioactive substance. Once the agent is out of your body, you are no longer a risk to others; but your bodily waste, such as sputum, might be. You might be discharged from the hospital the same day or very soon after.

For some lung cancers, brachytherapy is repeated a few days or a week later to maximize tumor shrinkage.

Interstitial brachytherapy

Permanent implantation of low-dose radioactive material might be done during the surgery intended to remove the tumor. If not inserted at that time, implants can be inserted using a bronchoscope while you're sedated. Radioactive agents chosen for this type of treatment are those with an active range of just a few centimeters, which ensures the safety of nearby healthy tissue and of others around you.

See Chapter 10, *Experiencing Hospitalization*, for more information about receiving interstitial radiotherapy.

Radioimmunotherapy

Radioimmunotherapy is a new treatment, still in early clinical trials for lung cancer, but promising.

Radioimmunotherapy involves linking a radioisotope, such as iodine-131 or yttrium-90, to a binding substance, such as a monoclonal antibody or a somatostatin analogue. The proposed benefit of radioimmunotherapy over existing radiation treatments is that a smaller amount of healthy tissue is exposed to radiation because the antibody attaches preferentially to, but not only to, cancerous tissue. Some healthy tissue is affected because the radioactive substance decays as the antibody travels to the tumor and because monoclonal antibodies also will attach to some antigens on healthy cells; but it is thought that this effect is less than that sustained during external beam therapy. Radioimmunotherapy is administered into a vein as in chemotherapy.

The correct dose of radioimmunotherapy must first be determined. To calculate this dose, a small "tracer" amount of the substance will be injected first and visualized using a CT scan or other imaging device. Based on what is seen, the doctors in charge will determine the total dose you should receive.

You will be kept in a lead-shielded hospital room throughout this treatment, and your body wastes will be disposed of in accordance with rules for handling hazardous waste. Face-to-face family visits will be very limited or denied entirely. The nurses who care for you might wear protective clothing and will limit contact with you.

If the radioisotope iodine-131 will be used, your thyroid gland will be shielded first, unless it has been infiltrated with lung cancer. The radioactive isotope I-131 will destroy the thyroid gland if it is absorbed.

To shield the thyroid, large doses of *nonradioactive* iodine, iodine-123, are given to you first. This substance is taken up by the thyroid in excess compared to other body tissues. After the maximum amount has been absorbed, the thyroid cannot absorb more iodine for several days. This protects the thyroid gland from absorbing subsequent doses of I-131.

This method of treatment is not likely to be used for those who have had previous allergic reactions to iodine in shrimp or other foods or in other medications.

Summary

Radiation therapy confuses and frightens some people. An advance glimpse at what it's like might help to alleviate this stress. This chapter is intended to address your concerns and fears.

As always, you should ask your doctor about any issues that concern you and immediately report any untoward effects to the medical staff.

Key points to remember:

- Simulation and preparation usually take longer than the treatments do. Treatments take just a few minutes.

- Treatment is painless, unless a head brace is used for one-time inpatient stereotactic radiosurgery (gamma knife).

- Fatigue, mental dullness, or confusion can accompany whole-brain radiotherapy and might become more pronounced as treatment progresses.

- Ask the staff before using skin products that might irritate skin made sensitive by treatment.

- Esophagitis (pain in the throat) or nausea are possible following irradiation of the chest or neck. Notify your doctor if you're experiencing pain or nausea.

CHAPTER 13

Adverse Effects of Treatment

The worse about medicine is that one kind
makes another necessary.

—Elbert Hubbard

REMARKABLE PROGRESS HAS BEEN MADE in alleviating the suffering associated with cancer treatment. This chapter describes the adverse effects of lung cancer treatment and what can be done about them.

Because some lung cancer patients are treated only with surgery, we first discuss the most common adverse effects associated with surgery. Then we discuss the adverse effects of chemotherapy, radiotherapy, and photodynamic therapy, ordered by symptom.

Although oncologists have reviewed this chapter, the author of this book is not a medical doctor. Symptoms that patients sometimes attribute to their treatment actually might be caused by worsening disease, as we discuss in Chapter 1, *Symptoms of Lung Cancer*. The information this chapter provides should never be substituted for your doctor's knowledge. Report to your doctor any adverse reactions that arise during or after treatment immediately, and direct all questions to your doctor, regardless of other sources of information available to you.

Terminology

What distinguishes the side effects of treatment from delayed or late effects, complications, or the effects of tumor activity? The somewhat arbitrary definitions are that side effects of treatment are those that occur within days or weeks of treatment; delayed effects are those that occur within weeks or months of cancer treatment; and late effects are those that occur months or years after treatment. Some side effects, such as shortness of breath or chest pain induced by surgery or radiological scarring, drift into becoming delayed or late effects. The medical community distinguishes between effects and complications by defining effects as expected and complications as somewhat unexpected.

Incidence and severity

Please be encouraged by the fact that, although we list many adverse effects here, you might have very little reaction or no discernible reaction at all to treatment. Keep in mind that you can reduce the side effects of treatment by avoiding smoking and drinking alcohol during treatment.

Even commonly used treatments for mild illnesses are known to have numerous adverse effects. Aspirin, for instance, is known to cause any of the following in certain people: vomiting; diarrhea; confusion; drowsiness; severe stomach pain; unusual bruising; bloody or black stools; gastrointestinal bleeding; dizziness; hearing loss; ringing in the ears; swelling of the hands, face, lips, eyes, throat, or tongue; difficulty swallowing or breathing; or hoarseness. It's noteworthy as well to remember that, as pharmacists sometimes say, any drug you swallow can cause nausea, and almost all drugs can cause dizziness in certain people. Larry Coffman, five-year survivor of SCLC, offers wise advice:

> Things do definitely improve with time. The side effects of treatment are not the same for any two people—don't forget that. I always expect the worst and am happy as a lark when I get the best.
>
> Please understand that not everyone scars extremely badly from radiation. Some scar very little: think positively.
>
> It is natural for your appetite to be reduced during treatment, that will get better as things taste and smell better.
>
> Weakness? Well, you are kind of going ten rounds with a boxer. Even they are weak for a while after a bout!
>
> I have since gained control of my life again. The longer I get from treatment finishing, the more of my life I reclaim. It may take some time and adjustments—let's face it: your body has actually been poisoned to keep it alive, so your body may be functioning differently. After a while, it may repair itself and return to normal.

Many side effects of treatment are normal and pose no danger to you. A change in the taste of food, for instance, is a common side effect of some treatments that does not necessarily herald serious problems. Your oncologist should give you fact sheets to provide you with information about side effects that are very serious, about which you should telephone as soon as you notice them. If your doctor doesn't offer this information, ask. Max Baldwin tells us:

> I received Taxol and carboplatin once a week for three weeks, then rested a week, then started the cycle again. This was repeated for four months. I also was given pain and nausea medicine.
>
> I didn't need to take the prescribed medicine for pain nor for nausea. I had small amounts of each, but I prefer not to take medicine unless absolutely necessary. Of course I lost my hair, but so what? I was starting to get bald anyway. My biggest problem has been numbness in my feet and hands. It sees to have gotten worse since treatment ended. The doctor says it may or may not go away. If you have ever had your feet frozen, that is how mine feel most of the time.
>
> My "bad days" consisted of slight nausea, bones aching and a general feeling of "getting the flu." This was usually two days after treatment for two or three days, and then I would have a couple of "good days" before treatment again. The treatment was under a clinical trial conducted at the Ellis Fischel Cancer Hospital in Columbia, Missouri. While I was receiving treatment, CT scans and x-rays showed my tumor had been reduced in size by almost two-thirds. (Fantastic!) I am presently being tested every 30 days, and so far the tumor is not growing at all.

Why do adverse effects happen?

Certain adverse effects, such as difficulty breathing or cardiac dysfunction, can follow treatment for lung cancer because lung cancer patients often have preexisting illnesses, such as blocked arteries or emphysema, that compromise heart or lung function. Treatment for cancer can worsen the functioning of these organs.

During surgery, some healthy tissue must be removed when the tumor is removed in order to ensure that the tumor is entirely gone. This is likely to reduce further one's ability to breathe. In other cases, surgery can cause scarring (sclerosis) that restricts healthy tissue, or the surgeon's tools can disturb nerve pathways.

Chemotherapeutic and radiotherapeutic treatments commonly used for lung cancer affect not only cancerous cells, but many healthy cells as well. Chemotherapy and radiotherapy regimens target cells that divide rapidly, as many cancer cells do. This means that many healthy cells that divide rapidly—cells in the mouth, intestinal tract, hair, fingernails, and others—will be affected, too. During treatment, these cells die all at once, instead of passing through the life cycle just a few at a time. This rapid turnover of cells causes some of the most common adverse effects of cancer treatment, such as diarrhea, mouth sores, unusual nail growth, or hair loss.

Still other adverse effects come about because of the body's attempt to heal itself. Tumor lysis syndrome, for instance, is a side effect of the body's attempt to clear itself of dying tumor cells after certain treatments. The immune system's reaction to radiation therapy can cause scarring (fibrosis) in the lungs and chest that takes months or years to develop.

Please note that such steroids as prednisone or Decadron, which you might be taking to control coughing, pain, or breathing problems, can cause a wide variety of adverse effects. Consider reading "Steroid-related effects," later in this chapter, if you are taking one of these drugs.

Kathleen Houlihan considers her upcoming chemotherapy :

> *Most of the people I had treatment with who were on chemotherapy did great—maybe a little loss of appetite or a little nausea, but nothing major. Of course, different people are on different chemicals, but I plan to sail through the week.*
>
> *I'll be taking Taxol and carboplatin, the same drugs I had one day per week during my radiation treatments. I did fine with them then, but I'll be getting approximately five times the amount I had then. Taxol makes most people lose their hair, usually after two or three weeks. I'd gladly give up my hair to get rid of every single remaining cancer cell, but I won't complain if I can get rid of the cancer without giving up my hair.*

Adverse effects after surgery

Complications and adverse effects arising from surgery vary enormously in type and frequency because of the variety and complexity of surgeries, which are always tailored to the patient's specific circumstances. Your surgeon can and must inform you of all possible risks you might face as a result of the surgery planned for you, but it's highly unlikely that you'll experience most of them. Some postsurgical adverse effects are:

- Abnormal tubelike formations between two organs (fistulae)
- Air leaks from the lung into nearby tissue (pneumothorax)
- Blood clots in the lung or veins
- Bone pain of long duration if ribs were cut
- Bruising (hematoma)
- Fluid (edema) in the lungs
- Heart arrhythymias
- Hemorrhage
- Herniation at incision sites or in the heart
- Infection or internal abscess
- Leaking lymphatic ducts (chylothorax)
- Lung collapse (atelectasis)
- Nausea
- Nerve damage, causing pain or dysfunction
- Pneumonia
- Pus in or near the incision or in the lungs (empyema)
- Reduced breathing capacity caused by reduced lung tissue
- Respiratory failure or acute respiratory distress syndrome (ARDS)
- Scar tissue (adhesions)
- Stretching, constricting, or weakening of supportive tissues
- Twisting of lung tissue (lobar torsion)

Adverse effects by symptom

The following sections discuss specific adverse effects, late effects, and complications of surgery, chemotherapy, and radiotherapy. The most common adverse effects after treatment for lung cancer are difficulty breathing, coughing, sore throat, infection, nausea, diarrhea, mouth sores, hair loss, pain, soreness or numbness in hands and feet, psychological effects (such as anxiety and depression), and fatigue. The most common late effects are shortness of breath, chest pain, coughing, fatigue, and psychological issues, such as anxiety and depression.

Cross references in the list of adverse effects by symptom refer to other items in the list, unless another chapter is specified.

Abdominal pain

Abdominal pain might occur following treatment with certain chemotherapy regimens that utilize vincristine, methotrexate, prednisone, or Decadron.

VRE, vancomycin-resistant enterococcus, is a bacterium that is found more frequently in hospitals than elsewhere. Characterized by diarrhea and general intestinal distress, it is difficult to treat because it is resistant to strong antibiotics. VRE is more likely to affect those who are hospitalized while having excessively low levels of white blood cells and suboptimal kidney function.

Typhlitis is a serious infection of the portion of the large bowel called the cecum and usually is associated with high-dose chemotherapy. Typhlitis results from unusual bacteria thriving in vulnerable parts of your intestine when your white blood cell counts are abnormally low. Your doctor can confirm this diagnosis with an ultrasound. Typhlitis also is known as neutropenic enterocolitis, necrotizing enterocolitis, or ileocecal syndrome. Phone your doctor immediately if you experience these in combination: nausea, vomiting, swollen abdomen, diarrhea, fever, and soreness in the lower right side.

See also "Bowel changes" and "Metabolic imbalances."

Abscess

Following surgery or radiation therapy for lung cancer, an abscess within the chest might develop. This abscess usually occurs as a late effect, if at all, but might develop earlier in certain people. If you have unusual or pronounced pain or an elevated temperature, notify your doctor immediately.

Allergic reactions

It's possible to have an allergic reaction to almost any drug, depending on a host of poorly understood factors. Allergic reactions are more likely to occur with high doses of a drug that is administered rapidly.

Allergic reactions are highly individualized to substance type, but the symptoms are similar and include any of these: hives, itching, racing heartbeat, low blood pressure, difficulty breathing, tightness in chest or throat, sore throat, fever, or chills. Symptoms of allergic reaction must be reported to the medical staff at once. Severe allergic reactions can be fatal.

Anemia

See "Fatigue and sleep disorders" and "Breathing problems, coughing, hoarseness."

Alopecia

See "Hair loss and growth."

Appetite or taste changes

Chemotherapy and radiotherapy can affect your taste buds. Some people can no longer taste food, or it tastes metallic or disgusting.

Adequate nutrition in spite of food aversion is a very important part of your recovery. Eat what you like, but eat as much nutritional food as you can. Ask your doctor about vitamin supplements and liquid supplements, such as Nutrical or Ensure. Avoid smoking and drinking alcohol during treatment. A lung cancer survivor describes changes he has made:

> I've been making changes in my eating. My appetite has been real good again. I'm drinking a high-protein dietary supplement and trying to gain back some weight.

Some lung cancer survivors note that, rather than craving particular foods, they are repelled by them, particularly by meats. Foods that once were favorites now have a repugnant taste and scent.

Bladder damage

Contact your doctor immediately if you have pain or pass blood while urinating, or if your urine remains dark.

Doxorubicin (Adriamycin) temporarily turns urine red or dark. This is harmless.

Drugs such as cyclophosphamide (Cytoxan), ifosfamide, vincristine, and such platinum-containing drugs as cisplatin can cause pain or damage the bladder. Hydration by mouth and IV is in some cases critical to protect the bladder from painful and sometimes chronic cystitis. Simultaneous administration of a drug called Mesna (mercaptoethane sulfonate) might be employed to protect the bladder when certain drugs are used. Sometimes this combination is administered during a brief hospital stay to allow close monitoring and guard against bladder damage.

Bleeding

You should report any unexpected bleeding following surgery or bronchoscopy to your doctor at once. Bed rest, codeine, blood transfusions, ceasing anticoagulant medication, or sealing blood vessels (embolization) might be recommended.

Bleeding during or following chemotherapy or radiotherapy might be caused by an inadequate number of platelets because treatment suppresses bone marrow. Contact your doctor, who might prescribe a transfusion or a drug or injection that stimulates the production of platelet precursors in bone marrow. As of this writing, Neumega has been approved by the FDA for this purpose.

Blood clots

If you have had surgery, have a central venous catheter, or have a large tumor and have just started treatment, be especially aware of chest, abdominal, or leg pain or difficulty breathing. These might signal a dangerous blood clot dislodging and capable of traveling to the lung or brain, causing suffocation or stroke.

Geri Capasso describes her brother Anthony's blood clots:

> The doctors used the term "diffuse lymphangeal spread" with my brother Anthony. He is back in the hospital. After he received Taxol, he became very short of breath, and they found two blood clots in his calf and one in his lung. He is now on blood thinners. They put umbrella stents in his veins, and he is on oxygen. We are hoping that as the clots dissolve his breathing will improve. He also has a largely unproductive cough, but sometimes he coughs yellow sputum.

Extended immobility after surgery might cause blood clots to form in the legs. Blood clots also might form around a central catheter at any time during treatment. At the beginning of treatment with chemotherapy, a large tumor might shrink rapidly in response to therapy and might dislodge a pre-existing blood clot.

Blood clots might be treated with anticoagulants, stents to hold the blood vessel open, or sieves placed in the blood vessel to capture clots.

Bone damage

Radiation therapy or the progression of disease can damage bone, particularly the spine, ribs, legs, and pelvis. Radiotherapy can cause pain and fracture six months to four years after treatment. There is no cure for this damage, although using such biphosphonate drugs as Aredia might be effective in limiting bone fracture. See "Pain" for ways to deal with this long-term effect.

Bowel changes

Certain drugs can cause black, tarry stools or bloody stools. Notify your doctor immediately if you're having chemotherapy and notice these changes.

Constipation can be a very serious problem during lung cancer treatment because inactivity, other illnesses, and certain drugs—such as the newer nausea drugs, vincristine, painkillers, antidepressants, or antihistamines—might slow or paralyze the intestine or mask the urge to move one's bowels. Constipation in its most serious form, a total blockage of the intestine called fecal impaction, can present as circulatory or respiratory distress. Call your doctor immediately if you feel constipated for more than three days or if you have difficulty breathing or symptoms of heart failure. Fecal impaction can be fatal even in the absence of a tumor.

If your doctor agrees, experiment with small amounts of different foods until you have a sense for what will maintain a balance between constipation and diarrhea. Increased fluid intake, regular exercise, increased dietary fiber, warm or hot drinks, privacy and quiet time in the bathroom, easy access to toilet or bedside commode, and stool softeners might be tried to ease constipation. Do not make dietary changes or greatly increase your fluid intake without first verifying these choices with your doctor.

Breathing problems, coughing, hoarseness

Breathing problems in lung cancer patients are common. Tumor growth; post-treatment infections, such as pneumonia; treatments for lung cancer; and drugs that affect the heart, such as cyclophosphamide or doxorubicin, all have the potential to cause coughing or difficulty breathing.

Call your doctor immediately if you have chest tightness, chest pain, coughing, hoarseness, fever, or trouble breathing. Lung collapse, for instance, either after surgery or following obstruction by a tumor or phlegm, is a medical emergency following surgery that can be fatal if not treated immediately.

Geri Capasso describes her brother Anthony's breathing problems:

> *I've been going through the breathing scare with my brother. He finally*
> *left the hospital this past Friday and yesterday he (wheeling that oxygen*
> *tank with him) went to his daughter's softball game and home for dinner,*
> *and then to his son's roller hockey game. (Thank God he didn't have to*
> *play!) We don't know if he will always need O², but "there is life with a*
> *tank." I just wanted to say that the breathing problem is stressful and*
> *nerve-wracking to say the least, but it can be dealt with.*

Surgical removal of lung tissue can result in difficulty breathing for several reasons. First, lung cancer patients often have decreased heart, circulatory, or lung capacity prior to surgery caused by other illnesses, such as heart disease or emphysema; removal of some healthy lung tissue along with the tumor further reduces one's ability to breathe. In addition, adverse effects of surgery, such as fistulae (see later), fever, an accumulation of fluid in the chest cavity (pleural effusion or, less often, chylothorax), or hemorrhage, can cause difficulty breathing. A man who had most of a lung removed observes:

> *Evidently the remaining lung tissue will take on some additional*
> *activity to make up for the loss. I have some capacity on both sides; the*
> *side where they took out most of the lung has grown to take on more*
> *function. One doctor told me that except for a lot of scar tissue, that lung*
> *looks better than the one on the other side that was never operated on.*
> *I still can't breathe very well.*

Damage to nearby healthy tissue also can contribute to breathing problems. Formation of scar tissue (fibrosis) in airways can narrow them, causing pain and breathing problems. Remaining healthy tissue can twist out of shape (torsion) during the healing process. Air can leak out of the lungs and lodge in nearby chest spaces (pneumothorax), reducing the lungs' ability to expand.

Rapid breathing (tachypnea) can be the body's effort to lower levels of excessive acid, called acidosis. Acidosis is a very early sign of certain conditions, such as serious infection, kidney damage, or diabetic complications, that should be treated immediately.

Difficulty breathing can be one of the earliest signs of an allergic reaction to chemotherapy. Certain chemotherapy drugs (such as cyclophosphamide and doxorubicin), however, can cause difficulty breathing days, weeks, or months after use.

Following radiotherapy, difficulty breathing associated with fibrosis is more likely to be a late effect occurring months or years after treatment. Various treatments, such as prednisone or captopril, have been studied, but none has been proven very effective. A lung cancer survivor recalls:

> I was so sick, I could hardly put one foot in front of each other for nine
> or ten months. When I got through with chemotherapy I felt pretty good.
> I was pushing myself, walking, and had pretty good breath. That radiation
> burn threw me back to where I didn't have air and could barely walk
> across the room. I've been on and off of prednisone.

Following photodynamic bronchoscopic therapy, coughing, cardiac dysfunction, or stroke might occur. In some cases, air is introduced into the circulatory system, which might explain cerebral or cardiac symptoms; in other cases, the light-sensitive drug used might be the cause of coughing.

In many cases, chronic shortness of breath or coughing after lung cancer treatment can be lessened with oxygen therapy or corticosteroid therapy. Oxygen therapy can include either portable tanks of pressurized oxygen (O^2) or an electronic unit that plugs into house current and extracts oxygen from room air. If drying of the throat or mouth results during oxygen therapy, ask for a humidifier bottle to attach to the oxygen line. Larry Coffman describes his lung damage and use of oxygen:

> I had 27 radiation exposures to my right lung, which worked. Although
> I live with some pretty severe effects from that radiation, if I had it to do
> all over again . . . in a heartbeat.
>
> I have developed severe chronic obstructive pulmonary disease (COPD)
> as a result of radiation and am oxygen dependent, as well. I also suffer
> from extreme fatigue and weakness; my heart has enlarged slightly and
> has moved toward the right side (as my right lung has lost mass). My left
> lung was clear from the fibrosis of pneumonia or COPD until about six
> months ago.
>
> You can regulate the moisture content of the air supply using the fluid
> bottle attached to the oxygen line. I am on oxygen 24/7 and I don't have a
> bottle for fluids attached. My nose is dry a little, but not too bad.
>
> My problem is not as much getting oxygen in as it is getting carbon
> dioxide out. Without oxygen, my ratio of carbon dioxide to oxygen is
> pretty much out of whack.

Chest pain

Chest pain can be caused by tumor growth, heartburn, surgery, or angina. Report this symptom to your doctor immediately if chest pain is severe.

See "Breathing problems, coughing, hoarseness" and "Heart and cardiovascular changes."

Chylothorax

See "Breathing problems, coughing, hoarseness" and "Fluid retention."

Cognitive changes

Many patients report that treatment with chemotherapy or cranial irradiation makes them feel fuzzy-minded, moody, forgetful, nervous, or unable to choose the right word. This lung cancer survivor agrees:

> Chemotherapy kind of affects your brain, even though the doctors sometimes won't tell you that. My treatments were three quarters of an hour to get an IV bag for nausea, then about three hours of Taxol and carboplatinum (Praplatin).

These symptoms might go away over time, but for many cancer survivors, cognitive effects have a long course. More serious cognitive changes also might occur.

Vincristine and platinum-containing drugs are capable of causing delirium or dementia. The antinausea drug metoclopramide can cause agitation. Steroid drugs, such as the glucocorticoids prednisone or Decadron, are particularly notorious for causing a wide array of aberrant mental processes, ranging from minor and rapid mood swings to severe mania or depression. These changes usually develop within the first two weeks of steroid use, but this is only a general guideline, because these changes may occur at any time, including during subsequent use following an uneventful first use. Often the actions of these drugs or the cancer itself interfere with normal levels of minerals and metabolites that can in turn affect cognitive function. See "Metabolic imbalances."

Treatment consists of modifying drug dose, controlling symptoms with sedatives or neuroleptic drugs, or just waiting for the effects of the drug to wear off.

Call your doctor if these symptoms are very disturbing or if you or a loved one feel that these side effects represent a danger to the patient or the family.

Dehydration

If you suspect you are dehydrated, call your doctor immediately. Dehydration is a very serious side effect of vomiting or diarrhea. Cancer patients must have adequate fluid to remove from the body toxins, as well as proteins released by dying cells. Moreover, the quantities of electrolytes and minerals, such as phosphorus, calcium, potassium, magnesium, and sodium, might be disrupted in the lung cancer patient, both by disease and by treatment. Dehydration exacerbates this imbalance.

The most reliable symptom of dehydration is thirst. Other signs include the inability to urinate about once an hour, the production of very little urine, or the production of urine that is both dark and low in volume. Other symptoms, such as faintness, dry lips, thick saliva, or loss of appetite, resemble the adverse effects of some chemotherapies too closely to be reliable indicators of dehydration.

Take in as much fluid as possible, but do not drink products containing electrolytes (such as the products marketed to sports enthusiasts) unless your doctor says that your kidneys are in good condition and these drinks will do you no harm.

Diarrhea

Chemotherapy can cause diarrhea, as dying cells are shed from the intestine. Phone your doctor immediately if diarrhea is combined with a fever more than 1.5 degrees higher than your normal temperature, general malaise, severe chills, abdominal pain, night sweats, burning or pain while urinating, headache, neck stiffness, coughing, or trouble breathing.

Your doctor can recommend antidiarrheal drugs, which you will have to balance carefully with such other drugs as stool softeners to control constipation. Experiment with small amounts of different foods until you have a sense for what will maintain a balance between constipation and diarrhea. Kathy tells us:

> He stopped taking MS Contin (morphine), which he had been on since July. We didn't think too much about him stopping the drug, but the day after, his bowels were loose, then it turned to diarrhea for several days. It finally dawned on me that in addition to the morphine he was taking laxatives because the painkiller made him so constipated. Anyway his bowels must have freaked out when he stopped the morphine (and the laxative). The doctor gave him some antispasmodic medicine for the bowels and something else to help the heartburn he was having, and he began to feel better.

Dizziness, fainting, lightheadedness

Although dizziness, lightheadedness, or fainting are known benign side effects of many drugs, these symptoms can be serious adverse effects of chemotherapy. Notify your doctor immediately if you experience these symptoms.

Edema

See "Fluid retention."

Extravasation

See "Vein problems."

Eye changes

Methotrexate, Taxol, or vincristine administration is associated with blurred vision in some patients; vincristine administration can cause drooping eyelids. Lung cancer survivors who use prednisone for a long time to control cough or who have had whole-brain irradiation, might develop cataracts that can be removed surgically. Larry Coffman describes his eyesight changes:

> During my chemotherapy, I constantly complained of a change in my eyesight, only to be told "not to worry." Like others I know, my eyesight returned to "normal" after chemotherapy was completed.

Fatigue and sleep disorders

Those being treated for cancer list fatigue as the most debilitating symptom they experience. Ninety-five percent of those being treated for cancer report fatigue. Kathleen Houlihan tells of a sudden episode of fatigue soon after treatment:

> I felt quite good all week during treatment and walked two or three laps around the building every morning and evening I was there. But the trip home did me in. I was okay when I got to the airport, but the walk to the gate totally wiped me out. And the plane ride added to the slightly sour stomach I had. Thank goodness my dear friend SP met me at the airport for the plane change, and thank goodness we were able to catch one of the

electric carts to take us to the gate in the next terminal, instead of having
to go downstairs, get on the airport train, and then go back upstairs.
I don't think I could have made it.

Symptoms of fatigue should improve after treatment ends; however, many cancer survivors report fatigue years after treatment. For far too long, many cancer survivors weren't believed when they reported fatigue that lasted for years following treatment. The opinion used to be that one should feel tired only while red blood cell counts remained in the abnormally low range. The NCI now recognizes fatigue as one of the three most serious long-term effects of cancer treatment. A survivor concurs:

Coping with fatigue is so hard. The person who came up with some
medication that would get rid of this fatigue would be a millionaire.

A common cause of fatigue during treatment is low red blood cell counts. Transfusion of whole blood or packed red cells is commonly used to correct anemia. Drugs to stimulate production of new red blood cells in bone marrow can help with this anemia-related fatigue. As of this writing, erythropoietin (Procrit) is approved by the FDA for this purpose.

While being treated, you might be able to offset some of the effects of fatigue on well-being and performance by getting as much rest as possible, eating well, and exercising moderately. Nonetheless, you might do best to adjust your demands on yourself to these new circumstances: let the less critical things go, attend only to what matters the most, and seek reliable and sound emotional support. This lung cancer survivor describes his perseverance against fatigue:

I try to get out golfing. I play with a foursome. If I get tired, I'll just stop
walking and ride on the cart. I played about twelve holes today. Keep
pushing along.

Sleep disorders among those being treated for cancer also are common, and in some cases persist years after treatment. Insomnia, "night horrors," and corresponding daytime sleepiness plague many lung cancer survivors.

Often, medicine cannot tell us why fatigue occurs, nor what to do about it, although fatigue seems to increase as the duration or intensity of treatment is increased. Because cancer-related fatigue can have so many causes, it is difficult to treat cancer-related fatigue with other than trial-and-error methods. Some causes of cancer-related fatigue are:

*   Nutritional deficit
*   Low blood counts

- Decreased lung capacity

- Chemotherapy- or radiation-induced damage to the heart, liver, or kidneys

- Depression and anxiety that accompanys cancer

- Tumor activity

- Tumor death (necrosis)

- Changed sleep patterns

- Whole-brain irradiation

- Chronic pain

A web site staffed by oncology nurses for cancer survivors suffering from post-treatment fatigue can be found at *http://www.cancerfatigue.org*. A discussion group for those suffering from cancer fatigue also exists on the Internet. Visit *listserv.acor.org* to enroll in the Cancer-Fatigue discussion group.

Feet

Sore feet can develop after certain chemotherapies. See "Neurotoxicity" and "Pain."

Fever, chills, sweats

Fever should always be reported to your doctor, especially if other signs of illness accompany fever. Fever can be the first symptom of life-threatening infection when white blood cells have been destroyed by therapy. Unattended fever in the absence of sufficient white blood cell numbers can be fatal and is a medical emergency requiring immediate attention.

Fibrosis

See "Breathing problems, coughing, hoarseness" and "Pain."

Fingers

See "Nail changes" and "Numbness, tingling, dizziness, deafness."

Fistulae

After surgery, chemotherapy, or radiation therapy—or simply as a result of disease—an abnormal tubelike connection called a fistula can form between internal organs. If you notice unusual phlegm, discharges, or odors, notify your doctor at once.

Fluid retention

Fluid retention can occur during or just after treatment, or even years after treatment. An excessive collection of fluid in various parts of the body can be caused by surgery, radiotherapy, certain chemotherapy drugs, or by tumor activity. Fluid retention in the chest may signal a recurrence of disease in the form of malignant pleural effusion. Fluid retention elsewhere, especially in the legs, might signal lymphedema or heart, liver, or kidney failure.

If you have a swollen abdomen, swollen legs, pouches or bubbles under the skin, or difficulty breathing, notify your doctor at once.

Hair loss and growth

Radiotherapy and many chemotherapeutic agents cause hair loss—alopecia—although there is a wide range of individual responses to treatment in this regard. Some people lose just a little hair. Others lose all hair, including body hair, eyebrows, and eyelashes. Others report losing gray hair earlier than hair that contains pigment. Those receiving radiation therapy might lose hair only on the spots irradiated, such as arm pit hair. Kathleen Houlihan ruminates on how she'll handle hair loss:

> They say I will probably lose my hair. That seems minor in the grand scheme of things, but several women have approached me and told me to try to prepare for it—that it ain't easy. So I've been trying on wigs and looking at hats and trying to be prepared. I guess it could happen any time starting about three weeks after the first chemotherapy treatment. Sometimes it comes back a different color. Maybe I'll be a redhead next time around!

Later Kathleen tells how it came about:

> I've had a bad hair week. It started coming out on Monday (especially when I washed it), which was right on schedule—two weeks to the day after I started the week of chemotherapy. By Wednesday, I could pull out

a good handful any time I ran my hand over my hair. I didn't wash it yesterday, but when I did this morning, it came out faster than I could shake it out of my hands. It's a strange feeling. Anyway, I figured I'd just wear a hat when I went out today, but the little hair that's left looked so pathetic even under a hat that I opted for a wig instead. And then, all of a sudden, it's not a bad hair day anymore!

This wig is another freebie I got at the American Cancer Society. It's short but not too short, wavy, and brown/auburn. I like it better than the freebie I got at the treatment center, but not as much as either of the ones I have picked out in salons. It's hard to choose between them, not being able to see them at the same time. Maybe I'll get both.

New hair should regrow in the weeks or months after treatment. In some instances, it might not regrow, although this is more common after radiotherapy than after chemotherapy. Kathleen's hair loss was less than she expected:

My hair loss has slowed way down, and I still have a little bit of hair left. I don't know if it will stay, or if it will come out after the next round of chemotherapy, but right now I have a very thin hairdo. You can see my scalp through it all the way around, but at least I'm not totally bald yet. And I don't scare my animals or myself when I look in the mirror. My friend DB cut my hair fairly short, and now it looks okay under a hat— bangs in front and a little fringe all around. When I go out, I wear either a hat or the wig. I've been getting a lot of compliments on the wig. It's nice having color in "my" hair again.

I continue to lose a little more hair every time I shampoo, but I still have enough to look decent under a hat or scarf, and I have found that they are much more comfortable than a wig. I'll be delighted if I can keep this thin hair covering throughout the whole course of chemotherapy and not have to use wigs much at all.

Methods to spare the scalp from exposure to chemotherapeutic agents, such as ice-packing or tourniquets, are not recommended because small amounts of cancer might be sequestered in the skin or blood vessels of the scalp. Denying chemotherapy the opportunity to kill all lung cancer cells might result in failed treatment or recurrence.

Headache

Headache can be associated with administration of certain chemotherapy drugs used for lung cancer, such as cyclophosphamide. Although headaches usually are not considered serious, you should notify your doctor, particularly if pain is severe.

Hearing problems

See "Neurotoxicity."

Heart and cardiovascular changes

Heart or cardiovascular damage can occur during or just after treatment, long after treatment, or as a result of tumor growth.

Call your doctor immediately if you experience any symptoms that resemble a heart attack, such as chest tightness or pain, difficulty breathing, unusually slow or rapid heartbeat, irregular or missed beats, or numbness in the left arm or shoulder.

Surgery for lung cancer can affect heart function in numerous ways—some obvious, such as decreased lung capacity or removal of blood vessels affected by disease, but some more subtle, such as uneven heartbeat or a breach (herniation) of the sac that contains the heart.

Doxorubicin and cyclophosphamide can be cardiotoxic. Their effects are more severe when these drugs are used together, but are more likely to cause late rather than immediate cardiovascular damage. Paclitaxel can temporarily lower blood pressure and slow the heart. Gemcitabine can increase heartbeat and raise blood pressure. Notify your doctor or the nursing staff if you have headache, feel dizzy, or if your heartbeat seems faster or slower than normal. Radiotherapy can induce acute pericarditis, with symptoms of racing heat, fever, and pain. Radiation can affect cardiac function with scarring and thickening of vessels months or years after treatment.

An echocardiogram, a stress electrocardiogram, or MUGA testing can detect heart damage. In some cases, medication or surgery can help alleviate heart disease.

Hemorrhage

Internal bleeding after surgery is abnormal and can be fatal. If you vomit blood, if you notice blood in your sputum, or if you have a collection of fluid in the chest, difficulty breathing, or any symptoms of blood loss (such as weakness or coldness), notify your doctor at once.

Hypercalcemia

See "Metabolic imbalances."

Infection

Infection can follow bronchoscopy, surgery, chemotherapy, or radiotherapy. Chemotherapy in particular can lower the number of infection-fighting white blood cells (normal counts can be found in Appendix C, *Test Results*.) Late complications, such as pneumonia, can sometimes follow lung surgery, especially in those over age 65. In any age group, formation of internal abscesses might occur well after surgery.

If you have a fever of more than 1.5 degrees higher than your normal temperature; pain, redness, or pus at the surgical site; general malaise; severe chills; night sweats; burning or pain while urinating; headache; neck stiffness; coughing; or trouble breathing, phone your doctor without delay.

Some patients' bodies are unable to elevate temperature when they are very ill or recovering from treatment. If you suspect you are infected, call your doctor immediately, even if you have no fever.

Kathleen describes what she expects after chemo:

> *We got home from my monthly treatment last night, and I'm doing quite well. I haven't felt sick at all—just a little off, a little spacey. So I'm just taking it easy and waiting to see what the rest of the month will bring. Apparently the effects last much of the month, and just when they ease up, it's time to go back for more. The main concern for now is to monitor my white cell counts and hope they don't go too low. They suggest staying out of crowds and trying to avoid germs—for the next six months! I'll be hopelessly behind on the movies.*

Infection can result when leukopenia, a lowering of white blood cell counts, occurs after treatment. The danger period for most patients is five to ten days after treatment. In general, chemotherapy is more likely to cause decreased white blood cell counts than is radiotherapy. Larry Coffman describes his approach to handling infection:

> I was hospitalized about nine times, every other month, over an eighteen-month period. I eventually came out of that rut. It was a rough road to travel, but it got better for me. I think my biggest concern was the tolerance that my body was building to the antibiotics, and it still is my biggest concern.
>
> I have been busy with school and battling pneumonia again. So far I have been able to remain out of the hospital. Of course that wouldn't have been the case had my primary physician known about an off-and-on 104.5 temp over two days. It almost seems that I'm back to that every-other-month schedule for pneumonia. Hope not!

While your blood counts are low, preventive measures include hand-washing; avoiding scratches and cuts with gentle skin care, such as using an electric razor and patting skin dry, rather than rubbing; thorough cooking of food; reducing human contact; avoiding crowds or wearing a mask when in a crowd; avoiding gardening; and avoiding handling kitty litter and other pet wastes. Avoid lung contaminants, such as tobacco and wood smoke. Studies with mice and rats have shown that even the minimal amount of smoke present in a family room with a wood fireplace in use can change the seriousness of a respiratory infection to a fatal infection. Some studies have shown immune system impairment by nicotine.

If an infection develops, your doctor will examine you. You might be admitted to the hospital, placed in an isolation room, and given a combination of immunoglobulin therapy, antibiotics, antiviral agents, or antifungal agents.

Insomnia

See "Fatigue and sleep disorders."

Jaundice

See "Kidney damage," "Liver or gallbladder dysfunction," and "Metabolic imbalances."

Joint pain and swelling

Disease or certain chemotherapies, such as Taxol, can cause pain and swelling in the shoulders, spine, or leg joints. Notify your doctor of these adverse effects.

If pain is disease-related, it will probably improve as treatment shrinks the tumor. If pain and swelling are drug-related, they might be treated with ibuprofen, steroids, opioids, antidepressants (which can act as painkillers), or anticonvulsives. Kathleen describes her joint pain, caused by tumor activity:

> I have now survived my second week of treatment. Some of the time I can barely walk because my joints have been swelling up, but most of the time I've been feeling reasonably okay. I still have my hair, although I have acquired a wig (free, from the American Cancer Society) and a scarf, just in case.

After a few more chemotherapy sessions, Kathleen says:

> Right now I feel good and strong. My joints are **much** better—just a minor nuisance now. My energy level is good. Some evenings I'm done in, but most of the time I feel like my energy is at 100 percent. I haven't succeeded in regaining the weight I lost at first during treatment, but that should be okay. I'm at a good, lean weight for me, but it's nice to have a little extra during these treatments. Basically, I feel just like my old self.

Kidney damage

Notify your doctor immediately if you have symptoms of kidney failure, such as unusually high or low levels of urination, difficulty urinating, swollen limbs, yellowing skin, decreased sweat, or heart or circulatory symptoms. Temporary or permanent damage to the kidneys might occur from tumor activity or with administration of certain drugs, such as carboplatin or methotrexate.

Leukopenia

Leukopenia is a drop in white blood cells counts that can reduce the body's ability to fight infection. Kathleen Houlihan describes the path of her blood counts:

> My white blood cell count has been low, which is an expected side effect of the chemotherapy. Last week it was down to 1,000 (normal is 4,000 and up). We were hoping it would come up by this week, but it didn't. It went

> down to 900, so my doctor has started me on injections of Neupogen, every other day for three doses, then recheck. It's supposed to stimulate the bone marrow to produce more white blood cells. In the meantime, I'm taking an antibiotic to stave off any bacterial infection and hoping no viruses come my way. I've got to get the count up to some (unknown to me) minimum level, or I won't be able to start my next round of chemotherapy. A lot of other cancer patients I know have been put on Neupogen, and it worked just fine for them, so I expect it will for me, too.
>
> I still feel good, just a little tired sometimes in the afternoon, but I feel pretty much normal and have pretty much a normal schedule—walking dogs mornings and evenings, doing things around the house, driving into town for shopping, errands, etc. I asked my health care case manager if I should stay home and avoid crowds while my white count is low, and she said no. She said they used to recommend that, but now they tell people to continue their normal routine. She says you feel better and get well sooner—just avoid sick people and small children. So I'm planning to see a movie with my friend DB this weekend.

Later, she describes her good reaction to Neupogen shots:

> The Neupogen worked, and my white blood cell count is off the chart. Normal range is 4,000 to 11,000. Mine went from 900 last week to 12,000 this week, after three Neupogen shots. So I'm off the antibiotic and there will be no problem starting the chemotherapy next week. Guess the Neupogen was worth the $347 it cost, after the insurance paid it down from $1,500! But that's for ten doses, so if I need it again in coming months, I have seven doses left. I still feel good—even better, actually, since I heard that my white count is up. I'm ready to go back to the treatment center and get it knocked down again!

See also "Infection."

Liver or gallbladder dysfunction

Mild liver or gallbladder problems sometimes develop when you are fed only by IV line (TPN, total parenteral nutrition). These problems usually go away when you resume eating normally. Certain drugs used against lung cancer, however, such as carboplatin, can damage the liver. Liver problems also can be a sign of a return or worsening of disease.

You should notify your doctor immediately if you notice any combination of symptoms of liver dysfunction: nausea, jaundice, swollen abdomen, pain in the upper abdomen, or mental confusion.

Lung damage

Cyclophosphamide, doxorubicin, bleomycin, mitomycin, methotrexate, vinblastine, vindesine, or radiotherapy can cause pulmonary fibrosis or pneumonitis. When radiation therapy is combined with chemotherapy, damage can be more pronounced. Certain complications of surgery, such as twisting or narrowing of tissue that remains, can reduce breathing capacity. Notify your doctor if you have any symptoms of lung impairment, such as chest pain or difficulty breathing.

See also "Breathing problems, coughing, hoarseness," "Radiation pneumonitis," "Radiation fibrosis," and "Pain."

Malaise

Many cancer patients, regardless of the kinds of drugs or radiation therapy they receive, report a general malaise—they say they just feel sick. Although this is fairly common, it should not be ignored. You should report any and all symptoms you have during treatment to your treatment team, being as specific as possible about what feels wrong. Kathleen describes feeling "off":

> Overall, I had a pretty easy time again with the chemotherapy. I started feeling a little off/spacey the last two days of it, and I had a touch of nausea in the car on the two-day drive home. Since I've been home, I still felt "off" for a few days—kind of a cross between feeling like I'm about to come down with a cold and feeling like I have a hangover—but I've been taking it pretty easy the last couple of days and feeling fine. I guess I just don't have as much stamina. But I'm certainly not complaining. I feel great compared to some of the stories I've heard about people getting chemotherapy. I think the delivery technique my doctors use and the vitamins make a big difference.

Memory loss

See "Cognitive changes."

Metabolic imbalances

The drugs used to treat lung cancer, sometimes in combination with the action of the tumor itself, may disrupt natural levels of electrolytes, minerals, insulin, or antidiuretic hormone. Hypercalcemia, an excess of calcium in the body, is associated with certain hormone-producing lung tumors. Disorders such as diabetes or syndrome of inappropriate antidiuretic hormone (SIADH) also may develop, or symptoms of delirium or adrenal disease may emerge.

Tumor lysis syndrome, arising from the death of large tumors, might arise shortly after chemotherapy is started. Symptoms of kidney failure caused by excessive amounts of calcium, phosphate, and potassium being released by dying tumors are noteworthy and can be offset with oral or IV hydration, alkalinization of the urine prior to chemotherapy, careful monitoring of electrolytes, use of diuretics, and low initial doses of chemotherapeutic agents.

If you or your loved ones notice any unusual symptoms, especially excessive thirst, unusually high or low levels of urination, swollen limbs, yellowing skin, decreased sweat, abdominal pain, bone pain, seizures, heart or circulatory symptoms, severe mood changes, dementia, delirium, cognitive changes, or psychotic behavior, call the doctor.

Mouth, throat, rectal changes (stomatitis, mucositis)

Chemotherapy, radiotherapy, or oxygen therapy for lung cancer may cause dry mouth and sore throat. Contact your doctor so he can determine whether this side effect is serious in your case, especially if sore throat is accompanied by symptoms of allergic reaction or by fever. Ask your doctor for pain medication if you're having difficulty eating or swallowing. Severe mouth or throat pain can be treated with IV feeding and pain medication until healing occurs. Some oncologists prescribe a rinse called Magic Mouthwash that contains a painkiller, an antibiotic, and an antifungal. Larry Coffman tells of his swallowing problems:

> I had a problem eating after the radiation treatments. I'm not a doctor, but it sounded as though the esophagus had been irritated pretty badly. My oncologist didn't call it acid reflux, but they gave me a mixture of Maalox and 2 percent lidocaine to numb the esophagus enough that I could eat. The bad effects lasted about four to six weeks.

I still have some minor effects lingering, acid reflux and the like, but overall, my esophagus is back to its usual abnormal self! Which means that I'm back to eating again.

Because normal saliva contains an antibiotic, dry mouth can lead to serious dental problems that result in whole-body (systemic) infection and tooth loss. Gentle but scrupulous dental care is a must. Avoid spicy, sour, or acidic foods. Examine your mouth daily for fuzzy white patches that might be a fungal infection. Ask your doctor for drugs to increase saliva flow or for instructions for a homemade mouth rinse that can be used several times a day.

If dry mouth and throat accompany oxygen therapy, ask for a humidifier bottle to attach to the oxygen line.

If you experience rectal pain that feels like hemorrhoids or painful or bloody bowel movements, don't suffer in silence. Painkillers and suppositories will help immensely.

If pain management doesn't work, intravenous feeding for about a week might be suggested. IV feeding for this purpose might be started in a doctor's office and managed at home

Muscle cramps and spasms

Some lung cancer survivors report muscle cramping, especially in the legs and particularly at night, during and after chemotherapy. Often the chemotherapy regimen in use contains vincristine or doxorubicin. Others report muscle spasms in the neck or elsewhere, following use of the antinausea drug metoclopramide.

Various remedies, such as quinine, calcium, potassium, or magnesium, exist. Because calcium, potassium, or magnesium can damage the kidneys, none should be used until you have discussed this issue with your doctor. Some patients report that heat treatment or alternating heat and cold treatment temporarily reduces pain. Others report that vibrators, massage, or acupuncture help.

Nail changes

Many lung cancer survivors report differences in the quality of fingernail and toenail growth during and after treatment. This problem is temporary and will resolve on its own after treatment ends.

In some cases, tumor activity or other diseases can affect tissue growth in fingertips, a finding known as clubbing. See Figure 1-4, "Clubbing of digits," in Chapter 1, *Symptoms of Lung Cancer* for an illustration of this phenomenon. If you suspect you have nail clubbing, notify your oncologist.

Nausea and vomiting

Nausea and vomiting are the result of some, but not all, of the drugs used for lung cancer treatment. Sometimes just the aroma of food can bring on nausea. If so, you might try eating foods that have been chilled.

Phone your doctor immediately if nausea and vomiting are combined with any of the symptoms described in the section "Infection," or if you notice blood or a coffee-ground appearance in vomitus.

It's important that nausea and vomiting be controlled, not just to reduce suffering, but also to allow your body to absorb nutrients to heal, to keep you well hydrated (and thus able to flush chemotherapy drugs from the body), to support your kidney function, and to allow for uninterrupted sleep (during which the immune system is rebuilt). You should not suffer nobly through nausea and vomiting as a mark of strength: you might harm yourself if you do.

Fortunately, excellent drugs are available today to control nausea and vomiting. Zofran (ondansetron) and Kytril (granisetron) are two such antiemetics, and anti-anxiety drugs, such as Xanax, a drug similar to Valium, might work for brief episodes of nausea. Some steroids (such as Decadron) also work, for reasons that are unclear. Older, less effective drugs, such as Compazine, are also still in use, sometimes in combination with newer drugs.

Take your antinausea medications on time, even if you feel well. They work by priming your body *before* nausea sets in. Moreover, if you wait to take them until you feel bad, you might lose them as you vomit. Keep your doctor informed about the success of these drugs because they can be recombined and substituted with others until a good solution is found.

If you are unable to keep food down in spite of nausea medication, feeding by IV line for a period of time will give your stomach a chance to recover.

Anticipatory nausea also is normal for many cancer patients. If you had treatment in the past that made you ill, during subsequent visits, your central nervous system might react with nausea to visual cues or odors in the doctor's office before treatment is begun. You're not crazy: many people report this reaction, even years after treatment. Chapter 15, *Stress and Stress Reduction*, describes this subconscious and unbidden learning process more fully.

Neurotoxicity

Adverse effects related to the central nervous system are sometimes seen during and after chemotherapy or radiotherapy for lung cancer. In some cases, the damage is very long term or permanent.

The platinum-based drugs cisplatin and carboplatin can cause muscle or tendon weakness, ringing in the ears, hearing loss, or seizures. Cisplatin can cause damage to hearing in one or both ears in about 30 percent of patients, sometimes after just one dose. For some patients, the damage to hearing is irreversible. Notify your doctor if you experience any of these adverse effects.

Neuropathies, including numbness, tingling, or pain in hands and feet, are sometimes seen after platinum-based or vincristine therapy or following therapy combining vincristine with etoposide. These neuropathies are usually, but not always, temporary. No treatment exists yet for these adverse effects, although a clinic that specializes in pain management might be able to offer relief. Larry Coffman experienced peripheral neuropathy after chemotherapy:

> I was given four courses of Navelbine. It had the effect of numbing my
> extremities and causing severe irritation to my veins.

Neuropathies of the chest or spine might follow radiation therapy for lung cancer, including pain or loss of sensation.

Seizures may follow use of such drugs as methotrexate, cisplatin, or ifosfamide. Only about three percent of patients receiving these agents experience seizures, and it is more likely to occur in patients who have had cranial irradiation, but it is also possible that seizures will occur in a patient whose metabolic balance has been affected by lung cancer or its treatment. Seizures can be controlled with antiseizure medication and are usually transient,if related to medication.

Some lung cancer patients who receive cisplatin or vincristine report odd head, neck, or leg symptoms when they tilt their head or twist their neck. This is called Lhermitte sign; some report it as dizziness, some as an electric shock, and others as an odd sensation that spans the gap between noise and movement. This symptom should abate in several months, but in some cases is a sign of permanent neurologic damage.

Treatment with the aminoglycoside antibiotics gentamycin, tobramycin, amikacin, or with vancomycin for infections that arise during cancer treatment can result in temporary or permanent hearing loss, vertigo, dizziness, or ringing in the ears. These disorders can be treated with surgery, drugs, rehabilitation exercises, or noise-blocking devices.

See also "Metabolic imbalances."

Neutropenia

See "Infection."

Nonhealing wounds

Some treatment regimens call for chemotherapy, radiotherapy, or both before surgery to reduce the size of the tumor, thus enhancing the chance of a more successful surgical removal. Both chemotherapy and radiotherapy can cause delays in wound healing by compromising the ability of healthy tissues to multiply and form scar tissue. Speak with your doctor as soon as possible if you suspect your healing is not progressing as it should.

Numbness, tingling, dizziness, deafness

See "Neurotoxicity."

Odors

See "Fistulae," "Infection," "Appetite or taste changes," or "Mouth, throat, rectal changes (stomatitis, mucositis)."

Pain

Pain is a common short- or long-term effect of lung cancer and its treatment. Pain in various parts of the body can result from damage attributable to surgery, the healing following surgery, chemotherapy, radiotherapy, or from the pressure of tumors on nerve pathways. Pain can affect the healing process, your overall health, your sense of well-being, and your ability to sleep. Moreover, chronic pain, even low-level pain, has an effect on mood and performance that you might not notice if pain gets gradually worse or if you've been dealing with it for a long time.

Pain during or after cancer therapy should always be reported immediately to your doctor. Do not use any pain medications without checking first with your doctor, because certain pain medications, even such over-the-counter drugs as Tylenol and ibuprofen, can interact dangerously with certain chemotherapy drugs.

Jaw, hand, foot, back, joint, stomach, or testicular pain can be associated with vincristine therapy. Other drug therapies can cause bone pain. Call your doctor immediately if you experience any of these symptoms.

Postsurgical pain might persist for months or years following treatment. Although advanced surgical techniques are used to reduce pain, chiefly by avoiding nerve groups, the surgeon's primary concern is the curing of cancer by removing all diseased tissue. At times, healthy tissue must be sacrificed to achieve this goal. As a result, lung cancer survivors might experience a variety of persistent painful phenomena, such as rib pain that spreads to other parts of the chest, pain from nerves that were accidentally severed, or a tightening of the airways at the point of suture.

Severe back pain might be associated with spread of disease or with degenerative changes to the spine following radiation therapy targeted near the spine. Surgery to fuse spinal discs might alleviate this pain.

Painful lung fibrosis, or fibrosis in nearby chest tissue, is a reaction of the immune system after exposure to radiation or cyclophosphamide. Fibrosis usually emerges months or years after treatment as a late effect, rather than a side effect. Fibrotic tissue changes can be permanent, however, unless anti-inflammatory drugs are administered along with radiotherapy.

Pain might occur during therapy that involves radiation implants. Ask for pain medication immediately if the implants or the position you must hold causes pain. Report any unusual symptoms, such as burning or sweating.

The injected colony stimulating factor G-CSF (Neupogen, Filgrastim), oral doses of prednisone, or paclitaxel can cause aching bones and joints. Ice packs might relieve this pain; if not, ask your doctor if the dose can be lowered. Bone pain associated with G-CSF is temporary.

For pain during urination, see "Bladder damage." See "Neurotoxicity" for pain in hands or feet. For pain associated with sexual activity, see Chapter 14, *Sexuality and Fertility*. For stress reduction to lessen pain, see Chapter 15.

If you have persistent pain of any magnitude, don't try to ignore it. There are ways to address pain so it does not become worse or cause permanent damage. You might consider consulting a pain specialist or pain clinic for a multimodal approach to pain control that may include excellent long-acting pain medications; surgery; behavior modification; pain control devices, such as implantable nonaddictive morphine pumps or electrical stimulators; ultrasound treatments; or relaxation training. All of the following groups offer support or referrals for pain management:

- American Academy of Pain Medicine (708) 966-9510
- American Society of Clinical Hypnosis (847) 297-3317
- American Pain Society (847) 966-5595
- American Society of Anesthesiologists (847) 825-5586
- National Chronic Pain Outreach Association (301) 652-4948
- Agency for Health Care Policy and Research (800) 358-9295

A discussion group for those suffering from cancer pain exists on the Internet. Visit *listserv.acor.org* to enroll in the Cancer-Pain discussion group.

Pancytopenia

Pancytopenia is a lowering of all blood counts. It's treated with growth factors, such as Neupogen, Procrit, or Neumega, or with transfusions of red cells, platelets, or irradiated whole blood. See "Infection" for additional information.

Peripheral neuropathy

See "Fingers," "Feet," and "Neurotoxicity."

Pneumonitis

Intravenous administration of cyclophosphamide, mitomycin, vinblastine, or vindesine can cause pneumonitis, appearing as painful or difficult breathing. Report these symptoms to your doctor immediately.

When the lungs are irradiated, pneumonitis may develop within the first year following treatment. Usually, the area damaged coincides with tissue that was irradiated, but on occasion, other lung tissue is affected as well. The symptoms of pneumonitis resemble pneumonia, and it must be distinguished from pneumonia. Pneumonitis is treated with steroids.

Postsurgical confusion

Anything from mild confusion to overt psychotic behavior occurs in some people following general anesthesia, especially in those over age 50. Although time is the best cure, a change in pain medication or room location might also help.

Post-treatment constitutional syndrome

Some patients who have had lung surgery experience a collection of symptoms—pain at the surgical site, malaise, appetite and weight loss, and decreased lung capacity—known as post-treatment constitutional syndrome. The symptoms might persist for weeks or months after treatment. Rest, exercise, and good nutrition may help overcome them.

Psychological damage

Post-traumatic stress disorder, depression, and anxiety are recognized as frequent short- and long-term sequels to cancer's stress and can be addressed by a professional experienced in handling the psychological issues of cancer survivorship. See Chapter 16, *Getting Support*. A lung cancer survivor notes that anxiety impacts breathing:

> *In the pulmonary therapy group I'm part of we have a doctor who has lung cancer. His depression and nerves have been a real problem. He's found an anti-depressant pill that helps him. If you get anxious, you don't breathe as well or as deeply.*

Pulmonary thrombosis

See "Blood clots."

Pus and discharge

See "Fistulae" and "Infection."

Radiation fibrosis

Radiation fibrosis is the formation of fibrous scar tissue within the lung, caused by the immune system's reaction to radiation. It develops months or years after radiation therapy and might or might not be preceded by pneumonitis. This fibrous tissue is knotty and stiff and interferes with an organ's ability to do its job. Fibrosis in the chest structures or lungs can interfere with breathing. Larry Coffman, five-year survivor of SCLC, deals today with scarring from radiation therapy:

> *I happen to be one of those people who scars a lot, and when I received radiation therapy, my lung was damaged extensively. The resulting scar tissue has pretty much prevented its use, so I am on oxygen at the present time. Not because I can't get enough air, but because of the carbon dioxide buildup in the blood stream, as the blood still flows to the damaged lung and the gases are not exchanged as they normally would. I still suffer tiredness and weakness to an extent. I thank the Lord for my survival and enjoy each and every day. I'd rather be a little scarred than—well, we know what the alternative would be!*

There is some recent evidence that administering steroid drugs or certain experimental agents, such as interferon, simultaneously with radiotherapy can reduce the immune reaction that causes fibrosis. Administering steroids after radiation therapy must be done promptly upon noticing the onset of fibrosis because delay causes steroid therapy to be ineffective.

Recent research with hyperbaric oxygen has shown some promise in reducing the negative effect of radiotherapy on certain tissues, such as blood vessels in the brain.

Radiation pneumonitis

See "Pneumonitis" and "Lung damage."

Recall sensitivities

Radiation therapy and certain chemotherapies can damage tissue in a way that leaves it reactive to further treatment for months or years afterward. Radiation to an area can cause tissue in that area to react with pain and dysfunction when chemotherapy is administered afterward, even if the chemotherapy is injected elsewhere.

If you have experienced extravasation (see "Vein problems") during IV chemotherapy, the damaged tissue might remain sensitive to the drug used for years after.

If you believe you're experiencing recall sensitivity, contact your oncologist.

Scar tissue

Scar tissue can form in chest structures following surgery or radiation therapy, causing pain or constriction of organs. There is no treatment yet for this condition.

Second cancers

One of the most serious late risks associated with lung cancer is the risk of developing a second cancer; that is, a tumor whose development is distinct from a recurrence or metastasis of the first tumor.

The chief risk of second cancer that lung cancer survivors face is development of a second lung tumor. It is thought that the same environmental or genetic aberrations that triggered the first tumor, especially tobacco smoking, remain to cause a second primary cancer. If you still smoke, you should quit.

Some lung cancer survivors are more likely to develop second primary tumors in other organs than are the general population. The most common sites of second tumors are the breast, esophagus, head, or neck.

Radiation therapy is linked to the development of second solid tumors. Second tumors that arise following radiotherapy almost always arise in or very near sites of previous irradiation, called radiation ports. The incidence of radiation-induced tumors begins to rise about fifteen years after treatment.

Lung cancer survivors who were treated with high-dose chemotherapy that contains such drugs as etoposide might be at increased risk of developing treatment-related leukemias. Too few lung cancer patients have been treated with high-dose chemotherapy to quantify the risk, although this finding is well documented among lymphoma and breast cancer patients treated with high doses of etoposide.

For all lung cancer survivors, regular surveillance with some combination of chest x-rays, CT scans, MRI, blood tests, or mammography is mandatory.

Seizures

See "Neurotoxicity" and "Metabolic imbalances."

Sexual problems

A variety of problems with fertility, sexual performance, and sexual enjoyment can arise during or after surgery or chemotherapy for lung cancer. These problems are discussed in Chapter 14.

A discussion group for those dealing with issues of sexuality following cancer treatment exists on the Internet. Visit *listserv.acor.org* to enroll in the Cancer-Sexuality discussion group.

For an excellent and compassionate discussion of sexual issues after cancer treatment, see *Sexuality and Fertility After Cancer* by Dr. Leslie Schover (John Wiley & Sons, 1997).

Shingles

All who had chicken pox as a child harbor within their nerve cells a herpesvirus called varicella zoster, the virus that causes chicken pox and shingles, two manifestations of the same illness. When the immune system becomes suppressed or dysfunctional, varicella zoster may re-emerge from nerve endings, causing quite terrible pain and blisters called herpes zoster, or shingles. The virus can affect any or all nerve endings within the entire body, but it is most likely to appear along the side of the face, neck, arm, or side of the body. Although ten to twenty percent of those with shingles may never produce blisters, they will still experience itching, pain, or both. The blisters tend to appear in a line, following the path of nerves. Shingles that affect the eye can cause temporary or permanent blindness.

There are many human herpesviruses; varicella zoster is just one. It should not be confused with the genital herpesvirus that is transmitted sexually.

As soon as symptoms appear, call your doctor. An antiviral medication, such as acyclovir, and perhaps pain medication, as well, should be started promptly. It is not unusual to require codeine or even morphine briefly for severe shingles episodes. Shingles normally heal within four to six weeks, but some patients experience lingering pain for years afterward. If this happens, a procedure called a nerve block or glycerine block can be performed by a neurosurgeon. It should alleviate pain for several months and can be repeated if needed.

Skin problems

A variety of skin problems—pain, burning, discoloration, thickening, sweat gland changes, scaling, wrinkling, dryness, rash, hives, redness, peeling, sun sensitivity, or ulceration—are associated with radiation therapy, photodynamic therapy, or certain chemotherapies used for lung cancer.

> *Radiation burn really slowed me down, on the spot just above my breastbone. I was told it wasn't uncommon, because they want to make that area doggone hot. There is burning and scar tissue. The scar doesn't let oxygen into my bloodstream.*

The change in skin color that might accompany treatment is often a tanned effect, but this is not a true suntan that will protect you from the sun's rays. In fact, your skin might be overly sensitive to sunlight and prone to wrinkling, freckling, or premature aging, and should be protected accordingly.

Call your doctor about skin reactions. Dermatologic problems can be complex and hard to diagnose, and certain skin symptoms might be a sign of tumor spread to other organs. Common remedies, such as lotions that contain alcohol, might make the problem worse, especially if itching is your chief complaint or if radiotherapy is still underway.

Steroid-related effects

Prednisone and Decadron, the most commonly prescribed glucocorticoids for controlling cough or inflammation associated with tumor activity or radiotherapy, can be responsible for many adverse effects if given in high doses, especially after long-term use. Adverse effects associated with high doses or long-term use can include a suppressed immune response, appetite increases, rapid mood changes, insomnia, stomach pain, gastric ulcers, pancreatitis, diabetes, depression, weight gain (especially in the trunk and face), changes in blood chemistry, menstrual irregularities, impotence, facial redness, thinning of skin, stretch marks, acne, bruising, changes in bodily hair, cataracts, glaucoma, protrusion of the eyeballs, weakening of muscles, osteoporosis, avascular necrosis of bone, high blood pressure, seizures, and, rarely, psychosis.

Fortunately, there is an excellent book available about Prednisone and its side effects. *Coping With Prednisone* (Griffin, 1998), written by patient Eugenia Zukerman and her sister, Julie Ingelfinger, who is a medical doctor, can answer just about all questions you might have about using this drug.

Thirst

Cyclophosphamide, prednisone, or certain hormone-producing lung tumors can induce diabetes in certain people. Notify your doctor immediately if you experience prolonged, unexplained thirst.

See "Dehydration" and "Metabolic imbalances."

Tumor lysis syndrome

The waste products of a tumor as it dies might disrupt natural levels of body substances, such as electrolytes or antidiuretic hormones. Tumor lysis syndrome, arising from the death of large tumors, might arise shortly after chemotherapy is started. Symptoms of kidney failure caused by excessive amounts of calcium, phosphate, and potassium released by dying tumors are possible and can be offset with oral or IV hydration, careful monitoring of electrolytes, and use of diuretics.

If you or your loved ones notice any unusual symptoms, especially excessive thirst, unusually high or low levels of urination, swollen limbs, yellowing skin, decreased sweat, abdominal pain, or heart or circulatory symptoms, call the doctor.

See "Kidney damage" and "Metabolic imbalances."

Ulceration

Following radiation therapy, healthy skin that was in the path of the radiation beam might ulcerate. The condition might become chronic.

See "Nonhealing wounds" and "Skin problems" for more information.

Urinary problems

See "Infection," "Bladder damage," and "Kidney damage."

Vein problems

At times, chemotherapy that is administered intravenously can leak out of the vein into surrounding tissue, an adverse event called extravasation. The reaction of the body to a high concentration of chemotherapy in the skin or other tissue can be serious and painful. The vein might be unusable for chemotherapy thereafter; the skin might die, slough off, and fail to regrow. Symptoms of extravasation include pain, redness, swelling, or burning at the IV or catheter site, during or after the administration of chemotherapy. Notify the medical staff immediately if you have these symptoms during or just after treatment.

If administered into the arm veins, certain drugs—such as cisplatin, vincristine (Oncovin), vinorelbine (Navelbine), or doxorubicin (Adriamycin)—may cause pain, stiffness, redness, or swelling of veins; in some cases, even if no leakage has occurred.

If you notice lengths of rigid, painful, swollen, or red veins in the days or weeks following chemo, tell your doctor. Geri Capasso tells of her brother Anthony's reaction to chemo:

> Monday night my brother felt pain in his left arm just above the elbow and it looked a little swollen. Yesterday he went in for his fourth round of Gemzar (he had his fourth round of cisplatin a few days earlier). The doctor thinks it might be an infection, and prescribed Keflex. Last night and this morning he had no temperature. Early this morning the pain got bad, and it is redder and more swollen.

Ice packs or warm (not hot) compresses may relieve the pain associated with veins that have reacted to chemotherapy. To spare your veins from additional damage, your doctor may recommend that you have a venous access device, such as a PICC line or central catheter, inserted.

Water retention

See "Fluid retention," "Kidney damage," and "Heart and cardiovascular changes."

Weight gain

Long-term use of steroids to control coughing or pain might cause weight gain. Usually, this weight is lost when steroid therapy is reduced or ended. Larry Coffman describes his weight gain:

> I was told that in some cases, the weight gain after treatment is a defense mechanism to ensure survival. I know that in my case I started at about 190 seven or eight months before diagnosis, and when I was diagnosed I weighed in at a hefty 235. After treatment, I gained up to a paunchy 252.

Weight loss

Most chemotherapies, as well as radiotherapy for lung cancer, cause rapidly dividing cells to die more frequently than other cells. The cells lining the gastrointestinal tract are rapidly dividing cells, so when they are exposed to anticancer drugs, they die sooner than their natural cycle would dictate. As a result, it might become difficult to absorb nutrients during treatment for lung cancer; the effect is made worse if nausea and diarrhea are present. Larry Coffman tells how he dealt with weight loss:

> *"Just goes to show that just when you think you got it bad, somebody else has it worse." I can't remember the author of that phrase, but it sure does apply to lung cancer and its treatment.*
>
> *I actually began to gain weight (235 pounds) before my diagnosis (imagine that), and that in itself was a small miracle, although I was unaware of this at the time. I was a 5' 10" butterball—okay, folks, no turkey jokes.*
>
> *I dropped over 70 pounds during treatment. I was given some concoction of Maalox and 2 percent Lidocaine to numb my esophagus for up to 30 minutes in order that I could drink my dietary supplement (Sustacal). Well, it worked, for about 30 seconds, then they tried straight 2 percent Lidocaine, one teaspoon before a meal. That lasted long enough for me to put the bottle away. I tried to tell them that I had a very high pain threshold, but alas, they wanted to try it their way   go figure. Therefore, I just quit trying to eat altogether.*
>
> *I believe to this day that the weight gain, albeit not advisable for everyone, is the single most important reason for my survival, not to in any way diminish the importance of the radiation therapy or chemotherapy. It re-enforces my notion that health care professionals can talk statistics all they want, but the body, mind and spirit will know things that we are unaware of . . . well, let me put my matchbox (my very small soapbox) away.*
>
> *You know, come to think of it, I have met very few patients or survivors that would actually fit into one of the health communities' statistical categories anyway. Especially me!*

If you are losing weight during treatment, notify your doctor and see the suggestions included under "Appetite or taste changes," "Diarrhea," and "Nausea and vomiting."

CHAPTER 14

Sexuality and Fertility

Any scientist who has ever been in love knows that he may
understand everything about sex hormones but the actual
experience is something quite different.

—Dame Kathleen Lonsdale

FOR SOME OF US, SEXUALITY AND FERTILITY take a back seat during the cancer experience, but for others, these are very emotional issues—almost as emotionally charged as cancer itself.

In this chapter, we discuss ways to recognize, prevent, correct, or adjust to problems with sexuality and fertility. First, we discuss specific issues of sexuality, including treatment-induced menopause, then harvesting ova and sperm and fertility treatments.

In spite of the increasing incidence of lung cancer among women, pregnancy coinciding with lung cancer remains rare, and we do not discuss it here.

A full discussion of techniques to enhance sexuality and fertility after treatment for lung cancer is beyond the scope of this book; only certain techniques are mentioned in the text that follows. You can find many references in the *Notes* and in Appendix A, *Resources*, so you can verify facts or do further reading.

Sexuality

It's not unusual for lung cancer survivors to report decreased or frustrated sexual desire during and after treatment. Fortunately, issues of sexuality during and after cancer treatment are common and treatable. If you're unhappy with your sexuality, discuss with your oncologist a referral to a gynecologist, urologist, or andrologist who specializes in post-cancer care and consider consulting a sex therapist if you feel it's warranted.

Many good medical solutions are available today for those who suffer neurologic or other physical impairments from cancer treatment. Various therapies are available, for instance, to sustain erection and to relieve vaginal pain. If sexual hormones are out of balance, sexual pleasure and satisfaction may improve with hormone replacement therapy or vaginal estrogen creams. An extraordinary array of medications and devices is available to help those who have sexual side effects from cancer or its therapy.

It's important to bear in mind that most sources of support for sexuality after cancer deal with *all* cancers and that subtle neuropathologic problems may remain after the use of specific neurotoxic therapies for lung cancer, such as vincristine or cisplatin. Consequently, your efforts to find help might have to target multiple resources. For example, your libido may suffer when treatment-related chronic fatigue or chemically induced depression is present.

As a lung cancer survivor, you need to be aware that separating the psychological effects of disease from the physiological effects of treatment may be difficult or impossible. Purely emotional perceptions and misconceptions regarding sexual drive and satisfaction are always a possibility, of course, but they may be compounded by frank physical damage. This means that, should you decide to seek help *only* from a sexuality counselor, it's possible for physical difficulties to be misdiagnosed as psychological problems. Medical history is full of such errors, such as the "Fakers' Disease" of the nineteenth century, which we recognize today as the autoimmune disorder multiple sclerosis. In short, if you're convinced that your problems have a physical basis that outweighs any psychological component, avoid those who attempt to label you as emotionally ill and seek help elsewhere.

Sexuality and cancer treatment

Certain neurotoxic drugs used during chemotherapy can affect the sexual organs temporarily or permanently, thus affecting sexual pleasure. Fibrosis formation after radiotherapy can limit oxygen metabolism, inducing fatigue. Irradiation of the brain can interfere with brain signals to ovaries and testes, affecting fertility and libido. Surgery can reduce lung volume, induce fatigue, or cause scarring and other adverse physical phenomena that in turn affect sexuality.

Difficulty gaining or maintaining an erection, vaginal and vulvar pain during intercourse, loss of sensation in the genitals, loss of the sexual urge (libido), and failure to ovulate are not uncommon among cancer survivors.

Many medical and surgical remedies exist for these problems. Consulting a reproductive endocrinologist, a gynecologist, a gynecologic urologist, or an andrologist for advice would be wise. Ask for details regarding devices or medications to gain or maintain erection, hormone replacement therapy, or lubricating or hormone creams to ease vaginal or vulvar pain during intercourse.

Your oncologic treatment team should first approve any drugs prescribed. This is particularly true for hormone replacement therapy if you have a neuroendocrine tumor, because these tumors might be stimulated by hormone therapy.

Treatment-induced menopause

Female lung cancer survivors who are treated with chemotherapy or cranial irradiation might experience temporary or permanent menopause.

The hallmark event that scientists note in menopause is cessation of ovulation and the end of fertility. To the female experiencing it, though, the corresponding symptoms often are much more disturbing than the inability to conceive:

- Hot flashes
- Vaginal dryness
- Urinary tract infections
- Insomnia
- Facial hair
- Loss of libido
- Continual or irregular menses
- Breast tenderness
- Mood swings
- Hair thinning
- Bone loss
- Increased risk of cardiovascular disease

Symptoms associated with abrupt menopause may be more severe than the symptoms occurring with natural menopause.

In some cases, hormone replacement therapy (estrogen, estrogen and progesterone, or any of these with testosterone) might be appropriate to reduce or eliminate the overall symptoms of treatment-induced menopause. This should be verified with your oncologist.

When hormone replacement therapy is not appropriate, local estrogen-containing creams, estrogen rings, or water-based lubricants that are used in the vagina and on the vulva can provide relief from vaginal dryness and pain during intercourse. Moreover, topical estrogen-containing creams and estrogen rings are to some degree absorbed by the body and may provide some relief from other symptoms.

General points

Although full coverage of sexuality after cancer is not possible in this brief chapter, a few general points are worth mentioning:

- Communicate about sex. Communicate not just during or after attempting sex, at which times emotions are too highly charged, but always. In particular, tell your partner if you're experiencing pain.

- Cuddle, touch, and be affectionate, even if you're temporarily not up to sex as you used to know it. A sexual relationship based on love can be described as one of continual foreplay. Just walking side by side touching can be an act of lovemaking.

- If you're male, bear in mind that male orgasm without erection and without ejaculating is possible. Moreover, many partners consistently report sexual pleasure that does not require penetration by an erect penis. Good options for achieving an erection, such as medication or hydraulic implants, exist if failure to obtain or maintain an erection continues to be a concern.

- Be patient. Expect new sensations and keep an open mind about new experiences. Sex may be very good after cancer, but it might not be exactly the same as it was before cancer.

- Ask your doctor if the partner who is under treatment should protect the other partner from chemotherapeutic drugs that may persist in sperm or vaginal secretions. The amount of chemotherapeutic agents present in body fluids is likely very low, but it may be best to be careful. Wearing a condom or vulvar shield might be recommended. (Radiotherapy poses no similar risk.)

- Lung cancer cannot be "caught" during sex, although some viruses that may cause certain other cancers can. In addition to HIV and one of the herpesviruses, Human T-cell Lymphotropic Virus I (HTLV-I) is transmitted by sexual contact, as is the human papillomavirus thought to be linked to most cases of cervical cancer.

- The endorphins released during sexual pleasure reduce pain elsewhere in the body.

Sources of information about sexuality

Several sources of information, discussed in the following sections, are available to you in dealing with decreased or unsatisfactory sexuality after cancer treatment.

Doctors

Your doctors can be sources of basic information regarding how cancer and treatments are affecting you physically and how those physical changes are impacting your sexuality. Your doctor might not be able to address all your concerns, though. She might lack knowledge in this specialty; she might have less time than you need for discussion; she may incorrectly interpret what's important to you unless you're very clear when communicating. She might feel uncomfortable discussing sexuality, or she may feel it's "just a psychological problem." She should be able to refer you to counselors, however, who can guide you in separating the physical and psychological components.

Counselors

Purely psychological discomforts may be more difficult to address, and success in this area may depend on one's access to good counselors. The best choice is a sexuality therapist who is familiar with both the physical and psychological effects of serious illnesses such as cancer. Large urban centers are more likely to have specialists in sexual counseling than rural areas. Contact the American Association of Sex Educators, Counselors, and Therapists at (319) 895-8407 or visit *http://www.aasect.org*.

Support groups

Support groups, either those focused on cancer or on the sexual problems following other illnesses, are an excellent way to discover tactics, insights, and clinical information regarding sexual problems after cancer.

Support groups for those dealing with issues of sexuality or fertility after cancer therapy exist on the Internet. Visit *listerv.acor.org* to enroll in the Cancer-Sexuality or Cancer-Fertility discussion groups.

Books

An extraordinarily good resource that deals with these issues in a sensitive, fair way is Leslie Schover's 1997 book, *Sexuality and Fertility After Cancer* (John Wiley & Sons). Especially impressive is her sensitivity toward those over age 65, whose sexual needs sometimes are neglected by the medical community. As those over 65 are well aware, people remain sexual beings for their entire lives.

Dr. Schover describes the techniques and technologies available for sustaining erection, reducing vaginal pain, and many other problems that are all too often borne silently. She discusses sexual adaptation for those minus genitals or breasts and those living with an ostomy or scarring. Childhood cancer survivors and their unique adaptations are covered. Her discussion of the possible divergence in sexuality caused by cancer is grounded in a thorough introduction to sexual function in the absence of cancer.

Two books about cancer in general that contain chapters on sexuality are *Everyone's Guide to Cancer Therapy*, edited by Dollinger, Rosenbaum, and Cable (Andrews McMeel, 1998); and The American Cancer Society's 1997 publication, *Informed Decisions*.

Fertility

If you were treated with chemotherapy or brain irradiation for lung cancer and are still in your reproductive years, you may experience temporary or permanent fertility problems, such as failure to ovulate or reduction in sperm counts. Lung surgery and chest irradiation have no direct effects on fertility. Use of pelvic irradiation for lung cancer metastases is rare, but has a well-studied dose-related negative effect on fertility.

Treatments to boost fertility and aid in conception are available, but it's very likely that an attempt to conceive will be discouraged by your doctors until you have been disease-free for a meaningful amount of time.

The medical literature contains little information about lung cancer, fertility, and pregnancy. The effects of treatment for such cancers as Hodgkin's lymphoma and childhood acute lymphoblastic leukemia (ALL), which occur primarily in children and adolescents, offer some insights, though. Often young patients with these cancers are successfully treated, which means that many are now long-term survivors who have experienced subsequent fertility problems. Some of the drugs used to treat these cancers and lung cancer are identical, and dosages of these drugs in some combined chemotherapy regimens are similar. This means that certain comparisons can be made between the findings of the more plentiful fertility studies following those cancers and lung cancer.

Nevertheless, because of the scarcity of information regarding fertility directly related to chemotherapy for lung cancer and the ongoing development of new treatments for lung cancer, you should discuss with your oncologist the potential risk to fertility that your specific chemotherapy treatment might entail.

Harvesting sperm, ova, and stem cells

Often, lung cancer symptoms are acute and treatment is urgent. If treatment isn't urgent, though, and becoming a parent is a future concern, harvesting of sperm or ova might be wise for patients about to receive certain chemotherapies. With newer fertility techniques, even sperm reduced in number or of lesser quality can be used to produce a pregnancy. You should consider harvesting and storing sperm in spite of its quality or quantity.

Ova are harvested by inserting a fine needle through the abdominal or vaginal wall, guided by an imaging tool, such as ultrasound. In some cases, hormones that stimulate egg production are given in advance so that many eggs will mature simultaneously. These abundant eggs are then harvested in one procedure and frozen (cryopreserved). This is usually an outpatient procedure for which you'll be given anesthetic and sedation.

It might be difficult to find a center that freezes ova that are unfertilized because the technology to successfully fertilize ova (also called oocytes) after thawing is fairly new. Most centers prefer to harvest ova, fertilize them, and freeze the resulting embryos. Ask your doctor about this before the procedure if you don't have a partner or sperm donor or ask the center to proceed with freezing anyway, assuming the enhanced fertilization techniques will be readily available when you decide to use the oocytes you've stored.

Sperm can be harvested in several ways. The simplest method is the collection of ejaculate either following masturbation or following sexual intercourse, during which a special collecting condom is worn. Harvesting via masturbation or sexual intercourse usually must be done in a private room in the sperm banking facility, not at home. Because sperm die so quickly, they must be frozen immediately.

Fertility treatments

Infertility that occurs after cancer treatment might be treatable by fertility specialists called reproductive endocrinologists. A full discussion of techniques to enhance fertility is beyond the scope of this book, but several general methods are mentioned here:

- Stimulation of ovulation (ovulation induction)
- Concentration of sperm
- Selection of healthy, motile sperm
- Assisted penetration of the ovum by sperm
- In vitro fertilization/embryo transfer and micromanipulation techniques
- Insemination
- Sperm retrieval techniques
- Egg or sperm donation

Ask your oncologist or the American Board of Medical Specialties for a referral to one or more reproductive endocrinologists in your area. Additional resources are available in Appendix A.

Summary

Issues of sexuality during and after cancer treatment are common and treatable. Take advantage of the resources available by finding a gynecologist, gynecologic urologist, or andrologist who specializes in post-cancer care, and consider consulting a sex therapist, if needed.

Temporary or permanent infertility might arise if you were treated for lung cancer with chemotherapy or cranial irradiation and are still in your reproductive years. Effective treatments to boost fertility and aid in conception are available. If treatment need not start immediately, you might consider harvesting of sperm or ova before treatment begins because the effects of some treatments on fertility are not completely understood.

Drugs prescribed to relieve sexual problems should be approved first by your oncologic treatment team. This is particularly true for hormone replacement therapy if you have a neuroendocrine tumor because these tumors might be stimulated by hormone therapy.

CHAPTER 15

Stress and Stress Reduction

A good laugh and a long sleep are the best cures
in the doctor's book.

—Irish proverb

SOME PEOPLE BELIEVE that their cancer was caused by stress, that it will be made worse by stress, or that perhaps they have a cancer-prone personality. Many research studies have attempted to discover links between cancer, stress, depression, personality, and coping skills. The connections are complex:

* First, there is no consistent evidence that stress causes or worsens cancer. Studies done using animals and humans do not consistently show a positive association between stress and cancer, not even when underlying disease already exists. In fact, in some animals, some forms of stress cause tumors to shrink. More details are provided under "Stress and cancer?" later in this chapter.

* Second, the few studies that hint at a link between personality and cancer are not conclusive for various reasons, such as the design of the study. Details are discussed in the section later in this chapter titled "A cancer personality?"

This chapter describes the known associations—or the lack of them—between stress, the immune system, illness, and cancer. It offers a definition of stress, then discusses physical and emotional responses to stress, as well as the tenuous evidence regarding stress as a cause of cancer. The chapter concludes with ways you can minimize stress or make stress a useful experience.

What is stress?

Experts in various fields of medicine and psychology recognize many different circumstances and events as stressful. Depending on the circumstances or point of view, we can view stress as a threatening object likely to cause stress, the actual reaction of stress to the threatening object, the physical reaction within our bodies to the threat, or the state of mind that precedes our taking some action in response to threat:

- For the psychiatrist studying brain chemistry, our awakening in the morning and the corresponding rise or fall in levels of several hormones may be viewed as a stressful event for the constantly adapting brain.
- For the psychologist, overcrowding of humans in urban areas can be viewed as a stressful event.
- For an orthopedic surgeon, the impact sustained by cartilage within the knee when one runs on concrete is viewed as stress.

The psychoneuroimmunologist, however, views the interaction of the immune system with the central nervous system as an adaptation to stress. This interpretation, which can accommodate both physical and emotional stress, will be the chief focus of this chapter.

For the sake of readability, we won't differentiate between responses and reactions, nor between anxiety and worry. We will assume that the stress of a cancer diagnosis causes distress, although some authorities maintain that not all stressors cause distress.

Responses to stress

Our bodies and minds respond to stress in many ways. These adaptations may change with the type and intensity of the stressor, the amount of time the person has been exposed to it, his previous experiences trying to adapt to similar stressful events, the person experiencing stress, and his physical and emotional state at the time.

Although many emotional responses to stress, such as anger and withdrawal, are possible, the responses most often reported by cancer survivors are fear, anxiety, and depression. The National Cancer Institute reports that, both during and after diagnosis and treatment, almost half of cancer patients report anxiety and about a quarter report significant anxiety; 20 percent experience transient or long-term depression; and 15 percent are diagnosed with post-traumatic stress disorder. Estimates by other researchers are sometimes much higher.

Fear is sometimes useful

Several bodily changes occur as a reaction to a fearful event. During fear, hormones that prepare us to adapt to stress are released in a chain reaction, first from the brain, which in turn triggers the release of antistress hormones from the adrenal glands. Our heart rate increases, blood is redirected to body parts associated with fight or flight, and extra sugar is made available in the bloodstream via the liver.

Fear can be a useful, goal-oriented reaction to a stressor. Each of these physical changes is aimed either at our fleeing from danger or conquering it bodily.

Fascinating research into brain structure and function has shown that the amygdala, part of the "old brain" conserved in most creatures from reptiles up through the primates, including humans, is the brain organ responsible for finding safety quickly when fear arises. Direct connections between the amygdala and our sensory organs bypass the higher brain centers of decision making, allowing us to react very quickly to threats, sometimes without our being aware that we have perceived them. For instance, if you hike in the woods, have you ever stopped abruptly after sensing just a muted change of color or pattern and, upon closer inspection, realized that the subtle difference is a snake? This brain connection is probably responsible for the immediate, calm, highly effective, goal-oriented behavior that some people exhibit in unbelievably horrifying situations.

Although fear doesn't feel good, it can be a useful, goal-oriented reaction to a stressor. It galvanizes us and prepares us for action. The extreme and immediate physical reaction to fear, however, does little or nothing to prepare us to deal intellectually with a fearful situation that requires extensive analysis, planning, and decision making, such as absorbing the technical medical information about our cancer diagnosis. On the contrary, research has shown that both very low and very high levels of the antistress hormones from the adrenal gland interfere with learning new tasks. Short of our ability to jump up and flee the doctor's office or our sudden acquisition of strength to throttle the bearer of bad news, we have been poorly prepared by evolution for dealing with cancer as a stressful event. As a result, an out-of-phase mismatch of events is what many of us experience when being told of the cancer diagnosis—with a strong likelihood that we will remember forever and with great acuity the perceptual cues that were present, instead of the key points that the doctor attempted to relay.

Anxiety is unhealthy

Most adults have experienced the difference between fear and anxiety. Fear is an acute, strong, visceral response to stress. Anxiety is a nagging, chronic, or generalized fear response. Although some would choose the chronic physical distress of anxiety over the pronounced physical distress of fear, anxiety might be the more physically harmful of the two experiences.

Unresolved fear may convert to anxiety as we begin to grow accustomed to a threat. When we're anxious, the same physical changes that accompany fear occur at lower levels, with deleterious effects on our body. Sustained increased heart output and constriction of blood vessels to rechannel blood to certain organs can contribute to the development of high blood pressure and cardiovascular disease. Altered sugar metabolism can worsen diabetes. The tendency for digestive activity to increase in times of stress can exacerbate underlying gastric ulcers.

Worry and anxiety involve recycling the same fear, repeatedly examining the outcomes and evaluating interventions. We sometimes use this activity to justify worry, assuming that repeated scrutiny will result in knowing what to do if worse comes to worst, but this continual rehearsal of negative events in search of solutions may not benefit us should danger actually arise. The two thought processes, worry and planning, center in different parts of the brain. On magnetic resonance imaging, those who worry show activity in the emotional part of the brain, whereas those who plan show activity in the opposite hemisphere, the so-called logical half of the brain. This may mean that, from the standpoint of providing a good solution in the face of danger, worry is not the best strategy. Worry does not determine the best solution and move on to the next problem. It prevents us from detecting and dealing with new problems in a timely and effective way.

Physical symptoms of anxiety may include any of the following: shortness of breath, sigh breathing, dry mouth, inability to swallow, trembling, weakness, incessant crying, circular or obsessive thoughts, inability to concentrate, paralytic or manic movements, insomnia, headache, recurrent nightmares, or extreme fatigue.

Pseudoanxiety

What feels like anxiety is not always caused by worry. Sometimes anxious feelings can have physical causes. In some cases, symptoms that are indistinguishable from anxiety can be caused by the tumor itself or by its treatment:

- Lung cancer tumors in or near the lung can cause shortness of breath.
- Tumors in certain parts of the kidney or in the adrenal gland can stimulate the adrenal gland to overproduce cortisol, a hormone released during fearful episodes.

- Tumors of the brain near or in the pituitary can stimulate hormones that in turn stimulate the adrenal glands to overproduce cortisol.

- Surgery for lung cancer can reduce lung volume, causing shortness of breath that both masquerades as and can induce anxiety.

These medications also can cause anxiety:

- Corticosteriods, such as prednisone

- The newer antidepressant drugs used to control nausea and pain, such as Prozac

- Cessation of the use of the quick-acting antianxiety drugs, such as Valium or Ativan

Certain physical changes that accompany incipient medical conditions are heralded by feelings of anxiety:

- Pneumonia

- Heart attack

- Electrolyte imbalance

- Angina

But the chief cause of anxiety among cancer survivors is worry and sustained, unresolved fear: fear of pain, abandonment, dependency, financial ruin, professional ruin, recurrence of disease, or fear of death.

Conditioned responses

When we worry for a long time about one problem, new electrical circuitry is laid in our brains. Sometimes conditions resembling or related to our problem will trigger anxiety symptoms or symptoms of physical distress. Many cancer survivors report anticipatory nausea just smelling the rubbing alcohol used to clean the skin over a vein before chemotherapy is administered. Studies have shown that this response can cause their blood counts to drop—even if they are not given chemotherapy in that session.

Obviously, this reaction, called a conditioned response, can have a direct impact on the immune system, as has been demonstrated many times in animals. For example, one study demonstrated that when rats were fed a combination of immune suppressant and saccharine dissolved in water, their white blood cell counts dropped afterward, as expected. When the experiment was repeated using only saccharine in water, white blood cell counts still dropped. This outcome demonstrates that the association of event and outcome does not require knowing, for example, what chemotherapy is intended to do. Physiological cause and effect can occur absent the cognitive processes as we know them today.

This does not imply, of course, that you can skip chemotherapy because just thinking about it may have some of the same effects. There's no evidence that a conditioned drop in blood counts coincides with an attack by the immune system on tumor cells.

Depression

Research has shown that those who are depressed often have suboptimal immune system function.

Most cases of depression that coincide with cancer are called situational depressive episodes, directly related to the stress of adjusting to cancer. These depressive episodes differ from organic disturbances, such as manic depression or unipolar depression, unless the person has had episodes of these diseases in the past, well before the cancer diagnosis.

Depression may be diagnosed if one or more of the following symptoms persist for more than two weeks:

- Despair
- Excessive sleepiness
- Insomnia
- Appetite disturbance
- Irritabilty
- Inability to function
- Loss of interest in sex and other pleasurable activities
- Thoughts of suicide

Learned helplessness

Cancer-related problems that seem to have no solution can cause depression. When one experiences repeatedly that efforts to solve problems don't work or are punished, often one ceases trying. This is called learned helplessness, which can lead to despair and is linked to depression. Subsequently, when new problems arise that could indeed be solved or when new methods of dealing with old problems emerge, those exhibiting learned helplessness fail to act. A therapist trained to deal with depression can help you overcome despair.

Chemically induced depression

In addition to the psychological factors surrounding cancer that can cause depression, some chemotherapies that are neurotoxic or toxic to the thyroid, such as Taxol, prednisone, or interleukin-2, can cause chemically induced depression. Please note, though, that these possible side effects do not necessarily occur in every person who uses these drugs.

The effects of stress on the immune system

The stress hormones released by the adrenals during episodes of fear and anxiety also affect white blood cells, the infection-fighting army within one's blood. Initially, the surge of brain and adrenal hormones that accompanies stress causes an increase in circulating white blood cells. When cortisol remains high, however, white blood cell numbers are reduced. As stress, anxiety, or depression continues unabated over weeks or months, output of the adrenal hormone cortisol is consistently high and white blood cell numbers remain reduced.

Larry Coffman describes his approach to reducing stress:

> *I have turned the whole mess over to the Lord and changed my way of life. I used to stress at everything, smoke, drink, and eat the worst diet. I quit smoking and drinking, and am continually battling the diet thing. I now only worry about the things that I can change. I no longer stress over things that are out my control: those I turn over to the Lord. Many times I will visualize the internal battle with the cancer and I always see the immune system winning. Many time I would lose myself in the visualization, sort of like day dreaming, then after a while wake up.*
>
> *Belief is a strong weapon and the mind can cause enormous changes in the body. If you think about it, why not will yourself well. It is an accepted notion that you can will yourself sick.*

Stress and cancer?

If prolonged stress and resulting anxiety affect the number of white blood cells in one's body, does this mean that stress can cause cancer or make it worse? The answer, based on animal and human research, is unclear.

Animal studies support what many recognize intuitively: if stress had an unequivocal link to the development of cancer, just about everyone would develop cancer. If stressful life events within the last three years were responsible for the emergence of cancer, then everyone who survived imprisonment in Auschwitz and other Nazi annihilation camps ought to have been diagnosed with cancer soon after being freed by the Allies. Continuing with the same analogy, all people who are diagnosed with cancer should either develop a second cancer triggered by the stress of the first diagnosis or should never be able to recover from the first cancer. Likewise, all loved ones of those diagnosed with cancer should then develop a cancer from dealing with the stress of their loved ones' suffering.

In fact, animal studies show a very wide range of tumor responses to stress, depending on:

- The type of stressor used
- The ability of the animal to modify or escape the stressor
- The species being tested
- Gender
- The animal's previous experience with this stressor
- Whether the tumor was chemically induced or transplanted
- Whether the tumor is primary or a metastasis

In some cases, stress causes animal tumors to shrink.

Human studies performed so far have been less direct than animal studies in measuring stress and tumor response because few humans would tolerate having tumors chemically induced, transplanted, or deliberately subjected to stress for science's sake while terribly ill. The best study design would follow cancer-free people for years, recording stressful events and subsequent cancer diagnoses.

Most human studies performed so far have relied on retrospective self-reports of stress levels prior to the cancer diagnosis. This method of collecting information is often criticized as of dubious reliability. For instance, a person who has just been diagnosed with cancer and who has agreed to fill out a questionnaire on life factors might report that other recent stressful life events were not very stressful. Compared to this newest problem, cancer, indeed these events may in retrospect not seem stressful. Yet at the time the previous stressful events occurred, they may have been perceived and reacted to as very stressful events.

In short, although stress has been undeniably linked, over and over, to increased rates of some illnesses (such as upper respiratory infection and certain autoimmune diseases), there is no clear causative link between stress and cancer. Several excellent texts on the topic of stress, the immune system, and cancer are listed in Appendix A, *Resources*.

A cancer personality?

If stress causes both emotional and physical changes, but does not consistently have a part in the development of cancer, what other factors might be responsible? Can the ways a person adapts to stress affect his or her health? Do habitual ways of adapting hint at a "cancer personality"? The evidence, based on animal and human research, is conflicting.

Obviously, animal studies on this topic are difficult to perform because we can't know with certainty what animals are feeling, so most studies are done on humans. Often the design of these studies has been criticized.

For instance, melancholia, or what we would call depression today, received attention in the past as a personality trait possibly linked to cancer; but we know today that depression is less a personality trait or coping mechanism than an imbalance in brain chemistry that has many different causes, including genetics, situational adjustment, influenza, heart attack, and stroke.

Breast cancer is relatively well studied with respect to personality type. One study of breast cancer survivors assessed personality and coping styles, using a questionnaire and an interview the day before breast biopsy. They concluded that women who were stoical and "psychologically morbid," rather than expressive and emotional, were more likely to have malignant findings in biopsied tissue. Here are some reasons why the design of studies of this kind, and this study in particular, are criticized:

- Those of us who have had biopsies know that this experience is often stressful and are likely to derail our responses, if we are able at all to take such an interview seriously in this very emotionally charged setting.

- Suppose those found to have a malignancy already had a good idea of what their diagnosis might be? Suppose this idea had time to develop for a week or two while they waited for the surgery? Would the women questioned be likely to display more evolved, thought-out, stoical coping styles, perhaps not consistent with their usual more spontaneous reactions? In fact, some of the women in this study indeed had been informed by their radiologists that the lesions appearing on mammography most likely were malignant.

- How can we know that the answers on a questionnaire, even when the anxiety surrounding a biopsy is not an issue, reflect how someone really behaves?

- Suppose coping styles early in life predispose us to breast cancer, but our coping styles at maturity are what is measured by these questionnaires?

- What kind of person volunteers to fill out a questionnaire? (Questionnaire studies always face this criticism.) Would emotional women be more likely to decline and stoical women more likely to comply? Or, if a small honorarium is offered, say about $30.00, as is common for many psychological studies, will less affluent women be overrepresented because, for an affluent women, the invasion of privacy and the time lost isn't worth $30.00? If so, do less affluent women have other life conditions that would predispose them to breast cancer, such as living in an air- or water-polluted neighborhood?

- Suppose the behavior described as stoical is an artifact of some other circumstance, such as working long, exhausting hours under artificial light for several years? Other plausible theories of breast cancer development suggest that the increasing rate of breast cancer is linked to increasing lifetime estrogen exposure. Studies have demonstrated that estrogen exposure begins earlier now, for the age of first menstruation has steadily decreased in industrialized countries since the use of electric light became widespread in the twentieth century.

- And, finally, if this study had been designed in an era when being stoical was admired and being expressive was considered psychologically morbid, would the researchers have attempted to prove that expressive women were more likely to develop breast cancer? A woman whose family members have had a range of cancers points out that their personalities did not determine outcomes:

> In my family, we have had five cancers: one male denier who has survived nine years, a female outspoken fighter who has died, an emotional, expressive man who has died, an introverted female who has died, and an outspoken, complaining female who has survived more than twenty years. In each case, type of cancer—lymphomas, prostate, breast and colon cancers—and stage of disease at diagnosis were far more meaningful to survival than personality type.

No doubt everyone can think of similar cases within his own experience, in spite of the findings of studies published on this topic. Indeed, some studies have found no association between personality, coping style, and breast cancer.[1,2]

As you can see, the supposed link between personality and the development of cancer is a tenuous one.

Why stress should be reduced

If fear is not very useful in dealing with cancer, and anxiety and depression pose risks for long-term health problems, what reactions and responses deal effectively with cancer-related stress? And if stress is not linked conclusively to the inception or growth of tumors and may in fact shrink tumors in some cases, why attempt to reduce the stress that is associated with the cancer experience?

First, most people prefer feeling good to feeling bad. Stress reduction techniques can help you feel better.

Second, increased levels of stress clearly are tied to the worsening of certain illnesses, such as upper respiratory infections. If you've decided on a course of chemotherapy or radiation therapy, your immune system may be compromised for a few days or a week during each cycle. It's best to avoid infections and to minimize those that may arise during these troughs. Stress reduction techniques may help you keep secondary health problems at a minimum while undergoing anticancer therapy.

Third, high levels of stress for long periods of time can contribute to the development of high blood pressure, gastric ulcers, migraine headaches, certain autoimmune diseases, and other stress-related illnesses.

Larry Coffman elaborates on his beliefs:

> My lung cancer was in the upper right lobe and my nodes were involved, yet I'm still here writing about it as many, many more are, as a result of advances in drugs and advances in the support that people receive due to education and technology. I am a true believer that medicine alone cannot defeat cancer. It takes the strong will of the human spirit, as well.

Stress-reduction techniques

A chapter of this length cannot do justice to the history of theories of stress and stress reduction and the ways of life that arose to accomplish this. Nonetheless, stress reduction, albeit under different names, has always been of interest to humans and has received close scrutiny in the twentieth century after the chemical link between stress and hormones was delineated. Thus, various ways to reduce stress have been discovered—or rediscovered.

Kathleen Houlihan describes her plans for reducing stress and bringing her entire body into the healing process:

> I'm scheduled to have my next round of chemotherapy a week later than usual to give my white cells a little longer to recover. Meanwhile, we're back into our routine here, and I'm trying to add some meditation, visualization, and journaling to all the normal day-to-day stuff.

The following sections list, in alphabetic order, techniques that many have found useful for reducing stress. Not all of these will work for any one person; in fact, it's possible that none of these will work for you during particularly stressful times, such as periodic checkups, or if you have a symptom that might indicate recurrent lung cancer. We hope, though, that the following ideas will help you discover your own ways to unwind.

Acupuncture

Acupuncture is a versatile way to reduce stress and pain and is particularly good at relieving certain kinds of pain.

The ancient Chinese mapped the flow of energy in our bodies through pathways called meridians. These pathways are thought by Western medicine to be neuroelectric, although there continues to be discussion about the exact nature of these meridians. Eastern medicine believes that the misdirected flow of energy through these meridians accounts for most of the imbalances that occur within our bodies and that these imbalances cause illness and can be detected in twelve pulses.

The central nervous system produces hormones for which receptors exist on the surfaces of white blood cells. Recent gains in knowledge regarding this interaction of the central nervous system and the immune system may explain more fully some of acupuncture's mode of action.

An experienced acupuncturist will spend at least an hour taking a comprehensive medical and emotional history; will use few needles, perhaps no more than six; may prefer Japanese to Chinese needles because they're thinner; and will be skilled at using the needles in a way that is not perceptibly painful, or barely so.

The needles come in packets for single use only. You'll be able to see your practitioner opening these packets, which is reassuring if you have well-justified doubts about the reuse of needles. All body surfaces on which needles are used are cleaned first with rubbing alcohol.

Certain acupuncture treatments call for the burning of an herb called Moxa that may irritate your lungs. Tell your acupuncturist if you prefer to avoid this phenomenon.

Shoes should come off last and go on first. The easiest and most regrettable way to find a tiny, thin, lost acupuncture needle on the floor is with your bare foot.

It's becoming increasingly common for health insurance companies to pay for part or most of an acupuncture treatment, although they generally pay less for psychological diagnoses (such as stress) than they do for medical diagnoses (such as migraine or endometriosis).

In some states, an acupuncture practice must be supervised by a medical doctor. Verify the licensing and credentials of your practitioner with your state health department. Organizations and resources that license practitioners or give people information about acupuncture and oriental medicine are listed in Appendix A.

Biofeedback

Biofeedback is a way to relearn how to relax, usually monitored by a psychiatrist or psychologist.

During initial biofeedback sessions, sticky sensors are attached to various muscle groups on the part of your body that seems tense or is in pain, and a graph of muscle tension is displayed on a screen that is similar to a home computer screen. Relaxation tapes or the guiding voice of a therapist are used to establish a calm atmosphere.

When you have relaxed these muscle groups, you can tell you've succeeded because the indicators on the screen have changed.

After a few sessions with the sensors and the screen, you no longer need them for echoing success, and you switch to doing relaxation exercises on your own. It is important to rehearse this stage of independence over and over with a therapist so that soon you can do the exercises independently in any setting.

As with acupuncture, it's becoming increasingly common for health insurance companies to pay for part or most of biofeedback treatment, although they generally pay less for psychological diagnoses (such as stress headache) than they do for medical diagnoses (such as migraine).

Counseling

Counseling sessions with a mediator or therapist who is experienced in cancer survivorship issues have proven very helpful to many people. Three randomized studies, including Dr. Spiegel's work with breast cancer survivors, have shown increased survival among melanoma and breast cancer survivors who received counseling.

Group counseling or support with other cancer survivors is a wonderful way to reduce stress. The group generates camaraderie, reduces feelings of isolation, offers practical as well as sympathetic support, and can become the source of many new friendships. See Chapter 16, *Getting Support*, for more information.

A counselor might be a psychiatrist, a psychologist with a PhD or a master's degree, or a licensed social worker. Some insurance companies pay a larger percentage of the cost for sessions with a psychiatrist or psychologist, but social workers often charge less to begin with.

Exercise

Modest regular exercise is a wonderful, well-documented way to reduce stress as well as improve overall health. Exercise also generates endorphins, the body's natural opiates, which reduce pain and ease depression.

Kathleen Houlihan wisely realizes that exercise will help her:

> *My husband Holt decided he wanted to go hiking in Utah last week. I was still feeling a little off, but I decided to go with him and just hang out and read or meditate while he went hiking. But he ended up choosing a trail we had been on before with our friends JS and LS, so we knew it was mostly level, along a mesa top. And there was a cloud cover and occasional light rain, so it was cool. So I hiked, too—1 hour out, rested and ate lunch for an hour while Holt did the scrambling at the end to check out the Anasazi ruin, and one hour back. I was a little tired, but quickly recovered after we got back to the car. That's about when I started feeling really good again.*

Be careful, though, not to be too strenuous, for very strenuous exercise, such as training for a marathon, can lower white blood cell counts for about 24 to 48 hours. Do only what feels good, stopping before the point of exhaustion. Check first with your oncologist before starting a new exercise regimen, especially if you have had radiation therapy in the chest area. This treatment, if given in high doses, entails a risk of cardiac damage.

Family

Of all social support factors that appear to contribute to the positive outcome of an illness, including cancer, the support of family or very close friends appears to be highest. This effect has been shown most clearly in studies of white males recovering from heart conditions, though. The beneficial effect is less clear when other illnesses, females, and members of nonwhite ethnic groups are studied.

Most people are both blessed and cursed with family. Cancer survivors report family members who range from saintly, indispensable soul mates to those seemingly hatched by Fate as an example of how not to behave. Nonetheless, at times there's something uniquely comforting about being surrounded by those who resemble you and share your body language and your mother tongue, regardless of their inclination, or lack of inclination, to offer support. If nothing else, the less helpful ones can unintentionally provide wry entertainment.

Occasionally, people have family members who need more support than the cancer survivor does or who are tooth-grindingly insensitive to what they're going through. And once in a while, stories surface about family members who actually blame the cancer survivor or family "rivals," such as a daughter-in-law, for the cancer.

Don't berate yourself if you find you frequently need a vacation from family members who put themselves first at all costs. Often, these unhealthy imbalances in family dynamics were present all along, but remained subtle and bearable until the cancer experience highlighted them.

Friends

Few other stress reducers are as good as having sympathetic, listening friends.

Kathleen Houlihan is very happy with the support she's received from friends and sees her cancer experience as a catalyst:

> *The brightest silver lining so far in this cancer cloud is that I am back*
> *in close touch with so many dear friends and relatives, many of whom I*

had been pretty much on a Christmas-card-only basis with for quite a while. One of these people is my dear friend MD. My husband Holt and I met M and her husband R at a party shortly after we moved to a new city. We became good friends after we learned that they were actually at the Game of the Century (Texas-Arkansas) in 1969 in Arkansas. Holt and I had watched it in Austin, and met the victorious Longhorns at the airport that night when they returned. Oh, that Cotton Spire! Anyway, M recently emailed me a great "visualization." She said, "Like a tug of war rope we are pulling hard against this cancer thing on the other end. I know you and Holt are at the front of the line and you have a huge string of people pulling real hard, so please visualize how strong you and we all are." I really like that image.

When friends offer to help, don't be too noble to say yes. Keep in mind that often they don't know quite what to say when they learn of your cancer, especially at first, so they may prefer to act instead.

If they're good listeners, let them know if you do, or do not, feel like talking about cancer today—and that tomorrow might be different. Undoubtedly there will be days when reducing stress means talking about cancer, and other days when one more word about cancer will make you want to run for cover. Try to sense or ask if they feel like listening, too.

Far too many cancer survivors report that friends, even very good friends, disappear when cancer appears. These friends are speechless, sad, frightened, self-righteous, or guilty that they're healthy—never mind that perhaps we're much more sad and frightened than they might be.

Each of us has to decide on a way to handle this abandonment that meshes with our system of ethics. Many cancer survivors say that they just don't need additional sources of sadness, stress, or blame in their lives, and they move on to find new friends, often in cancer support groups. Other cancer survivors try to keep their old friends by never talking about cancer. Bear in mind, though, that for those who are very fearful about cancer, just being around someone with cancer might be frightening.

If you have healthy friends who have remained a presence in spite of cancer—lawn-mowing, grocery-buying, baby-sitting friends; friends who have listened to you when you're scared; or friends who have just spent time with you if talking about cancer is not your style—you're very lucky. Show them that you're glad they're around.

Take solace, too, in the goodwill of those you may never meet. The daffodils that appear in hospitals during the American Cancer Society's Daffodil Days in March, for instance, are from someone who wants you to feel better.

Gaining knowledge

Not surprisingly, a book such as this supports the belief that gaining knowledge about your cancer, and thus gaining some control over your cancer experience, is an excellent coping mechanism. Learning about your illness and your options has been proven to reduce anxiety and stress and may be the crucial factor in your illness and its outcome. Not only can obtaining a correct diagnosis and learning about new, more effective treatments result in sound choices, but animal studies have shown that those who perceive that they have a means to escape stressful situations maintain higher white blood cell counts than those who perceive otherwise. Bear in mind as well that although our doctors often must master information about a broad variety of cancers or are immersed deeply in their own research projects, we have the opportunity to go narrow and deep, learning a great deal about our own illness.

If your doctor seems unreceptive about things you've learned, seek a second opinion or consider changing doctors. An excellent book on this topic, *Working With Your Doctor*, by Nancy Keene (O'Reilly, 1998), is available.

Worthy of mention is the observation that some doctors react badly to the idea that their patients find information on the Internet, because the information available on the Net ranges from abysmal to superb. If you use the Internet to research your illness (see Chapter 22, *Researching Your Illness*), avoid using the word Internet when discussing your findings with your oncologist. Instead, use terminology that credits the sources on which your findings are based: Medline, the PDQ database of the NCI, Cancerlit, certain reputable medical journals, and so on.

Hobbies, volunteer work

As a form of healthy denial and, in some cases, a form of exercise, hobbies are an excellent stress reducer. Immersed in an activity you enjoy, you're likely to forget cancer, breathe and laugh more easily, and feel capable.

Hobbies are especially important for reducing the stress that may be linked to the lowered self-esteem of those who are temporarily or permanently unable to return to work.

Laughter

In his book, *Anatomy of an Illness as Perceived by the Patient* (W.W. Norton, 1979), the late Norman Cousins says we should take humor seriously. Cousins was diagnosed in 1964 with ankylosing spondylitis, a degenerative disease of the connective tissue that causes disability and pain. He undertook to improve or cure his condition by focusing on positive, happy thinking, and he believed he succeeded.

Funny friends, books, and movies are good ways to forget about cancer for a while and can invoke some of the healthy bodily changes that come about when we laugh and relax. Two studies have found that mirthful laughter reduces blood levels of the hormones associated with stress.

Massage therapy

The backrubs and neckrubs given to you by loved ones will release endorphins that reduce pain and depression.

The lymphatic strokes practiced by massage therapists, on the other hand, are location-specific and might utilize a lot of pressure. Always check with your doctor before having deep massage therapy, because massage is thought by some researchers to hasten the spread of certain cancers through lymphatic vessels.

Your doctor may determine that professional therapeutic massage of certain parts of the body, those that appear unaffected by lung cancer, is acceptable.

Massage therapy is licensed by some states and recognized by a national organization, the American Massage Therapy Association (AMTA). In some states, massage therapy can be performed only under the supervision of a doctor, nurse, physical therapist, or chiropractor. Your local phone book will list the nearest chapter of the AMTA for verifying your practitioner's credentials. You can contact the national office by phone at (847) 864-0213, or at their web site *http://www.amtamassage.org*.

Meditation

Meditation is a way to interrupt negative, cyclic thinking by focusing on one soothing word or peaceful scene. Those who practice meditation regularly eventually are able to lower their blood pressure and levels of stress hormones. These reductions persist beyond the end of the meditation session and sometimes well beyond.

Lowering of blood pressure is beneficial for those who have cardiac or vascular damage.

Kathleen describes her meditation and visualization:

> *At this point, I hereby declare that our team has won the Tug of War against the cancer. In my visualization, my friends have pulled me so far away from the cancer that it has receded to a small speck in the distance. I think we can quit tugging. I thank all of them, from the bottom of my heart, for the major role they have played in the saving of my life. I thank them and pray for each of them every day. We do need to maintain some level of vigilance, though, to be sure and keep it at bay. Maybe some will remain on duty to see that the rope doesn't slip. Or maybe someone can suggest a new visualization I can use to keep me cancer-free.*

Minivacations, healthy denial, and escapism

Denial is a healthy coping mechanism as long as is doesn't cause us to neglect the care we need for cancer. Some healthy ways to take a minivacation from cancer are:

- Drive to work along a prettier route.

- Schedule day trips away from daily stress.

- Buy your favorite author's latest hardcover book instead of waiting for the paperback or library version.

- Grant yourself permission not to worry for one hour, one day, or one week.

- Take a nap on your lunch hour.

- Buy a pair of wild golf pants or lipstick that "isn't your color."

- Spend all day Saturday in your bathrobe reading old *New Yorker* cartoons.

- Write a limerick and mail it anonymously to a friend.

- Odd though it may sound, you might enjoy celebrating the parts of your body that still work.

Kathleen Houlihan tells of her techniques for putting cancer aside:

> *During my checkup at the Cancer Treatment Centers of America, I went to the nutrition class, taught that week by Dr. Quillan. I always find his talks inspiring and uplifting. He usually ends by telling us to get happy and surround ourselves with beauty, music, poetry, etc., and reminds us "it's not what you're eating, it's what's eating you that matters." Then lunch with my friends LW and AW, and we were off by about 2:00. A full schedule. We stopped at Red Rock Canyon State Park,*

just west of Oklahoma City, to look around, and spent the night in Elk City, OK, as we did last time. It's a nice little town with good Mexican food and reasonable motel rates. Friday we visited the American Quarter Horse Museum in Amarillo and checked out Conchas Lake State Park in New Mexico on the way home. We're trying to stop and smell more roses along the way.

Music, song, and dance

Dr. Albert Schweitzer once said that he couldn't imagine life without music or cats. Schweitzer was an extremely productive, altruistic, humorous man who lived and worked in a difficult setting well into old age. He was a strong believer in the doctor within each of us and thought of himself as only the facilitator of our own healing processes.

Music can lower stress and enhance emotions. You can experiment with music to see which type suits your needs at different times. Some people find the relaxing or soul-thrilling effects of classical music best; others find that loud pop or rock music numbs pain and that its relatively simple, repetitive rhythms and singable melodies interrupt incessant worries. Still others enjoy rediscovering the ethnic music they may have abandoned in the past. Listening to a type of music we've never heard before, such as the Australian didgeree-doo or Tibetan chord-singing, might distract us from the worries of cancer.

Singing can release cares from your soul, might realign anxious breathing, or might improve lung capacity. Singing out loud in the car when you're alone, like scream-ing, can lower tension levels.

Classes in dance for people of all ages and both genders are available in many community centers. If you feel that you need greater control in your life, ballet's dis-cipline, controlled breathing, and classic beauty may make you feel better. If, on the other hand, you feel there's too much control in your life, jazz or aerobics may allow you to set free some inhibitions. Flamenco might help you rediscover the sexuality that may have gone to sleep when you heard the word cancer. Yoga, t'ai chi, and Feldenkreis movement, all of which span the disciplines of exercise and dance, are fine ways to stretch and relax.

Nutrition

In general, the diet that is recommended for those without cancer—a diet high in vegetables, fruits, and whole grains—remains the best diet for those with cancer. Please note, though, that those who are losing weight, suffering from loss of appetite, or recently recovering from surgery should consult their oncologists before substituting vegetables for meat.

A few nutritional factors seem to have some effect on mood:

- A diet high in animal protein has been linked to anxiety and panic attacks. Other studies have found that certain flavonoids, compounds found in plant but not animal tissue, are similar to Valium in their relaxing action. This might mean that it's not reducing meat intake, but increasing vegetable intake that lowers anxious episodes in some people. If you're suffering from severe anxiety symptoms related to your cancer diagnosis, you might try modifying your diet to contain more vegetables and grains—but check first with your oncologist.

- Drinking milk at bedtime or eating turkey for dinner is known to help with relaxation. These foods are high in tryptophan, an amino acid that aids sleep. Tryptophan is used by the body to make serotonin, a neurotransmitter that affects mood and is the target of many of the newer antidepressants.

- Low blood levels of zinc have been correlated to treatment-resistant depression and to an increase in the undesirable immune system inflammatory response sometimes seen in depressive patients.

- Cachexia, the weight loss experienced by some cancer patients, has been linked to depression, which is thought to be triggered by nutritional deficits or by the tumor's commandeering of dietary substances otherwise needed for the manufacture of brain neurotransmitters.

Always verify a change in diet first with your oncologist.

Pets

You may find that your pets, considered family members by some, are a unique solace to you through the cancer experience. Animals seem to have a knack for knowing when we need help, and they don't care if we smell funny or if our hair is missing. They don't become instantly bashful because of our diagnosis, and they aren't afraid they'll catch cancer from us. How many humans will sit by us for an hour in the bathroom while we're sick, as our cats will? And who's funnier than the puppy who barks at the wig on the dresser?

Positive thinking and visualization

Positive thinking and visualization have been shown to increase immune system function in some studies. Oddly, one study has shown that when cancer survivors visualize an immune system attack of the tumor, using attack images that are incorrect according to what is known today about immune system function, immune system parameters still improve. This may reflect the "taking charge" phenomenon: the belief that you can escape stress tends to lessen the effect of stress on the immune system.

Visualization can be used as described above to attempt to direct inner forces against the cancer, or to relax by calling to mind pleasant experiences, places, or dreams. Initially, it might be useful to practice visualization in a quiet, relaxed atmosphere, but eventually you can do it anywhere.

Reading

As a form of escapism, reading is a good way to reduce stress. As a means of learning more about your illness, reading may make you feel more stressed temporarily, but this stress may be offset by long stretches of peace of mind after you're able to make better medical decisions based on what you've learned by reading.

If you have a personal computer, reading from and writing to the various lung cancer discussion groups on the Internet can provide a cathartic outlet for you. See "Support groups" later in the chapter.

Relaxation training

This technique is similar to biofeedback, and it incorporates visualization techniques described under "Positive thinking and visualization"

Sleep

Research shows that even one night of missed sleep lowers levels of natural killer (NK) white blood cells that attack tumors. Although NK counts recover quickly once sleep is restored, persistent lack of sleep is an opportunity for illness.

Animal research on the artificial shifting of the phases of lightness and darkness shows that the immune system is depressed by the shifting. Fishes that occupy parts of the ocean that receive low light in winter experience an additional breeding cycle if artificial light is increased, and simultaneously, their white blood cell counts decrease.

Snuggles and smooches

Being kissed, hugged, and patted by people who love you causes endorphins to be released within the central nervous system. Endorphins are natural opiates produced by our bodies, capable of reducing pain and depression and producing feelings of well-being.

Hugging and kissing your partner can be enjoyable and healthy, even if you're feeling too tired or pained at the moment to enjoy all of the sexual activities you enjoyed before diagnosis.

Spirituality, religious beliefs

Your religious beliefs may provide comfort when little else is making sense. Some people find that their spiritual beliefs sustain them in spite of a seemingly arbitrary infliction of suffering, either because their religion provides answers for the question of human suffering or because of independently developed theological beliefs.

A survivor describes how his faith helped them:

> *After surgery, the nursing supervisors tried to ask me how I felt about it being cancerous. It just kind of hits you in the face. The word cancer is a big thing. I have a lot of faith. I told the nurse, "It's in the good Lord's hands." She responded, "Well, the good Lord has sent a lot of doctors to help you." After I got out and was on pain medications, I depended a lot on faith.*

Other cancer survivors, however, experience a crisis of faith after their cancer diagnosis. They find it difficult, for instance, to reconcile the emergence of a seemingly undeserved, life-threatening illness with their belief in a kind, nonpunitive deity.

On a more human level, the support that fellow church or temple members furnish to those who need help is clearly an asset in stress reduction. Support might take the form of emotional support (cards, calls, hugs, or visits), prayer, practical support (drives to and from the doctor or casseroles for supper), or financial support for someone who is underinsured.

The May 1995 issue of the *Journal of the American Medical Association* contains an article showing a correlation between religious practice and prayer and increased good health. At least one other study has shown that a person who is prayed for improves when ill, even if he is not aware that prayers are being said.

Larry Coffman describes his strength through faith:

> *Remember that lung cancer is survivable, although I have to agree that I would be looking through rose-colored glasses if I didn't balance all this by saying that there are those that don't make it. I turned the entire matter over to the Lord a couple of weeks after diagnosis. I got very tired of living with the fear and have been at peace since. This has allowed me to concentrate on both my spiritual as well as physical and mental healing. Keep on fighting the "dragon" and empowering yourself so that you can make informed and educated decisions. I can't speak for others, but take each day as it comes and cherish the same.*

Support groups

For some of us, support groups can be the difference, literally, between life and death. The opportunity to exchange information with those who have already weathered lung cancer can provide you with everything from emotional support to the knowledge to question your treatment and seek medical help elsewhere. Support groups are an immeasurably useful way to do this, bringing together a variety of skills, sometimes including medical and legal knowledge.

Moreover, Dr. Spiegel's work with breast cancer survivors shows longer survival among those who were part of support groups, a serendipitous finding from a study intending to highlight other aspects of survival.

Support groups are offered locally in many areas by organizations such as the American Cancer Society, the Wellness Community, or local hospitals. If you have Internet access, support groups are also available on the Internet. See Chapter 16 for instructions about subscribing.

Water

In the 1930s, marine biologist Sir Alister Hardy noted that humans have features in common with water mammals, features not found in any other primates, such as a subcutaneous layer of body fat; hair that grows in one direction, which reduces water resistance; a protective dive reflex within the respiratory system; a nose that blocks water during a dive; residual webbed toes; and fully webbed toes in seven percent of humans. He argues that humans might have spent a period of evolution in water.

Anthropologists may settle this point eventually, but for our immediate use, it means that, for some of us, water is a wonderful way to relax. A good swim or a warm tub with salts and a good book can make you briefly more than just human.

Writing

If you have an urge to write, you'll be encouraged to know that those who write very honestly and emotionally about their frightening, negative experiences increase the function of their white blood cells. Writing can be in a range of formats. You can write for yourself in a journal, write letters to friends, write letters for your children to be read when they're older, or write email to cancer discussion groups on the Internet.

Stress medications

Stress associated with cancer responds well to antianxiety and antidepressant medication. Research has shown, though, that these medications are most effective when used in combination with counseling and behavior modification training.

There are many drugs to choose from to ease anxiety or depression or to aid sleep. The newer drugs available today have fewer side effects and are less likely to be addictive than drugs used just a few years ago.

Your oncologist should review all stress medications prescribed by any physician, including a psychiatrist.

Antianxiety medication

Antianxiety drugs (anxiolytics) fall broadly into two groups, the older, fast-acting drugs and the newer, slower-acting drugs:

- The fast-acting benzodiazepine drugs, such as Valium, Ativan, or Xanax, are potentially addictive and can cause rebound anxiety when they're stopped. The mood change following use of these antianxiety drugs is pronounced and rapid, similar to the effect of alcohol. It's unwise to drive or operate heavy machinery when using drugs in the benzodiazepine family. At certain doses these drugs can suppress the respiratory system.

- The newer antianxiety drugs, such as BuSpar (buspirone), cross the boundary between antianxiety and antidepressive drugs, are not addictive, and can be stopped abruptly with no ill effect. They take two to three weeks to work. The mood change following use of these drugs is more subtle and gradual, and sleepiness, if present, is less pronounced than with the benzodiazepines.

Please note that the antianxiety drug Ativan, a benzodiazepine, is often used just prior to chemotherapy to control nausea. In this limited usage it is unlikely to be addictive and can be an asset in anxiety and nausea control.

Antidepressant medication

The availability of today's more effective, safer antidepressants is a blessing for those coping with cancer. Unlike the antidepressants of a few years ago, which caused sleepiness, weight gain, or other undesirable side effects, today's antidepressant medications are far safer and less disruptive of weight and sleep patterns. Antidepressants are also good pain relievers, although their mechanism as such is not entirely clear.

Some of the newer antidepressants can cause restlessness and insomnia for the first two or three weeks they are used. You might discuss with your doctor the temporary use of a sleeping pill until your body has adjusted to the antidepressant.

Improvement in mood is gradual with most of the antidepressants used today, changing slowly over a few weeks or months. The fullest effect is gained if the drugs are used continuously for months. Always check with your doctor before stopping an antidepressant, lest gains in improved mood be lost.

The best source for antidepressant medication is a psychiatrist. This specialist is the one most likely to be familiar with all antidepressants and their side effects and can rotate you through several until the best one for you is apparent.

Sleep medications

Sleep medications range from the very mildest, including over-the-counter antihistamines and Tylenol, to the stronger medications necessary for those using prednisone or those coping with moderate to severe anxiety. Drugs prescribed for severe pain, such as codeine and morphine, also induce sleep.

The antianxiety drugs in the benzodiazepine family, such as Ativan, are also used as sleep aids. See "Antianxiety medication" for information about these drugs.

Some of the newest sleeping pills target those who have trouble falling asleep. They're cleared very rapidly from the body, so they are less useful for those having trouble staying asleep. For at least some people, these drugs might be addictive.

Some people use melatonin, a substance marketed as a food supplement, to aid sleep. Always consult your oncologist before using any drug, whether prescription, nonprescription, or a "natural remedy" marketed as a food supplement.

Summary

The effects of stress and personality on the inception and growth of cancer are unclear and are still being studied. Animal models indicate that a wide range of tumor responses to physical and emotional stress are possible, depending in some instances on the species, gender, stressor, season, previous exposure to stress, and biological state.

Regardless of the effect of stress on cancer, there are good reasons to reduce stress. Your sense of well being will improve, and you can lessen or prevent the chance of secondary illnesses.

Key points to remember:

- Your oncologist should be informed of, and approve, any change in diet, exercise, or medication that you might be considering to reduce stress.

- There are no proven links between cancer and stress or between cancer and personality types.

- Reducing stress can help you avoid stress-related illnesses, such as upper respiratory infections, gastric ulcers, or the worsening of such autoimmune diseases as lupus, diabetes, or ulcerative colitis.

- Reducing stress can ease your breathing and help you avoid digestive extremes of diarrhea and constipation, thus helping you maintain good absorption of nutrients through your digestive system.

CHAPTER 16

Getting Support

Falling down you can do alone, but it takes
helping hands to get back up.

—Yiddish proverb

LUNG CANCER CAN BE A TERRIBLE BURDEN in its physical aspects alone, but to face lung cancer without emotional support can be far worse. Cancer can be an isolating experience for the patient because for others, it calls to mind issues that many people dread, such as chronic pain, the surrender of physical or financial independence, or death. Lung cancer patients in particular feel stigmatized, isolated, and ostracized by the well-publicized association between smoking and lung tumors.

The goal of this chapter is to get you the emotional and instrumental help you need. This chapter first details specific issues that might require the help of others: the smoking stereotype, the emotional and practical support needed to deal with such issues as oxygen support, keeping positive, transportation, child care, housecleaning, medical care within the home, workplace issues, and so on. Next, we address a few general aspects of communication and support, such as some typical reactions that the "healthy unaware" have to serious illness. We'll examine in detail the groups of people you might ask for support. We'll discuss your strongest, most abiding relationships with family members and loved ones; children and teenagers; friends, coworkers, and social contacts; and cancer counselors and support groups. Some examples of challenging moments in communication and how you might handle them are discussed. Quitting smoking is addressed at the end of the chapter.

Various organizations offer an almost staggering variety of services to lung cancer survivors, most of them free. Appendix A, *Resources*, contains a full list of such services.

Two hurtful stereotypes

There are two serious misperceptions that lung cancer patients and survivors face when dealing with others.

The first is the snapshot that healthy people carry in their heads about cancer patients and survivors. People who have never dealt with cancer—and some who have—expect all cancer patients to look ill and thin and suspect that all cancer survivors are facing a greatly shortened life span, putting on a good face for the public. They might overreact, for example, to seeing you on supplemental oxygen. The wife of a cancer survivor recalls the hurtful comments of a coworker:

> During my husband's chemotherapy, a coworker remarked that she'd seen him in the neighborhood. "The poor guy looks soooo thin," she said, with a hangdog expression. I told her he'd gained seventeen pounds above his "healthy" weight while on prednisone.

The second dangerous public misperception that many lung cancer survivors face is that their illness was caused by smoking and that the patient has only "got what she deserved." No one deserves cancer, no matter what their genetic makeup, environmental surroundings, or lifestyle choices. No one deserves lung cancer.

Ten to twenty percent of those who are diagnosed with lung cancer have never smoked. Only about ten percent of smokers develop lung tumors (although at least eight other cancers and various cardiopulmonary diseases are linked to smoking). Often, lung tumors appear in those who quit smoking many years earlier. Certain airborne toxins not inhaled by choice are linked to lung cancer. There are genetic predispositions to lung tumors that are not fully understood at this time. A variety of other illnesses and certain medications can predispose one to lung cancer (see Chapter 5, *What Is Lung Cancer?*).

Karen Parles, creator of Lung Cancer Online (*http://www.lungcanceronline.org*) and diagnosed at age 38 with NSCLC, describes how she has been treated:

> Since my lung cancer diagnosis, I have been sickened by what I have learned about the politics, economics and realities of lung cancer.
> A constant reminder of the smoking stigma associated with this disease is the inevitable question I hear when someone learns I have lung cancer, "Did you smoke . . . ?" Despite having never smoked, I still resent what is implied by this question, and wonder why people with coronary artery disease aren't confronted in the same way. Many lung cancer survivors do feel guilty about "causing" their lung cancer through smoking. This guilt, combined with the public prejudice against people with lung cancer, serves to stifle and weaken those who could best speak out and advocate for this deadly disease.

Further illustrating the stigma associated with lung cancer is the absence of the celebrity endorsements "enjoyed" by all of the other major cancers. Seasoned lung cancer advocates tell countless stories of approaching celebrities to speak out against lung cancer. Time after time, celebrities refuse to participate in lung cancer events because they don't want to be associated with a "smokers' disease." The most striking evidence of the apathy towards those afflicted with lung cancer is the virtual nonexistence of awareness and fundraising events. I was incredulous to discover that there are no walk-a-thons, no golf outings, no wine tastings, no hospital gala events benefiting lung cancer research, or funding support services for people with lung cancer. Television, radio, and newspaper outlets offer special features on breast, ovarian, prostate, colon, and children's cancers, but virtually nothing on the number one cancer killer. This lack of public empathy and support is demoralizing— our personal battles against lung cancer are compounded by the added stigma of having a "smokers' disease."

As a never-smoker with lung cancer, I have learned a lot about people who smoke. I have learned that over 90 percent of smokers began smoking as teenagers. Teenagers do not take to heart the long-term implications of smoking and think that they can quit at any time. Teenagers are risk takers—they try alcohol and drugs, as well as smoking. I have also learned that alcoholics and drug addicts receive more public sympathy than smokers. The tobacco companies continue to play an unconscionable role in perpetuating this deadly addiction among young people.

Whenever lung cancer is discussed, "smokers" are cited as its victims. A "smoker" is an abstract notion, not an individual with a life-threatening disease who is worthy of our caring and support. I think that the public needs to know that these "smokers" are people with names and faces and families. They also need to know that, in fact, 50 percent of these "smokers" with lung cancer are not smokers at all, but former smokers and never-smokers. By standing up and speaking up, those of us with lung cancer can most effectively put a face on this deadly disease, and garner the public support necessary for adequate funding of lung cancer research.

Unfortunately, most of the public is not aware of these granular statistical details. Consequently, many people, perhaps even some medical personnel and other cancer survivors, are inclined to blame the patient for the disease. Blaming the patient might seem to be an inevitable point of view to some people—after all, even some lung cancer patients blame themselves for having smoked—but one's privately held opinions on smoking should never interfere with patient care or support. Larry Coffman, five-year survivor of SCLC, tells his point of view:

> It is sad that lung cancer is on the political back burner today. Please keep in mind that we, as lung cancer survivors, live with the stigma that we have created our own problem, even though a growing number of lung cancer patients have never smoked, either directly or by secondhand. I write letters to Congress day after day to provide tobacco-related illness and disease benefits for our veterans. I continue to hit the brick wall, as tobacco is a well-funded lobby.
>
> As great as the American Cancer Society is, they have become a political organization with an agenda that is to be "politically correct" and will continue to do as their largest contributors desire. We must continue to financially support the efforts of the Association for Lung Cancer Awareness, Support, and Education (ALCASE) for our voice. And if ALCASE becomes another ACS, then we'll find another more worthy organization.

Specific needs

The word "support" means different things to different people, or different things on different days.

Practical support

There are very tangible, instrumental ways that others can support you, such as:

- Offering to locate and interpret medical information about your illness
- Offering their points of view for your decision-making process
- Giving up smoking when you do to reduce your temptation to smoke
- Offering to donate a pint of blood for you
- Helping you move about at home after surgery
- Offering to do some of your cooking, cleaning, laundry, or shopping
- Driving you to and from treatment visits

- Acting as an advocate for you when you're not well enough to express your needs or demand better care
- Keeping track of medications you must take if you're too groggy to do so
- Monitoring your reactions to specific medications
- Helping you obtain or transport oxygen equipment
- Organizing fundraisers or offering financial support
- Calling insurance companies, medical offices, or employers to iron out misunderstandings
- Researching possible claims against tobacco industry settlements, or tax breaks offered by some states for those trying to quit smoking
- Babysitting your children or grandchildren
- Offering to stay overnight with you if you need nursing care
- Giving backrubs or other anxiety-lowering help when breathing is difficult
- Offering to assume temporarily some or all of your work
- Understanding that fatigue is the most common long-term effect faced by cancer survivors, often lasting for years

Kathleen Houlihan describes some of the wonderful support she had from relatives during her treatment:

> My father and my cousin KJ visited me while my husband Holt was
> away. It was probably a little boring for them, just following me around to
> treatments, doctors' appointments, and classes, and then hanging out
> while I napped, but they did get a good feel for what it's like around here,
> and I sure enjoyed having them. My dear friend CW and her daughter
> JW came for an overnight visit last weekend. It was very nice, and they
> were relieved to see me looking so good.

Emotional support

There are many ways that others can provide emotional support:

- Attempting to understand how you feel, however alien it may seem to them, while avoiding assuming that they know how you feel.
- Avoiding making inaccurate, frightening, and frustrating comparisons of lung cancer to other cancers.

- Cheering you on when you feel bad during quitting smoking.

- Being available when you want company.

- Sending gifts and cards if you're housebound or hospitalized.

- Attending to your children's or grandchildren's emotional needs.

- Avoiding asking nosy or inappropriate questions, offering instead to listen when you're ready to talk.

- Learning to say, "I'm sorry this happened to you. Please let me know what I can do for you," instead of avoiding you or asking nosy questions.

- Maintaining support over time. Many cancer survivors report receiving a great deal of support initially, only to see it diminish as time passes.

Kathleen Houlihan tells of her husband's emotional strength and presence:

> Holt is working out of town for a couple of weeks. He's missing the whole hair saga, but he said he will love me whether I have hair or not. I wouldn't have expected it to be otherwise, but it was wonderful of him to say it.

Support issues specific to lung cancer

Almost all cancer survivors face the issues listed above. There are also several issues lung cancer survivors face that other cancer survivors might not face:

- The stigma of lung cancer being associated with smoking. Those who do or did smoke experience stigmatization in ways that are different from those who have never smoked—but both often experience the ostracism of a disease ostensibly "caused by the patient."

- Lack of understanding about reduced pulmonary function's causing shortness of breath. Others might not understand that your activity is more restricted than it was, for example, or that certain things might take you longer to do because your lung capacity is diminished.

- Lack of understanding about your use of supplemental oxygen. Others might be uncomfortable around you, equating needing supplemental oxygen with life support or impending death. In fact, some people require supplemental oxygen for years and for diseases other than lung cancer.

- Lack of understanding about the chest pain that might persist long after surgery or radiotherapy.

- Lack of understanding about slow-growing forms of lung cancer and stable metastases. Because you might look and act healthy while knowing these tumors will require treatment sooner or later, others might think you're lying to them or just deceiving yourself.

Communicating about these needs

Those who have no experience with lung cancer might not understand intuitively what you're facing, yet the support you receive from others often is a result of how good you are at asking for help and saying thanks. You should consider communicating very clearly about the following issues:

- Your illness might recur years later because some lung tissue remains. This is often a second independent lung tumor, not a metastasis of the first tumor.

- Ten to twenty percent of those who are diagnosed with lung cancer have never smoked. The public cannot afford to indulge in the myth of lung cancer as a disease that needs no research funding because "the cause is already known" or "the patient brought it on himself."

- For some people diagnosed at any stage, but especially in stages II, III, and IV, the path is an uncertain one regarding recurrence of disease and the success of treatment.

- You might look and seem healthy, even while harboring a slow-growing type of lung cancer, stable disease, or a progression of disease.

- Lung cancer may travel to the brain, but this is not necessarily a hopeless circumstance. For detailed information about this issue, see Chapter 6, *Prognosis*, and Chapters 8 and 9, *Treating Non-Small Cell Lung Cancer* and *Treating Small Cell Lung Cancer*.

- Treatment and the fatigue that might follow can leave you unable to work for long periods of time. Fatigue is a common side effect of cancer treatment and can be a long-term effect, in some cases lasting for years.

- Long-term pain, shortness of breath, or coughing requiring medication or oxygen might result after surgery, chemotherapy, or radiotherapy. Sometimes these treatments are temporary and very effective; sometimes they are needed for a longer period of time.

Typical reactions to requests for help

In an ideal world, you would be surrounded by people who come forward as soon as you need help. They would know what you need before you need it, would give lovingly and unselfishly, and would never become exhausted. Money would flow without a second thought, and those who help you would expect nothing in return. Kathleen Houlihan tells us of her sister-in-law's very kind support:

> My husband Holt's sister AT is a dear. She was willing to drop everything and fly to be with me while I traveled out of town for treatment. She and I had a great time together, catching up on all the details of the last seventeen years since the year Holt and I spent out in LA. And she waited on me hand and foot, spoiling me even more than Holt does. She also drove us back all 683 miles home.

A three-year survivor of small cell lung cancer describes how wonderful her family and friends have been:

> I have lived to see many happy events in my family's life. My son graduated from college with an accounting degree after seven years of college in May of 1998. I am very proud and happy.
>
> I would not have been able to do any of this without my husband, who has been there every step of the way. I cannot drive anymore due to the nerve damage from my treatment, and this man drove me to every single treatment and doctor's appointment: 6 months of chemo, 28 daily chest radiation sessions, and 15 brain radiation sessions. This man has put up with more than any person should have to deal with, and I am very grateful.
>
> I will be 52 years young in August of this year. I am blessed with a wonderful family and a great network of friends.

But for others, it's not always this good. Often, healthy people are only partially aware of what you're going through. Nausea? Fatigue? Shortness of breath? While "the healthy unaware" might have had nausea and fatigue in the past, it's likely that they were quickly remedied. They might not realize what it's like to experience nausea for days each week, even before the chemotherapy treatment has begun. They don't truly understand what it's like to be tired all day, every day, as soon as they wake in the morning. Continual shortness of breath is a frightening development that very few healthy people have had to adjust to.

At times, others would like to offer support, but don't know what to do or say. They might say the wrong thing. In some instances, others find it easier just to avoid discussing the issue of your illness. They hope—it is presumed—that if they dwell on other topics, you (and they) will feel normal again. In very rare cases, the motives of others are not at all honorable, and they might say or do things that are despicable.

Frequently there are good explanations for what you might perceive as the failure of others to provide adequate support. Other people, being mortal, have finite logistic, emotional, and financial resources. They still have their own responsibilities and needs to address. Kathy describes her own health problems that had to be addressed while her husband Marty was ill:

> We all began seeing a counselor and I stopped taking care of everyone. I made Marty put together and keep track of his own pills, I didn't make appointments for him, and when he complained to me about pain, I just said I was sorry and that he needed to talk to the doctor—or I said nothing at all. I was beginning to feel like he blamed me for not healing him—it was easier to be mad at me than face reality, I guess.
>
> Anyway, I was going to be responsible for nobody but myself, which is when I decided to have the hysterectomy/oophorectomy that I had put off in the fall. Marty was horrible about it. I thought he wouldn't even be there to take me home. He seemed to dismiss my need to recover from the surgery. Finally, one day I said, "Look, I just had parts of my body cut out of me and I need down time to recover, and my medical needs are more urgent at this time." I literally laid in the recliner for three weeks.

If they are loved ones, they may have assumed some of your responsibilities, as well. They might be attempting to manage this on a reduced income, if the lung cancer survivor is unable to contribute financially. They might be concerned that the time they're missing from work to provide care will jeopardize the family's only remaining source of income. The thought of losing a loved one is probably highly threatening to them, perhaps causing anger, terror, sadness, and a host of other debilitating feelings. None of these issues justifies unkind behavior, of course, but hidden concerns might cause loved ones to seem angry, withdrawn, distracted, inattentive, overly controlling, or insensitive.

Fortunately, it appears that many lung cancer survivors receive most of the support they need, when they need it, with just an occasional bump along the way—if they make their needs known.

Cancer counselor and survivor Nan Suhadolc points out that those you must deal with for support tend to fall into three categories—nurturing, supportive, and toxic—whether they're family, friends, or acquaintances. In other words, your closest family members, upon whom you might hope to rely, might be at times negative and unsupportive: emotionally toxic to you. Those who are less close actually might be more nurturing at times than family members. In the discussions that follow, the term "loved ones" implies those who are nurturing, even if they are not related to you by blood or marriage.

How to communicate successfully

There's no one way to communicate successfully with others about your needs. Even among people who believe they know each other well, misunderstandings and hurt feelings arise because of daily variations in mood or because of circumstances of which they're unaware. Your own skills in dealing with lung cancer come into play, too, when what was not upsetting yesterday may be upsetting today if you're sick, tired, and discouraged.

Despite these ups and downs, many lung cancer survivors have learned by experience about communicating with others. Details regarding how to discuss your illness will be touched on in each section below, but some very general guidelines are:

- With your closest loved ones, be as honest as possible, as gently as possible.

- With those to whom you're not very close, use your judgment about what and how much to say, protect yourself and them from undesirable consequences, until you can assess the quality of their responses. You may choose, for example, to tell some family members, social acquaintances, and coworkers a few things about your treatment, while avoiding lengthy, painful discussions or topics they're likely to misunderstand.

- For that group in the middle comprising good friends and perhaps other family members, try to sense the boundary. Just as you have limits to what you can bear, few friends are able to absorb all of your pain all of the time. Asking, "Are you in the mood to listen to this today?" or "Do you have the time and energy to be my sounding board?" are two possible approaches. And the reverse is true: you need to be clear, but tactful, if you don't feel like discussing your circumstances, for instance, or if you aren't feeling sturdy enough to have visitors.

These general suggestions are probably no surprise to you. Nor will be the fact that there are exceptions to every rule. Many cancer survivors report very unusual reactive behaviors in even their very best friends and closest loved ones.

The general guidelines of telling your closest loved ones the most and with greatest honesty may not hold. For example, you might have a close relative who handles bad news better if you joke about it a little, but who will never be able to react appropriately to the rawer emotions. She may turn tail and run if you cry, for instance. Conversely, you might have a casual friend with a medical background who is a skilled listener and who can at times provide you with more objective support than your family can. From such an interaction a very deep friendship may grow.

Although most loved ones will support you, it's not unheard of for some family members and friends to blame the patient or disappear when they discover you have cancer. There's no one solution to this very painful problem. Often, lung cancer survivors just move on to find new friends, but some cancer survivors justifiably neither forgive nor forget. Sometimes the absentee relative or friend will reappear and apologize, perhaps not until years later.

The wife of a cancer survivor tells of two hurtful incidents, which were the exception rather than the rule:

> When my husband was in the hospital for surgery, my sister and her husband sent flowers. Afterward, we didn't hear from them during the six months of his chemotherapy, in spite of my telephone calls to them. My next-door neighbor phoned us one time during this six-month period—to ask me to babysit for her!
>
> Fortunately these oddballs were the minority of our friends and relatives. If anything, the experience made the good relationships even better…and we made new friends in the cancer support group.

Gender and cultural differences in communicating about illness also can affect the outcome of asking for help, especially in the US, because the population is composed of so many cultural groups.

Communicating with loved ones

Some families work better as a team than others. It's rare for any team of people to respond perfectly when it comes to dealing with a crisis. You might observe these lapses frequently in the workplace, but often one is especially hurt when one's family fails to respond appropriately.

Owing to the many variations in group behavior, it's not possible to cover in this section all family behaviors with which you might have to contend. Instead, we discuss the most common problems and solutions.

For many people of all ages, a new crisis initially tends to elicit behaviors that worked well in the past. These reflexive behaviors might include arguing, escapism, intellectualizing the problem, or taking control. For children or grandchildren in crisis, we might see a return to the dependent behaviors they had outgrown. The overall impression in a crisis might be that those around you are reverting to immature, maladaptive behaviors. Keep in mind that your cancer might be a brand-new experience for those around you and that learned coping behaviors can be hard habits to change, especially in a time of great stress.

It might be harder for your loved ones to help you if you don't communicate clearly about your circumstances. With this group, don't be shy or proud. Ask for all the help you need, even if it embarrasses you. Many family members express chagrin at the seeming reluctance of cancer patients to "trouble" them. They in turn hesitate to invade the patient's privacy by prying or being dominant. Consequently, the already upsetting cancer experience can transform into an even larger menace than it is because nobody will talk about it.

On the other hand, if your family is closely knit, sharing and verbalizing just about everything, the stresses associated with lung cancer might appear to be taking a greater toll than one might see in a family with fewer emotional ties and more independent members. The telling point is the success of your family's long-term adaptation, not any temporary disequilibrium, emotional flotsam, or distancing you might experience.

Geri Capasso's deep love for her brother Anthony is obvious in her support for him:

> Just today, as I was feeling the weight of my brother's cancer, I was wondering if it were me, would or could I feel any worse? But this has been a bad week. His doctor thinks he has bronchitis. I'm back to square one. Just when you think you've learned to live with it, it's like that Jim Croce song, "Operator," when he says, "give me the number so I can call and tell her I'm fine and show that I've overcome the blow, learned to take it well, I only wish my words could just convince myself that it just isn't real cause that's not the way it feels…."

> *I'm grateful that my brother is still full of fight, but I'm sure that he has his moments, and he is human and entitled. But what I have learned from my brother is that even though it's sad, unfair, scary, depressing, and frustrating, to say the least, it doesn't mean that this battle can't be won! The support, positive energy, and information that I have gotten has helped me to stay strong, move on, and see that my brother has a fighting chance.*

What you need from loved ones may change as your experiences evolve from diagnosis through treatment. Different relatives and loved ones may prove good at handling different things. Unlike coworkers and casual acquaintances, close family members and loved ones probably won't surprise you too often with their reactions because it's likely you already know their weaknesses and strengths. You might find yourself occasionally disappointed, but perhaps not surprised.

Larry Coffman, five-year survivor of SCLC, reflects on his support:

> *I am so glad that my family and friends were there for me. Many times, families remain, but friends disappear out of fear. Caregivers need to be treated by the practitioners as well as the patient and make sure that they treat you emotionally as well as physically. I have often thought that the treatment was far worse than the disease, albeit that modern advances in treatment are turning that around.*

Communicating needs to adults

Ideally, communicating with the loving adults in your life about your needs should be relatively easy. Honesty, gentleness, and especially gratitude should serve well. With a couple of exceptions, such as a relative who's mentally ill or physically frail, adults who are nearest and dearest should be trusted to handle every aspect, even the worst aspects, of your illness appropriately.

In reality, however, cancer might challenge a family's beliefs and myths about their family unit and might alter the established dynamics of the family. If the father, mother, husband, or wife has always been a wise and strong provider, for example, the balance of power might shift temporarily during treatment for lung cancer. Older people with lung cancer might have adult children who want to return to their parent the nurturing they received when they were young. If the partner without lung cancer has developed an untoward reliance on the strong one, it may be a difficult transition to assume control for a while. The partner with lung cancer might suffer lowered self esteem when roles shift. It's important to keep in mind that often these shifts are temporary.

Many lung cancer survivors note that their loved ones become ill, too, while trying to help them deal with treatment and emotional issues. Upper respiratory infections, such as sore throats; persistent GI tract problems, such as diarrhea; emergence of autoimmune disorders; and worsening of certain other chronic illnesses, such as herpes, diabetes, or heart disease often go hand-in-hand with the extreme emotional stress associated with a loved one's having cancer. At times, though, lung cancer survivors report that a relative seems to want to be sicker than the person with cancer. This does indeed happen in some families, and if it happens in yours, chances are you've seen this kind of behavior before from that individual. The deciding factor is whether the ostensibly ill person continues to provide help to the best of his ability or uses the illness as an excuse not to help—or even to punish you.

If you find that the adult loved ones in your life are reacting to your needs in unhelpful ways, do ask why. It might be a simple thing to put right. If they seem angry, it's possible some older unresolved issues are being forced to the fore by the stress of dealing with lung cancer. They may feel, for instance, that they owe you little because in the past you were not supportive of them when they needed help or because they asked you for many years to give up smoking.

If the issues seem to be about blaming you for smoking—particularly if your closest loved ones have never smoked or gave up smoking—you might try asking your partner to evaluate you as an entire person with a long history of being a loving, productive, reliable partner: to focus less on the feelings of betrayal or abandonment that might be part of his reaction.

If attempts to communicate don't make much difference, it might be a disappointment to realize that the strength you thought existed in the relationship does not exist—or at least not for this set of circumstances. Perhaps you could rely on someone else temporarily for what you need. Sometimes loved ones just need some time to settle down and get used to the changes and increased responsibilities that cancer brings.

Avoid asking a third family member to intervene if you have difficulty getting along with a loved one. Triangles such as this seldom succeed because they hint at two-against-one and talking behind each other's backs.

If reasonable attempts to get the help you need fail, you might discuss attending family counseling with the person who seems to be acting out of character.

If none of these attempts works, then finding alternate support or finding ways to live without such people, temporarily or permanently, is in your best interest. Because of the seriousness of lung cancer, your concerns must be put first, at least for the time being. You may be surprised to find that, in spite of lung cancer, your life is more serene and enjoyable in the absence of such difficult people. A decision not to deal with someone is also a means of dealing with them.

Communicating with good friends

You expect your good friends to stand by you while you're facing serious problems. Close friends can offer you such help as emotional support, occasional running of errands, some cooking, household chores, babysitting, or an escapist night on the town. As with loved ones, you might occasionally be disappointed or surprised if they fail to live up to your opinions of them. On the other hand, many lung cancer survivors have discovered that good friends earn their wings in heaven by way of loyalty and selflessness and that to some come to mean as much to them as their family members do.

Because they usually have a lower emotional investment in the relationship than family members do, good friends can be easier to deal with at times than family members. They can be more objective about some of your problems. A lung cancer survivor recalls kind gestures from his neighbors:

> When I lost my hair, people didn't know what to say. Some of them
> would say, "You look so good!" when I knew that I looked terrible.
> However, most of them were real supportive, especially in the
> neighborhood. It's the best neighborhood. We've all lived here so long.
> I don't know how I could have gotten through it without them. Little things
> really helped pull me through, like my Norm's lentil soup.

This objectivity is purchased with their relative distance. Good friends, in order to remain good friends, may need an occasional vacation from you and your problems. If you give them space to refresh themselves, they are able to return to you with more emotional vigor.

Most people will find that at least some friends or acquaintances will have responses that are disappointing, but you can't control how other people react to cancer.

Communicating with coworkers

What you can ask of your coworkers depends on the structure, size, and pace of the company's workforce, the level of competitiveness your profession experiences, and the degree to which your work relationships drift into friendships. The minimum you can ask of coworkers is patience and discretion, but frequently they give you much more. Often the feelings your coworkers express and the support they offer are a tremendous reinforcement for your well-being. To know you are needed and missed can be uplifting.

In general, though, exercise some caution asking favors of coworkers who are not also friends, because the request might seem out of bounds or might backfire if you're deemed too sick to perform well after revealing a weakness or need. As with some friends, coworkers might want to know everything about your illness, nothing about it, or some intermediate subset of information that's hard to define and may change daily.

The good news is that many lung cancer survivors report that coworkers pitch in and offer assistance without being asked: blood donations, bake sales, shopping, baby sitting, cheering visits, and so on might materialize without your having to ask. Many lung cancer survivors report that coworkers donate unused sick days to them or pinch-hit for them if they miss time or feel sick or tired.

On the other hand, if some coworkers are reluctant to recognize your illness, owing to their own fears or lack of social skills, they might never refer to it, not even to wish you well. You can feel free to say nothing to the potentially unsympathetic coworker if you choose, but there are disadvantages in not keeping your immediate supervisor informed about your health status. For example, if your supervisor is unaware of problems you're experiencing as a result of your illness or its treatment, you might have difficulty winning a favorable decision if a dispute about your performance arises.

Remember that cancer is considered a disability under the Americans with Disabilities Act (ADA), so you don't have to endure negative reactions in the workplace that result in demonstrable emotional or professional harm to you, such as denial of a promotion or censure for using earned sick time: you have legal recourse.

Communicating with social acquaintances

Social acquaintances comprise a wide variety of people. Some of these people, such as church or temple members, expect you to ask for help. Others, such as the spouses of coworkers, touch on your life only briefly or occasionally, and probably don't expect you to ask them to help. Many lung cancer survivors are pleasantly surprised, though, to find that people who they thought were practically strangers pitch in and help without being asked.

Unlike your family, friends, and coworkers, social acquaintances don't usually have the opportunity to see you doing everyday things; consequently, they might have more misunderstandings about what you're going through. On the other hand, people you choose to see socially might have more in common with you than, for instance, those you have no choice but to work with.

In general, what you can ask of social acquaintances depends on the context in which you know them. If they're fellow Junior Leaguers or Jaycees, you might expect help because these groups specialize in helping others. If they're the friendly couple with season tickets next to yours at the theater, perhaps you should not expect their help.

Communicating with children

Communicating with young children has different goals than communicating with adults. Although it's true that children sometimes provide major instrumental support if no other family members are available, generally it isn't necessary or fair to expect a great deal of help from children. More often, they can be asked to help with small, safe chores to make them feel part of the solution and to reinforce the honest relationship they've grown accustomed to.

Human children are inclined by biology to think the world revolves around them. Very young infants do not understand, for instance, that Mommy is a separate person who can leave them with Daddy and go grocery shopping, and they might become quite upset when they discover that Mommy is gone. This bonding trait is probably essential to survival for a species whose young have a long and vulnerable nurturing period such as that humans and some other mammals have.

This egocentric thought process lingers well through childhood, though, and causes children to think that bad things that happen are their fault. They might think that you developed cancer because they were very angry with you when you once punished them, for example. They might even have wished you were dead, and now it appears to be coming true. Depending on their religious upbringing, they might believe that God saw them misbehave and is punishing them.

For many reasons, children see us differently from our view of ourselves. Lack of experience with emotions, fear of abandonment, or just plain being shorter than adults means their perspective is truly different. Often small children can't distinguish a sad or aging adult face from a grouchy one, for example, and because adults are all-powerful from their perspective, unconsciously they hedge their bets by tailoring their actions to forestall anger instead of sadness, which from their perspective is the worse of these two in terms of the consequences for the child.

Difference of perspective between adults and children might also cause efforts to explain lung cancer to backfire. If you try to compare lung cancer to any illness they've had, it might create an extreme fear that becomes obvious when the next normal childhood illness strikes them.

It's also the case that children cycle through feelings more rapidly than adults. Periods of sadness might quickly be replaced by playful spells or intense involvement in activities outside the family. Keep in mind that these rapid shifts are normal, not an indication that they are uncaring or unaware.

For these and other reasons, honesty and patience with children about lung cancer is essential. Kathy describes her young daughters' surprisingly mature grasp of reality and their concerns if Marty were to die:

> Our then four-year-old asked a lot of questions about death, even though we never directly told her that dad could die. I'm sure she heard us talking. My then thirteen-year-old understood what was happening and that her dad could die. I explained the statistics to her. I learned later that she was very worried about our finances. We had to file bankruptcy, and I think she thought we would end up homeless or something. We talked about it, and I explained all the things available to us later on—life insurance, social security, and so on, and that you don't lose your home when you file bankruptcy.

Some children appear on the surface to be doing well, but their thought processes and worry become apparent in covert ways. They might draw heartbreaking pictures of a sick family member or re-enact an illness with siblings or friends. Parents can gain useful insight into the child's mental health by observing these events, accepting them as normal under these circumstances, reassuring the child as much as possible, and providing counseling, if necessary.

Karen Parles (*http://www.lungcanceronline.org*) describes how she helped her children weather her illness:

> The most overwhelming concern I had after my diagnosis was how my illness would affect my two children who were then seven and eight years old. My overriding priority was to keep life as normal as possible for them.
>
> In order to accomplish this, my mother moved in with us temporarily to help out on the home front, my friends drove the kids to activities, and teachers kept an eye out for any signs of stress during school hours. We told the children that I had lung cancer, but that surgery and chemotherapy would get rid of it.

Still, there were some heartbreaking moments. My daughter would ask me why I couldn't be like the other mommies and participate in her school activities. I did my best to explain that the side effects of my treatment would be temporary, something I knew to be true. What I could not promise her was that I would survive, so I left that conversation for another time.

During chemo and after surgery, I spent hours lying on the couch in our den—my kids always knew where to find me. When they played outside, my son would periodically come back inside just to give me a kiss. I experienced the guilt of seeing them take on extra responsibility and worry because of my illness.

The most helpful thing that I did was to give them each a special journal. The kids wrote to me in their journals, sharing their thoughts and feelings. This turned out to be a valuable exercise for all of us.

Communicating needs to teenagers

This is a topic on which an entire book could be written.

An adolescent trying to break away from the family and become independent is likely to experience quite ambivalent feelings if a parent or grandparent is diagnosed with cancer. Just at the time in her life when she'd rather avoid talking to any adult, circumstances may force her to become very intimate and empathic with an older person she views as all-powerful. She must be patient and caring toward one of the people most likely to make her angry by holding her to high standards, enforcing rules, denying her privileges, or restricting her freedom. She might, for instance, replace experimenting with cigarettes with experimenting with alcohol out of fear of smoking. Conversely, if you were diagnosed with lung cancer but have never smoked, your child might begin smoking as a surrender to apparent hopelessness against this disease.

Some find that teens turn surly, or run amok when faced with the physical, emotional, and financial hardships associated with cancer. Some experts say that boys are more likely to act out anger and grief in violent ways than girls are.

Nonetheless, some people find that their adolescent children or grandchildren are extraordinary in their ability to comprehend what's needed and that they follow through with a maturity that's well beyond their years.

But, even more so than younger children, teens can appear to be knowledgeable and well adjusted when in fact they are not. This group often has a physical or intellectual maturity that is way beyond their level of emotional maturity.

A willingness to overlook unexplainable lapses, a keen awareness of such dangerous symptoms as excessive silence, and an honesty that is geared to their level of understanding is wise. Frequent offers to chat candidly are a good tactic. These offers confirm their belief that they can approach you about difficult subjects.

If you have a teen who's developing behaviors that are a danger to herself or others, such as smoking, drinking, acting out rage, violating laws, or considering dropping out of school, find a counselor who specializes in the adaptation of children to serious illness. Attempts to handle these problems by yourself might risk compounding your health problems, or might make of you a psychologically abused parent or grandparent—and these attempts might fail anyway. A teen may carry "cancer anger" formed during these especially rebellious years well into adulthood.

If you have a teen who's doing housework and assisting with medical care while continuing to carry his academic responsibilities, thank him at least daily.

Dealing with the healthy unaware

Almost every cancer survivor has had a verbal exchange with one of the "healthy unaware" that has left her angry, hurt, or speechless. Unlike questions from your doctor, which are intended to elicit useful information that can be used to plan your treatment and control side effects, often the casual acquaintance is just a little too curious or honestly uninformed.

What you choose to do or say to remarks like these depends on what consequences you're willing to endure. In most cases, the classic reply from Judith Martin (also known as Miss Manners), "Now, why would anyone say such a rude thing?" is right on the mark, but not always socially adroit.

In instances where consequences do matter, you might want to try one of the following replies. These responses are listed only as suggestions; there are no answers that are right for all settings and all personalities. Your style might be completely different, but it's sometimes helpful to know that these kinds of rude questions have been asked of others and that a few people have found comebacks that were satisfying to them. If someone asks you a rude or outlandish question, there's no rule that says you must be serious in return. Nor do you have to stretch to comfort the person who asks it, as if her discomfort with your illness were the most important issue:

- **The profound thought.** A deliberately obscure reply, perhaps quoting something in a foreign language that sounds impressive, but is meaningless. Latin is a good choice because so few people speak it anymore. How many people know, for instance, the CIA's motto, "Veritas vos Liberabit" ("The truth shall set you free")? They needn't know you're having fun at their expense. They'll just think that cancer has made you a better person, a deep thinker. And they're right, aren't they?

- **The escape.** "Gotta go! Time for my bungee-jumping lesson." You can, of course, substitute basket-weaving or yodelling lessons if you think this person might actually be a bungee jumper.

- **The sympathetic noise.** You can say, for example, "That's an interesting point of view," or "You appear to have given this a lot of thought." These replies give the other party's ego the attention she's trying to get without committing you to agreement, continued dialog, or revealing intimacy. They're also good transitional phrases for shifting the conversation to a less offensive subject.

- **The reckless handling of truth.** Miss Manners also says that those who ask nosy questions deserve to be lied to.

- **The mysterious telephone disconnection.** If you're being annoyed by someone on the phone, wait until you're doing the talking, then press the disconnect button. Nobody would ever suspect you of hanging up on yourself until it happens several times, after which they might take the hint.

If you prefer the head-on approach, here are a few of the most disturbing and least informed reactions that some lung cancer survivors have encountered, and a few suggested replies, factual or saucy:

Q: *Do you smoke?*
A: About 80 percent of lung cancers are linked to smoking. This means that, statistically, you can skip the nosy questions with four out of five lung cancer survivors you meet.
A: Smoking is linked to several other cancers besides lung cancer. Do you ask people who have had pancreatic, bladder, esophageal, kidney, or rectal cancer if they've smoked?

Q: *How long does your doctor say you have?*
A: Why? (Beady eye contact and flared nostrils.)
A: She says I'm still safe buying green bananas.

Q: *You look so bad/thin/pale/et cetera.*

A: Actually, I've gained ten pounds, my blood pressure is down fifteen points, and last weekend I walked in a six-kilometer race.

A: My, what a lovely smile you have! Are those your own teeth?

Q: *What happened to your beautiful hair?*

A: Oh, *this* hair. I borrowed it from a friend.

Q: *God doesn't give us anything we can't handle.*

A: My God is too kind to be that petty.

Q: *It seems like it always comes back.*

A: It's not possible to make accurate generalizations about lung cancers because there are several types and several stages.

Q: *You deserve what you got because you smoked.*

A: I'm sorry to alarm you, but life has a 100 percent mortality rate. This means that your turn will come, too.

Sources of support

Many professional sources of support exist for cancer patients and survivors. Here are some suggestions.

Cancer counselors

Anxiety and depression are very common among cancer patients and survivors. If you'd like someone to speak with about the many issues you're facing but you don't want to join a support group, perhaps you should consider a counselor who specializes in cancer survivorship issues. Often, these licensed specialists are themselves cancer survivors or have family members who are. They have useful experience with grieving for lost health, anxiety, insomnia, chronic pain, dealing with disappearing friends, unsympathetic bosses, children who are acting out, medical personnel who seem detached, and many of the other issues you might encounter when faced with lung cancer.

Support groups

It would be difficult to say too many good things about the effect of a support group on a lung cancer survivor. In addition to the personal testimonials from people who feel they found sanity, love, and knowledge from the members of their support groups, research by Dr. David Spiegel has shown that emotional support can extend the lives of some cancer survivors. Some support groups are not moderated by professional cancer counselors, but when they are, it can be a better experience than an unmoderated group.

Support groups are the one place outside of your inner circle of loved ones where you can ask or say just about anything. In some cases, you can ask help of supportive group members that you would be afraid to ask of family for fear of overburdening or frightening them. Moreover, the setting is sometimes freer than the family setting regarding candid speech because everyone present understands all too clearly what you're going through.

For some, support groups can be the difference, literally, between life and death. The opportunity to exchange information with those who have already weathered lung cancer can provide you with the knowledge to question your treatment and seek medical help elsewhere. Support groups are an immeasurably useful way to do this, bringing together a variety of skills, including medical and legal knowledge. A lung cancer survivor now advises others to look for opportunities to talk with others who have cancer:

> The pulmonary doctor put me into an exercise and pulmonary therapy group. In the group, people have a variety of things. Four people in my group have lung cancer. It functions as a support group. We spend the first 45 minutes in class or telling our stories and the next 45 minutes in exercise. Looking back, I wish had been in a support group. They are great.
>
> Now I know many people with cancer. I might meet them sitting around waiting for my turn in the CT scan or in my pulmonary therapy group. I just listen to their problems and their stories. It's the best thing people can do for each other.

Support groups are offered locally in many areas by groups such as Alliance for Lung Cancer Advocacy, Support, and Education (ALCASE), the American Cancer Society, the Wellness Community, Cancer Care, or local hospitals. If you have a personal computer, support groups are also available on the Internet.

Local, telephone, and Internet support groups have their advantages and disadvantages. Many people use several.

Lung cancer support

Please note that lung cancer patients and survivors face special support issues because of the impact of smoking on the development of some lung tumors. In practice, this means that you might not find the support you need in a general cancer support group. Cruel as it might seem, survivors of other cancers might be so lacking in empathy that they'll blame you for "causing your own disease." They might assume you're a smoker even if you've never smoked. If your prognosis is not so good, they might not want to hear you discuss end-of-life issues. They might berate you for "giving up," even if your road has been a long, difficult one and you're just facing the future realistically.

Consider a support group specifically for lung cancer survivors or a general support group that contains at least one other lung cancer survivor.

In-person support groups

Local support groups are useful for those who are able to get about easily, have access to a car, and enjoy face-to-face discussion, even about topics that might be upsetting. If you're in a local support group, you're likely to have a stream of visitors if you're hospitalized and friends to offer you instrumental support, such as help with groceries or babysitting. Often, members trade phone numbers and form deep friendships.

The disadvantages of local support groups are that they usually contain only a small number of people, perhaps ten or less, and meet only at certain times of the week or month. The smallness of the group can affect the quality of the information shared. For example, if no group member has traveled for care, you'll have to make your travel plans with less foreknowledge; if nobody else in the group has had lung cancer, you might feel even more isolated. Some members of local support groups report that they feel excluded when things take a turn for the worse, as if some group members want to shield themselves from the possibility that similar bad things may happen to them, too. This is less likely to happen, though, if the group is moderated by a trained therapist.

ALCASE maintains a list of in-person support groups—this is a great resource that is available at 1 (800) 298-2436 or on the web at *http://www.alcase.org*.

Internet support

Internet support groups offer several hundred friends available at all times of the day. You can communicate at three AM when you have insomnia, and you can communicate with other survivors, even if you have trouble getting around for various reasons.

The people you meet will be from all over the country and, in some cases, all over the world and represent a tremendous amount of experience. If you're a little shy about expressing emotion in front of other people, an Internet group is a good choice because you can write a message and read what you plan to say before you decide to send the message. If you need to cry, you can do so without feeling conflicted about crying in front of other people. If you want to avoid irrelevant or upsetting messages for a spell, you can delete them unread.

Many of the Internet support groups schedule in-person reunions and gatherings. Often, members form personal friendships and write private email or trade phone numbers to form even closer friendships. Sometimes members discover that they're living quite close by and become very good friends.

Karen Parles says:

> The most important thing I found on the Internet was not a web site, but an online lung cancer discussion group called LUNG-ONC (listserv. acor.org). Through LUNG-ONC, I was immediately able to connect with hundreds of people with lung cancer.
>
> This was invaluable. There is really no substitute for talking with other lung cancer survivors. LUNG-ONC enabled me to connect with other young mothers with whom I could share the particular heartache of raising small children while fighting lung cancer. During chemotherapy, I shared information on dealing with various side effects. I also learned that other patients often had answers to practical questions like where to buy a wig or what type of pillow to use after surgery. Prior to my pneumonectomy, I was able to communicate with several people who had undergone pneumonectomies themselves and to benefit from their experiences.
>
> I do not know where this type of support could be found other than on the Internet. There are very few in-person lung cancer support groups. LUNG-ONC is available 24 hours a day, 7 days a week—and there is no commute! LUNG-ONC makes me feel less isolated. Because of LUNG-ONC, I know that I am not the only 38-year-old nonsmoker on the planet with lung cancer.

The Association of Cancer Online Resources, Inc. (ACOR) offers many lung cancer Internet support groups. The number of members given is approximate at the time of writing and will vary over time. A convenient automatic subscription feature is available for ACOR Internet discussion groups at ACOR's site, *listserv.acor.org*.

- LUNG-ONC is an ACOR group offering medical discussion and emotional support for all lung cancer patients, survivors, and their loved ones. It has about 472 members.

- LUNG-BAC is an ACOR discussion group for those diagnosed with bronchioloalveolar carcinoma. It had 54 members as of October 2000.

- LUNG-NSCLC is an ACOR discussion group for those diagnosed with non-small cell lung cancer. It has 171 members.

- LUNG-SCLC is an ACOR discussion group for those diagnosed with small cell lung cancer. It had 97 members as of October 2000.

- Cancer-Pain (249 members), Cancer-Sexuality (160 members), Cancer-Fertility (83 members), Cancer-Fatigue (210 members), and Cancer-Depression (107 members) are ACOR discussion groups for those with cancer-related side effects, late effects, and long-term effects.

The chief disadvantage of an Internet support group is that the loss of a friend can be very difficult when you cannot say good-bye in person and have no photographs to remind you of them and no grave to visit. Sometimes group members simply will never hear again from another member and they never learn what really happened. Some group members deal with their grief by creating a memorial web page dedicated to a lost relative or friend, containing photos and examples of wisdom learned about living with lung cancer.

Other disadvantages of Internet support groups include cultural differences that cause mistaken communication and needless arguments, heavy mail volumes about topics you may feel don't pertain to your circumstances, incorrect medical information, a range of social and communication skills, strongly held opinions about smoking, and, of course, the cost of a personal computer and access to the Internet.

Employee assistance programs (EAPs)

Increasingly, employers are finding that it's to everyone's benefit if they offer formal assistance to employees who have special needs at difficult times. Employee assistance programs are designed to help the employee weather life changes and become happy and productive again. If your employer has an EAP, you should ask what it has to offer.

You should be aware, however, that if a health-related dispute over job performance goes to court, employers can subpoena any doctor's records, and so are given access to records that accumulate when you use an EAP. This includes material that most people assume is confidential, such as the notes a psychologist or social worker takes during a therapy session, even if they don't bear directly on your job performance.

If you're seeing a psychologist privately, your employer might not know that you are or who you're seeing. Clearly, this makes serving a subpoena more difficult. But if you use an EAP, the wolf is guarding the chickens, so to speak. In spite of safeguards that supposedly shield irrelevant material from nonprivileged eyes, your employer may become privy to information, for example, about a dependent child or a grandchild who began using alcohol or drugs after your diagnosis. These confidential documents also may be admitted as evidence into the permanent and public legal record, should you have a workplace dispute that is settled in court.[1]

Support organizations

The Alliance for Lung Cancer Advocacy, Support, and Education (ALCASE), in Vancouver, Washington, is the only national group dedicated to supporting people whose lives have been affected by lung cancer, offering various forms of support for lung cancer survivors, including support group meetings, buddy systems, wigs, lodging for out-of-town treatment, and help with quitting smoking. You can reach them by phone at (800) 298-2436 or on the Web at *http://www.alcase.org*.

Your church; local chapters of the Elks, Rotary, or Shriners; or other civic groups may be able to offer you various kinds of help, including transportation for treatment, financial assistance, or pitch-in efforts for lawn care and cooking. Moreover, an enormous collection of nonprofit organizations exists to help you in various ways. Groups for general needs, children's aid, young adults' aid, home care or temporary hospice care, and pain management can be found in Appendix A.

Quitting smoking

Quitting smoking is hard. If it were easy, almost everyone would already have quit, because of the abundance of well-publicized information about the dangers of smoking. The presence or absence of willpower, intellectual gifts, or emotional strength doesn't seem to make that much difference when trying to quit: nicotine is a stalwart enemy.

But if you still smoke, you should consider quitting.

If your lung cancer was diagnosed at an early stage and your treatment is considered successful, you can improve your chances of remaining free of lung cancer (and many other cancers) significantly by stopping smoking.

If you were diagnosed at a later stage and your doctor says the success of your treatment remains to be seen, quitting smoking will improve your quality of life by improving heart function and that of remaining healthy lung tissue.

Quitting smoking will make treatment easier and more effective by hastening healing after surgery; by improving liver, kidney, heart, and lung function; and by making more oxygen available to metabolize certain drugs or interact with radiotherapy, which requires oxygen in irradiated tissue to be effective.

Lung cancer and lung capacity are not the only good reasons to quit smoking. The following information is distilled from the publications of the NCI.

Cigarettes contain over 3,000 chemicals, of which 60 are known to be cancer-causing (carcinogenic). The toxins in tobacco products are known to contribute to the development of cancer in at least eight other organs besides the lung:

- Pancreas
- Bladder
- Kidney
- Esophagus
- Oral cavity
- Larynx
- Pharynx
- Uterine cervix (in females)
- Rectum and colon

Some evidence exists for the development of other cancers linked to tobacco-related toxins in the stomach, liver, and prostate.

Environmental tobacco smoke might be responsible for these cancers in nonsmoking bystanders:

- Breast
- Nasal sinus
- Bladder

- Uterine cervix (in daughters of women who smoke during pregnancy)
- Uterine cervix (in wives of men who smoke)

Larry Coffman describes quitting smoking:

> Smoking is one of the hardest habits to break. After all, nicotine is a more powerful drug than cocaine, and more addictive.
>
> I tried many times in my life to quit smoking, but it took the words "go home and get your affairs in order" to make me want to quit. I smoked my last cigarette just 24 hours before my chemotherapy and radiation were to begin.
>
> If it helps to write about it, then by all means do so. Try getting a little memo pad that you can carry around, when the urge strikes; you just write down what you are doing, who you are with, the kind of weather you're having, and anything except about smoking. It might get you past the urge and help a little.
>
> Man, oh man, to think that someone with lung cancer would keep on with the smoking habit, not to mention a loved one continuing . . . but I do understand how hard it is to stop.
>
> You have to really want to put them down for good in order to be successful. You can say "I want to quit" a dozen times a day, but until your mind catches up with your heart, you will be on that roller coaster. I know: I was on that coaster for many years.
>
> I went into treatment in January 1996. In February, three other people came into treatment with limited stage SCLC. They were still smoking. By June of 1996, I was the only one of the four still not smoking. In October of 1996, I was the only one still alive.
>
> I only know three things: four of four had limited stage SCLC, three of four smoked, and one of four survived. My best guess is that had they quit smoking, they MIGHT have survived.

Reading material about quitting smoking and information on organizations that can help you quit smoking are listed in Appendix A. A particularly good resource can be found at Quitnet, *http://www.quitnet.org*.

Summary

Your experience with lung cancer might be the most vulnerable, powerless experience of your life. Getting the support you need is critical to adequate recovery, especially during and after surgery, chemotherapy, or radiotherapy.

Key points to remember:

- ALCASE, the American Cancer Society, and the Wellness Community offer various forms of support for lung cancer survivors, including support group meetings, buddy systems, wigs, lodging for out-of-town treatment, and help with quitting smoking.

- Deal overtly with issues of blame about smoking. If the person you perceive as assigning blame is a medical care provider, make it clear that you will seek care elsewhere if her opinion seems to be interfering with your care. Ask caregivers to entertain whatever opinions they will, but to evaluate you as an entire person, not just a smoker, and to give you the support you need regardless of their opinions.

- If you still smoke, consider quitting. Your recovery from treatment will improve and your chances of developing a second lung tumor or any of several other cancers will decrease. An enormous amount of assistance is available for those who want to quit smoking. See Appendix A for a list of organizations that can help.

- Various studies have shown that anxiety and depression are common among cancer survivors. Consider seeking help from a cancer counselor if you're having trouble with incessant crying, loss of appetite, insomnia, or other symptoms of anxiety and depression.

CHAPTER 17

Finances, Employment, and Record Keeping

Financial ruin from medical bills is almost exclusively
an American disease.

—Roul Turley

RECOVERING YOUR HEALTH should be all that requires your stamina and concentration after being diagnosed with and treated for lung cancer. Unfortunately, the side effects of cancer go beyond the physical, impacting your social, professional, and financial well-being. If you're an American with lung cancer, you're likely to become an instant, but unwilling, expert on finances, insurance, and workplace issues.

You can ease the nonmedical aspects of your cancer experience in some ways. By becoming familiar with the somewhat harsh business side of cancer, following the progress of tobacco industry settlements, keeping careful records, and anticipating problems, you may avoid hospital billing convolutions, insurance payment denials, employment pitfalls, and financial degradation.

This chapter discusses some of the more common problems you may encounter, gives tips to avoid problems, and steers you to up-to-date resources that provide detailed solutions to these problems.

It is not the intent of this chapter to detail all issues concerning health insurance benefits; federal legislation, such as ERISA; Medicare and Medicaid coverage; unemployment insurance; and financial issues. The *Notes* and Appendix A, *Resources*, list many excellent books and other sources of information that much more thoroughly explore each of these topics. Some issues covered in this chapter, such as estate planning or declaring bankruptcy to protect your house and car, clearly require the aid of professionals, such as financial planners or tax attorneys.

Insurance issues

For lung cancer survivors, problems may arise with health insurance, unemployment insurance, or life insurance. Of these, health insurance is the most likely to cause heartache, frustration, and anger, but first, we'll discuss the main impediment to purchasing all kinds of health, life, disability, and care insurance: medical underwriting.

Restrictive medical underwriting

State and federal authorities have begun to address the problem of health insurance being denied to those with serious illnesses (see COBRA and HIPAA, discussed later in this section). Purchases of life, long-term care, and other insurance policies, though, are still impossible or expensive purchases for those with a cancer diagnosis.

The impediment is the medical examination or medical history questionnaire. If the policy is indeed offered to you after the actuaries have examined the statistics for your illness, it may be offered only with very high premiums. Moreover, employers who have no annual open enrollment period may refuse ever to insure you if you did not elect certain insurance options at time of hire, which is their only open enrollment period. The wife of a cancer survivor describes a frightening insurance problem:

> When my husband changed jobs, we decided to just add his name to my employer's medical policy in order to save money and have one provider. What we didn't realize was that his employer did not have annual "open enrollment"—so the only time he wouldn't be asked about his health was when he was hired.
>
> After he was diagnosed with cancer, I wanted to change jobs. By then, I'd heard horror stories about changing jobs and losing coverage because pre-existing conditions were excluded. I asked him to follow up with his employer to see if he could enroll for their medical insurance. They referred him to the policy's underwriters. (That should have given us a hint of what was to come.) "We will never insure you," they said. This meant I could never leave my job.
>
> Since then, his employer's policy has been renegotiated for more leniency, and federal laws have been passed to look after the medical insurance needs of people like us. But it was a bitter experience.

If your insurance needs are unmet, you should consider any offer that states that medical underwriting—insurance jargon for a close scrutiny of your health—is not necessary. Some advertisements state very clearly that a medical exam isn't necessary or that pre-existing conditions will not result in refusal. Some medical questionnaires for insurance enrollment ask health questions but do not mention cancer, not even in the section titled "Other." It's always worthwhile to ask for an application to see just how rigorous the medical scrutiny may be.

Of course, while most of these offers may be aboveboard, a proportion of these policies may be very expensive. The usual considerations for shopping wisely still apply, but if your insurance needs are great, or your estate planning justifies purchasing a whole-life policy that might bypass estate and inheritance taxes, for example, the additional cost may be worth it. Insurance companies are evaluated by A.M. Best, Moody's, and Standard and Poor. Choose only those with top ratings.

Health insurance

Cancer survivors in the US identify health insurance as a problematic issue more than any other issue except cancer itself. The delays and denials of managed care are the most common complaint, but other insurance issues also arise. Larry Coffman, five-year survivor of SCLC, is disappointed by healthcare coverage in the US:

> I haven't met an insurance company that I liked, or one that would pay out on the things that I thought that they should. Medicare did cover my annual exam and my one pair of bifocals, which helped greatly. An old saying, "When in doubt, check it out," holds true, especially for cancer patients/survivors. You cannot put a price tag on peace of mind.

If your medical insurance plan is in some way lacking, find out if your employer offers more than one medical insurance plan or holds an open enrollment each year. Open enrollment is the time period during which you may change plans without a medical examination or questionnaire; that is, without having your pre-existing health conditions held against you. Use the open enrollment period to upgrade to a better policy. Examine all plans closely for what they cover, especially for coverage of care given under the auspices of a clinical trial. Weigh an indemnity or preferred-provider plan, which may offer more access to more doctors for a higher price, against a high-coverage HMO requiring referrals and gatekeepers. The indemnity plan may cost more per doctor visit, but may provide you with the freedom to get care wherever *you* think best, without the delay of preapproval, including out-of-state care within a clinical trial or at a distant, but excellent, cancer center.

If you have been approved for Social Security Disability Income (SSDI, discussed later under "Disability income,") you'll be automatically enrolled in Medicare after getting disability benefits for two years. Moreover, Medicare coverage is free for 39 months after returning to work, if you're still disabled. If your income is low, your state may pay your Medicare premiums as part of Medicaid benefits. Contact your local Social Security Administration office for more information.

Take care when answering insurance company questions about "other insurance." The wife of a cancer survivor describes a frustrating problem with answering such questions:

> *When my husband changed jobs, we changed medical insurance plans, too, but his plan didn't provide dental insurance that was as good as I'd had, so I kept my previous dental plan through COBRA. His new medical insurance company sent us paperwork to fill out that contained a question about whether we had other insurance. I wrote in "yes," but noted that it was just dental insurance.*
>
> *Big mistake. For months afterward, until I dropped my dental coverage with the previous company, all of my claims for allergy shots, blood tests, and gynecology visits were denied on the premise that I had "other insurance" that ought to pay for these services. When I called the insurance company and held their feet to the fire, the customer service rep said, "To be honest with you, this is happening because your claims are processed by many different people, and some of them just don't bother to check for what your other insurance really is." Suppose they had denied my husband's claims for cancer surgery or chemotherapy?*

Losing medical insurance coverage if you change or lose jobs is still a problem, but less of a problem than before. In addition to various state laws, several federal laws exist to help you retain coverage. HIPAA, COBRA, and ERISA are enforced by the US Department of Labor Pension and Welfare Benefits Administration, (202) 219-8776.

- **HIPAA.** The Health Insurance Portability and Accountability Act of 1996 is a federal law intended to prohibit the permanent denial of medical coverage based on pre-existing conditions. HIPAA covers only employers with twenty or more employees. In general, it states that if you have had continuous medical insurance coverage for more than twelve months, your new medical insurance company cannot refuse to pay for medical care for your previous health problems. If your previous health coverage was for less than twelve months, each month you were covered reduces by one month the amount of time your new medical insurance company can refuse to pay for your previous health problems. No medical insurance company, however, can refuse to pay for your previous health problems for more than twelve months. There are loopholes in this law, though, that medical insurance companies might exploit. Some companies define a change of coverage from husband-and-wife to family coverage, for example, as a switch to a new plan, which could, in theory, restart the twelve-month clock. In July 1998, President Clinton issued a warning to insurance companies covering federal employees that such denials of payment will not be tolerated. Some states have older, stricter laws that resemble HIPAA, but provide better coverage. Call your state insurance commissioner for details.

- **COBRA.** The Consolidated Omnibus Budget Reconciliation Act of 1985 provides for a continuation of your old employer's medical insurance coverage for a *temporary* amount of time: from 18 to 39 months, depending on your circumstances. Always elect COBRA continuation coverage if you lose or change jobs until you're certain that your new employer's policy will cover expenses associated with your care. HIPAA, discussed above, does not always provide the continuous coverage the law intended because of its design and various loopholes.

- **ERISA.** The federal Employee Retirement Income Security Act of 1974 was a piece of legislation intended to safeguard employee pension rights, but it also has impacted employee health insurance. Self-insured employers are governed by ERISA in ways that can override state laws. Large, self-insured employers may hire a medical insurance company, such as Blue Cross, to administer their plan, so the insurance forms you receive might contain the insurance company's letterhead, but your employer is bearing the exact and full cost of your care at the time it is incurred instead of paying large indemnity premiums in advance. Owing to the overlap of state and ERISA regulations, self-insured employers cannot be sued in state courts for failing to pay claims. For this and other reasons, disputes about health insurance claims with self-insured employers can become very complex and may require the assistance of an attorney.

Most states have insurance pools known as CHIPS, comprehensive health insurance plans, for those who cannot get coverage through typical channels. Contact your state insurance commissioner for more information.

Ask about group health insurance policies that might be available through civil and community groups, fraternal organizations, professional groups, churches, or your union.

Medicare and Medicaid

Medicare is not just government-supplied medical insurance for those over age 65. If you have been entitled to Social Security Disability (SSDI) benefits for the past two years, you are eligible for Medicare.

Although Medicare Parts A and B are the most well known of the Medicare plans, much fuller (and more expensive) coverage may be provided by purchasing Medicare Supplemental Insurance, often called MediGap insurance. Ten versions of MediGap insurance are available, identified as A through J, with J providing the highest coverage and costing the most.

Medicaid is a health payment program for the financially needy that is run jointly by the federal government and each state government. As such, its rules and benefits vary greatly, depending on where you live. Examples of those who may qualify are recipients of Aid to Families with Dependent Children (AFDC), those receiving the Social Security's Administration's Supplemental Security Income (SSI), or certain nursing home patients.

For more information on either Medicare or Medicaid, see J. Robert Treanor's *Mercer Guide to Social Security and Medicare*, which is published yearly and is readily accessible in libraries and bookstores.

Unemployment insurance

Always apply for unemployment insurance if you lose your job, are laid off, or have your hours substantially reduced. Never assume that you're not eligible. Apply even if you have a suit pending for wrongful discharge.

Unemployment law and the granting and calculation of benefits are very complex and vary from state to state. In order to find information that's appropriate for your circumstances, you'll need to research the laws for your state, either on your own or with an attorney who specializes in these cases.

Life insurance

Life insurance that you buy as an individual is likely to be terribly expensive, if at all available, once you have had cancer. As mentioned earlier in the section called "Restrictive medical underwriting," if you have an opportunity to buy a good life insurance policy at a reasonable rate without a qualifying medical examination or other penalty for having a cancer diagnosis, consider the opportunity carefully.

Some employers offer life insurance policies requiring no medical exam with face values in multiples of one's annual salary. Although this usually is term coverage instead of whole life coverage, it may meet your family's needs very well. Some such policies can be kept even if you leave the company.

Whole-life policies often can be borrowed against, or sold in a viatical arrangement to a company that will buy your policy from you at less than its face value to provide you with money now. This option is useful if your heirs don't need your money, but you do, to pay current bills. Generally, viatical settlements require proof of terminal illness.

Check your existing life insurance policies for a clause that states you needn't pay premiums if you're receiving disability benefits.

Long-term care insurance

Now, more than ever, you should consider a long-term care policy as a safeguard against financially crippling nursing-home or nursing-care costs. As with life insurance policies discussed above, however, you're not likely to be able to find or afford a long-term care policy once having had a cancer diagnosis, unless one is offered at group rates with no medical examination required.

One very good option is to ask your children and their spouses if their employers offer such a policy for parents or in-laws as well as employees. This recent trend in employment benefits offerings is an attempt to recognize the increasing responsibilities that families face in caring for their older relatives while trying to work outside the home.

Many long-term care policies are eventually dropped by the client because they are so expensive, and the probability of needing long-term care seems so far away. If expense is an issue for you, you might choose a policy that has a clause that allows you to stop paying premiums after a number of years in return for lower benefits or payments over a shorter time. This compromise, while not ideal, will afford you at least some protection against potentially devastating long-term care costs.

Long-term disability insurance

Long-term disability insurance is a must for lung cancer survivors who would be producing income and supporting a household if they were entirely healthy. If you don't have a long-term disability insurance policy, it's wise to consider buying one.

Employers often offer long-term disability insurance at reduced rates or for free. If you can elect or purchase such a policy, do so. Although the Social Security Administration can pay you long-term disability under some conditions, often it's temporary, and frequently policies available in the private sector pay a better monthly benefit.

Note that most long-term disability policies encourage you to apply for SSDI, and then pay you only the difference between SSA's monthly benefit and the higher benefit your policy authorizes.

Some long-term disability policies can be taken with you if you leave your employer. Choose only a policy marked "guaranteed renewable" so that your policy cannot be canceled if your health gets worse.

Tobacco industry settlements

Momentum is building to force the tobacco industry to bear the health costs of nicotine addiction. Over 40 states have sued tobacco manufacturers for compensation of health-related expenses.

Larry Coffman, five-year survivor of SCLC, says:

> I have always declared that I would not involve myself with the fight against the tobacco industry unless they were proven to have manipulated the nicotine levels. Bingo! The proof is in the pudding, so to speak.
>
> I have since become an advocate for the reinstatement of the tobacco illness and disease benefits for our veterans, based on the tobacco industry documents.

Contact your state's attorney general or your state health commissioner to determine whether your health costs can be offset by a share of an amount awarded by the courts.

The National Association of Attorneys General (NAAG) works to establish policy and maintains current information regarding tobacco settlements. Contact information about the NAAG can be found in Appendix A in the section "Legal, financial, and insurance resources."

Financial issues

In general, financial issues cannot be addressed adequately in one chapter of a medical consumer's book. Nonetheless, a few issues are discussed in this section to inform you, rather than advise you, about problems you may encounter.

Major points

Here's an encapsulation of some fairly prominent issues:

- Air travel for cancer patients and their families can be free. Organizations that can help with travel costs are described in Appendix A.

- It may be worthwhile to refinance your home mortgage for a lower interest rate. If the current market rate for mortgages is significantly lower than yours, refinancing may reduce monthly payments, increase equity more rapidly, and ultimately reduce debt.

- Contact the Social Security Administration to see if you, your spouse, or your children are eligible for Supplemental Security Income. They can be reached by phone at (800) 772-1213 or on the web at *http://www.ssa.gov*. (SSI differs from SSDI, Social Security Disability Income.)

- Fundraising in your community or your place of employment can be a very effective way to address debts related to medical care. The Organ Transplant Fund, for example, provides sound help with raising funds for organ transplantation. See Appendix A for a list of other organizations that can help with financial issues.

- Estate planning always should be considered, even for seemingly small estates. Some options, such as a supportive care trust or purchase of a whole-life insurance policy, may preserve some assets for yourself, your spouse, or your children—but may interfere seriously with your eligibility for Medicare. Estate planning is especially important if your spouse or a child has serious health problems of his own, requiring long-term financial support.

- A debt consolidation or home equity loan may be a useful device for reducing debt.

Bankruptcy

The two leading reasons for declaring bankruptcy are excessive medical expenses and credit card debt.

Declaring bankruptcy has changed from a last-ditch, unethical, and humiliating way to escape obligation to an honorable, if humble, effort to restructure or reschedule debt payment. Of the three forms of bankruptcy that individuals (as opposed to businesses and farmers) may use, only one, Chapter 7 bankruptcy, discharges the debtor of all debt. The others, Chapters 11 and 13, provide for a repayment plan in an hierarchical and agreed-upon way, eliminating or postponing foreclosure on your home or repossession of your car. Once you have declared bankruptcy, your creditors are forbidden by law from harassing or suing you.

Declaring bankruptcy still should be close to your last resort for solving financial problems and should always be done under the guidance of a professional financial advisor or bankruptcy attorney.

Disability income

Several means are available to replace your income while you are disabled.

Social Security Disability Income (SSDI)

The Social Security Administration may grant disability benefits under the Social Security Disability Income (SSDI) plan to replace lost income for an adult or to provide assistance with caring for a child with lung cancer.

To smooth the process of applying for Social Security Disability Income, take all medical records with you and let your doctors know you're applying, because they will need to give evidence.

If SSDI is denied—and frequently it is denied on the first application—ask for Publication No. 05-10041, "The Appeals Process." Sometimes just a request to have your case reviewed by the SSA's physicians will speed an approval.

In some cases, it's possible to return to work and continue to collect SSDI benefits. This is possible because of special incentives the SSA provides to rehabilitate the disabled. The formula used to compute disability benefits while working is complex, but in general, you may attempt a trial work period of nine months, not necessarily consecutively, during which benefits are unchanged. If the trial does not succeed, benefits may continue. Ask the SSA for the publication called "Working While Disabled . . . How We Can Help" (Pub. No. 05-10095).

Military (VA) disability income

If you served in Southeast Asia during the Vietnam War and were stationed in or near areas known to be exposed to the herbicide Agent Orange, your subsequent development of lung, bronchial, laryngeal, or tracheal cancer is considered by the Veterans Administration to be related to dioxin exposure. (Dioxin is a contaminant of Agent Orange.) You will likely be eligible for temporary, permanent, full, or partial VA disability income benefits. If you pass away, your surviving wife or dependent children might be eligible for benefits.

Benefits will be retroactive to your date of first treatment and will continue as long as any long-term side effect of treatment is present. Such effects might include diminished lung capacity from surgery or radiotherapy, residual neural damage from chemotherapy, or intractable fatigue that interferes with your ability to work.

Note that if you refuse veteran's disability benefits from a sense of pride, it will be almost impossible to reopen your claim later. For instance, if you suffer a heart attack years after being treated with radiotherapy and your doctors are convinced your heart was damaged by this cancer treatment, you will not be permitted by the VA to reopen your case and collect benefits. Because damage from cancer treatment—particularly radiotherapy—may develop years after it's administered, it's best not to refuse a VA settlement if it's offered, no matter how well you feel nor how able to work you might be.

Note as well that you can receive partial VA disability benefits while working full-time.

The wife of a US Army veteran exposed to dioxin in Southeast Asia tells about filing for benefits with the Veterans Administration Agent Orange Program:

> When my husband was diagnosed with cancer, we filed a claim with the VA's Agent Orange program, even though we knew they were not covering his type of cancer at that time. It was a matter of principle. We wanted to be a statistic to catch their attention.
>
> A few years later, the VA broadened its decision and determined that my husband's cancer was related to Agent Orange exposure. They contacted us, and he received a retroactive payment for one year of full disability. He now receives monthly checks for being, by their ruling, still about 30 percent disabled.

Lung cancer is not the only cancer considered by the VA to be associated with dioxin exposure. Lymphoma, myeloma, soft tissue sarcoma, and several noncancer diseases are also compensable. For the most current information about Agent Orange compensation for lung and other cancers, call the Veterans Administration at (800) 827-1000 or visit their web site at *http://www.va.gov/pressrel/99fsao.htm*

Employment issues

Having and being treated for lung cancer can disrupt your job attendance and performance. If you're very lucky, you'll have managers and coworkers who accommodate your ups and downs, perhaps holding fundraisers for you or donating their own unused sick or vacation time for your use. Many of us are not this fortunate.

Protection under the law

As with finance and insurance issues, an employee has certain protections under the law. Verify the details of these laws because they may change over time:

- The Americans with Disabilities Act (ADA) recognizes cancer as a temporary or permanent disability for which you cannot be penalized by demotion or dismissal. It's also illegal to deny a qualified candidate a job simply because of a disability, but it's difficult to prove this kind of discrimination unless you know every other job applicant and all of their qualifications intimately. Call (800) 669-4000 or visit *http://www.usdoj.gov/crt/ada.html*.

- The Federal Rehabilitation Act, enforced by Department of Justice Civil Rights Division ((202) 514-4609), covers some people not covered by the ADA:

  - Employees of the executive branch of the federal government

  - Employees of employers who have federal contracts or receive federal assistance and have fewer than fifteen employees

- The 1993 Family and Medical Leave Act (FMLA) guarantees to those who have worked 25 hours per week for one year the right to twelve weeks of leave annually, either for one's own healthcare or to attend to a sick family member. You must give 30 days' prior notice. During these twelve weeks, your job or a similar one must be held open for you and your benefits must be maintained. The FMLA applies only to companies with 50 or more employees within a 75-mile radius. Violations of this law should be reported to the US Department of Labor.

Getting a job

If you're a cancer survivor, the rules might change when you try to get a new job. The protections in place for current employees can be sidestepped by employers who are afraid of hiring a cancer survivor. Here are some recommendations:

- Work with a job counselor to prepare a resume and practice interview skills.

- Choose a large employer over a small company because their larger pool of employees will tend to absorb any additional health insurance costs they incur to cover you. Moreover, some federal antidiscrimination laws do not apply to small employers.

- Do not volunteer information about your cancer history during an interview. Your ability to do the job should be the focus of the prospective employer's questions. Do not lie if asked about your health—instead, attempt to redirect the focus of questions or suggest that personal questions are inappropriate (and then reconsider working for someone who asks nosy questions).

- Under the ADA, employers cannot ask about your medical history or require you to take medical tests unless they have offered you a job.

- Some guides suggest that you not ask about health insurance until you're offered a job, but if you have highly sought job skills, good health insurance might be considered an enticement, and asking would not be inappropriate.

- Visit the US EEOC web site at *http://www.eeoc.gov* for tips about finding a job and addressing health-related discrimination incidents.

Record keeping

The value of record keeping cannot be overemphasized. Having evidence in writing of your position is indispensable, should disputes or questions arise. You should obtain records for all treatment, employment, and financial circumstances and keep them in some organized way and in a place safe from fire, theft, or flood.

Karen Parles was diagnosed in her thirties with NSCLC. Karen created Lung Cancer Online (*http://www.lungcanceronline.org*). She describes how frustrating the business side of cancer can be:

> *One aspect of living with cancer that I find to be an ongoing source of stress is the time and effort involved in managing the logistics of medical*

care. There is a seemingly endless amount of administrative detail and financial insecurity brought on by the vagaries of a difficult health insurance system.

My husband and I learned to be our own advocates and to not take anything for granted. We always called ahead before appointments to confirm that all tests and paperwork were in order. We got copies of every test, every doctor's note, every financial document, and put them into a green notebook that my husband always carried with him. We put copies of scans and x-rays into an artist's portfolio. We often used the green notebook for reference during appointments. In fact, our doctors came to rely on our green notebook for information that had not yet made it into my chart! In the end, the notebook proved to be an effective organizational tool that saved us hours of time and aggravation.

Biopsy samples

A new and very important concern you should address is the permanent storage of your biopsy tissue samples. Because of the development of new treatment technologies, such as monoclonal antibodies and tumor-derived vaccines, your biopsy samples may be needed years after they are removed from your body.

Yet some hospitals limit storage time for such samples because their storage resources are finite. This means that, lacking instructions otherwise, they may discard your tissue samples after a number of years.

Ask the hospital to keep your samples forever. If they are not able to do so, make arrangements to store the samples elsewhere.

Establish a record trail

Simple though it may sound, getting copies of all medical information, including films, and getting written copies of all tangential records related to employment, insurance, and finance are sometimes overlooked. Here are some tips for obtaining records:

- Request and keep copies of all medical records and bills as you go through diagnosis and treatment. This will establish with the doctor's staff your expectations, set a tone of efficiency, and will permit you instant access to material if you need it for second opinions. Having copies made and mailed after the fact can add five or more days, even weeks, to the time you need to collect records.

- If you're requesting records that must in turn be forwarded to another health center, make a copy for yourself before forwarding the material.

- When you're hospitalized, or if your treatments are done in the hospital on an outpatient basis, ask for itemized copies of bills. General or summarized hospital bills can be astonishingly obtuse, and even an itemized bill can be unclear. Most errors in hospital billing are found only by using an itemized bill's relative clarity.

- Always address financial, employment, or insurance disputes in writing, and keep a copy of what you've written.

- Keep a detailed phone log of all calls made to insurance companies, mortgage companies, and so on.

- Any decision reached verbally to correct errors should be followed by a written confirmation from the company. Ask for this confirmation, and if they won't furnish a written reply, write your own reply, stating, "Based on our phone conversation, it is my understanding that the following will happen," listing what you perceive to be true.

- Keep a calendar of appointments. Do not discard it at the end of the year. Keep it as a permanent part of your medical and financial files.

- If space permits, your calendar can double as a log for phone calls, changes in medications or symptoms, blood results, and so on. Otherwise, school exercise books or blank journals, the kind from which pages cannot easily be torn, may serve well.

- Record outgoing correspondence. Send all correspondence that's even remotely important by certified mail, using the return receipt option. Unlike registered mail, which is logged at each stop in the postal system, certified mail does not travel more slowly than regular mail and isn't much more expensive than regular mail. When the return receipt arrives, staple it to your copy of the correspondence: it is your proof that the mail arrived at its destination. Use fax transmission for speed when needed, but follow up with certified mail. An example of an appropriate use for certified mail is correspondence with an insurance company that requires 30 days' advance notice in order to review and approve treatment plans.

- Have copies of all original endoscopy, CT, or MRI films, or digital imaging made for your own files if at all possible. While copies of the reports that describe and analyze these images are useful, a doctor's access to source films or digital images is mandatory for certain kinds of review and decision-making.

- If the original endoscopy, CT, or MRI films are loaned to other doctors for second opinions, follow up to be sure they are returned to the central library or original office. (Digital images, while easily transmitted to other medical facilities, are not as easily lost as films are because the original data generally are kept on the computer that first recorded the data.)

Larry Coffman has accumulated his medical records:

> *Most physicians will provide you with a copy of your records, although a fee could be charged. This fee is usually the expense of making copies.*
>
> *I typed a letter to each physician and the hospital that I had dealt with. I requested a full copy of my records and said that I would be happy to pay the fee, if applicable, when I picked them up. I requested them in order to update and maintain my medical history files at home. I didn't have a problem getting them.*

Organizing the record trail

How little or how much you choose to organize will depend in some measure on how well you feel, how much energy you have remaining, and your record-keeping habits in general. Don't be surprised if you find yourself, normally a well-organized person, suddenly without the health or energy to file medical reimbursement forms. Others, though, may find that they become more organized as a coping mechanism.

You may find that record-keeping is a task you can delegate to a family member, friend, or neighbor who would love to help you, but doesn't know quite what to offer. Although you may not care to have someone outside your family making phone calls to correct billing mistakes, having someone sort and file bills and receipts on a weekly basis may help you. Sorting mail into stacks for filing is a task that a child might enjoy; scanning and storing documents on a PC might be something that a computer-literate relative might want to do.

Whatever method suits your current needs, do attempt at the very least to store medical and payment records in some way. A minimal technique is to put all records in one place, such as in one or more grocery bags, in case you need access to them in a hurry. If you or your volunteers have the time and energy to do so, you may lean toward a fairly elaborate system of organization that gives you instant access to items by topic, health center, or date.

Summary

There may be the rare person with lung cancer who relishes a payment challenge from stubborn insurance companies or the character-building experience of financial hardship, but most of us facing these issues, along with poor health, may begin to feel overwhelmed.

This chapter attempts to highlight the most important, most potentially damaging of these issues and supplies many references for finding the best and most current information.

Before making irrevocable decisions or expensive purchases, please consider consulting professionals who are familiar with recent changes in the various laws that govern insurance, employment, and finances.

CHAPTER 18

After Treatment Ends

Remember to cure the patient as well as the disease.

—Alvan Barach

YOUR CANCER EXPERIENCE DOESN'T END as the door closes behind you when you leave the clinic. Most likely, normalcy will creep up on you in the months that follow. Some lung cancer survivors are surprised to find that the end of treatment brings a variety of new concerns and plans. A contradictory mixture of feelings, a changed relationship with the oncologist, perhaps a renewed immersion in one's job, a reassessment of long-range plans, a different physical self—temporarily or permanently—and different behaviors on the part of friends and loved ones all may come about.

This chapter will discuss the emotional and practical aspects of the end of treatment. We will share with you what others have found difficult, surprising, or exhilarating. First, we will outline the physical and medical aspects related to facing ahead at the end of treatment, followed by the emotional aspects, and finishing with the social and professional aspects of adjusting after treatment ends.

In some cases, of course, these concerns overlap. For example, it's difficult not to have an emotional reaction to either upsetting or loving things that happen in the workplace, to ambiguous test results, or to the realization that you might require oxygen support, for instance, for many months.

Kathleen Houlihan, a survivor of NSCLC, tells about her anticipation of a happier future:

> It's wonderful to be home. When we first got to the Cancer Treatment Center seven weeks ago, I didn't want to leave the building. I felt safe in there, and I couldn't imagine going home. But the last week or two, as I got better and better, I started looking forward to leaving. Now I'm thrilled to be home, with our friends, our "animules," and our kitchen, where I can make all my health foods and power drinks. There's no place like it.

The chest x-ray I had before I left showed the tumor has shrunk down to about the size of a lemon, after starting out looking to me like a tennis ball. And the doctors say it will continue to shrink over the next four to six weeks. I guess there will always be something there, but presumably all the cancer cells will be dead, and what remains will be basically scar tissue. The pulmonologist said the radiation should kill 98–99.9 percent of the cancer cells, and the chemo I'll have over the next five months is intended to kill off the rest. So everything looks good at this point.

Since there is a high recurrence rate for lung cancer, they want me to return for checkups every three months for three years after I finish the chemo. Then every six months for two more years, and then once a year after that. I believe the checkups will all include MRI, CT scans, and bone scans. Thank goodness for insurance!

We're just trying to get the house back in shape and get back into a routine. Actually, my husband Holt is doing most of the work around here. I'm just trying to take care of myself, and he helps me with that, too. But I'm feeling better every day. It's great to be through with the radiation. It really was tiring. Now I'm napping just once a day. Today I didn't nap at all, but I think I'll go to bed early.

Medical monitoring

Fifteen or twenty years ago, doctors and patients had few choices for verifying that cancer had gone away and was staying away. Now there are blood tests and imaging tools that allow a view—often just a glimpse—of what's going on inside one's body.

These testing tools are both a blessing and a curse. It's true that now we can follow the progression and regression of tumors much more clearly. There are, however, instances of both false positives and false negatives from imaging studies that can only be evaluated accurately within the framework provided by additional testing or a second biopsy.

Follow-up tests

All patients treated for lung cancer need follow-up surveillance for recurrent disease or the development of second cancers. As you finish your treatment, your doctor will discuss when to return for follow-up visits. Ask your doctor about the type and timing of these tests, which vary, depending on individual factors, such as the type of lung cancer you had and what organs were affected. Follow-up visits most likely will include a physical examination, a discussion period for you and your doctor to share concerns, and a series of tests to confirm that you are disease-free.

Kathleen Houlihan describes her follow-up testing and the continued support she's receiving from health professionals:

> During my follow-up visit last week I had my port "accessed" and blood drawn at the infusion center that night, followed by a chest x-ray and CT scan and appointment with the radiation oncologist Wednesday morning. My left shoulder is just now getting stiff from the radiation I had all those months ago, but stretching exercises and massage should correct the problem.
>
> Then we saw my main doctor, the medical oncologist who went over the films. The tumor has shrunk a lot even since last October! Great news. Looks like there's very little of it remaining. And the CEA tumor marker is still well in the normal range at 1.7. Couldn't be better! We also saw my pulmonologist, who agreed I was doing well, but who reminded me I'm at high risk for a recurrence, as well as for another primary lung cancer. That's the reason for frequent checkups, including the bronchoscopy he did the following morning, after which he said my bronchi looked "clean as a whistle!" After the bronchoscopy Friday morning, we had lunch and then I rested, recovering from the light anesthesia, while my husband Holt ran errands and loaded the car.
>
> On Thursday afternoon, I saw my naturopathic doctor and reviewed my diet and supplements and the various tests we're going to do now to see if I need any detox or whatever. That was followed by a visit to the physical therapist for my shoulder.
>
> I forgot to mention the nutrition class Thursday morning, given by Dr. Patrick Quillan, author of the book "Beating Cancer with Nutrition." Dr. Quillan developed the nutrition program in Tulsa and appears in the weekly nutrition class about once a month.

Sometimes tests and imaging studies are delayed until a few months after the end of treatment because radiotherapy and many anticancer agents continue to have a tumor-killing effect for several months after they're used. Thereafter, imaging studies, x-rays, bronchoscopy, or blood tests may be repeated every three months for a number of years, then every six months for a number of years, then once a year for a number of years, then every few years. These tests might also be performed after surgery, but before radiotherapy, and so on, to assess which treatments are working and to aid in changing the treatment plan, if need be.

A male survivor of lung cancer describes his testing and the long-term effects of his treatment:

> I get a CT scan every three months. Last two scans have shown me in remission. I'm still dealing with shortness of breath and fatigue.

Kathleen describes some new tests she feels she was fortunate to have:

> We're back from the trip to Tulsa for my checkup. I had a newfangled procedure called a NeoTect scan instead of a CT scan this time. My pulmonologist, who ordered this scan, says it's a "poor person's PET scan." It is supposed to detect malignant lung masses, but apparently it also detects inflammation. My scan detected "something" at the original tumor site and in the mediastinum, the area between the lungs. So what is it, malignancy or inflammation? Because I'm doing so well, with no other symptoms, and because the areas in question are within the field that was radiated, my pulmonologist and my medical oncologist both think that the scan is showing inflammation from the radiation treatment last year. I guess the only other diagnostic procedure that could address this question would be a PET scan, which is very expensive and apparently not indicated at this point. So we'll just wait and see. I'll have all the scans (CT of chest and abdomen, bone, and brain) at my next three-month checkup in October, and we'll see what they show. Hopefully they will all be clear. My tumor marker (CEA) was even lower than it has been, at 1.2 (normal is less than 3), which is more reason to think the scan was not showing any malignancy, so I'm not too worried about it. It would have been nice if the scan had been clear, though.

Kathleen had also read about another test, which her insurance covers, which she took for peace of mind:

> Today we got the best news we've had in a year and a half—the results of my latest cancer test came back normal! It's called the AMAS test, for Anti-Malignin Antibody in Serum (http://www.amascancertest.com). The claim is that all cancer cells produce the malignin antigen, and this test measures antibodies to that antigen in the blood, thereby detecting cancer up to eighteen months sooner than any imaging studies. So my

local doctor (a friend of ours) drew blood on Tuesday, and my husband Holt worked it up in his office (let it sit for a half hour to coagulate, then let it sit for an hour in the fridge, then spin it down in the centrifuge, then pack it in dry ice) to send via FedEx to the lab in Boston that is the only place that does the test.

The test was developed by Dr. and Dr. Bogoch, who also did all the research on it, and it's their lab that does the test. I read about it in several books on alternative approaches to cancer. I guess the test is not widely known or accepted because it is proprietary and only done at that one lab. But the research looks good to me and, more importantly, to Holt, my husband, the doctor. It's supposed to be 99 percent accurate. And mine came back normal! We take that to mean that I don't have any malignin antigens in my blood, which should mean I don't have any cancer cells in my body.

If all this is correct (please, God), I think this test is more meaningful than CT scans, brain MRIs, and the like. Just because they don't detect any cancer doesn't mean that it's not there in as-yet undetectable amounts. It seems that this simple $135 test (which my insurance covers, as does Medicare), plus FedEx shipping, should be able to replace all those other costly, uncomfortable, radiation-laden tests that are used every few months for monitoring cancer patients. I guess I don't have quite enough confidence in the AMAS test yet to abandon all those others, but I sure like it (with these results) as a supplementary measure.

It's possible to have questionable liver lesions appear on imaging studies after certain chemotherapies, or to have suspicious lung spots appear after irradiation of the chest. These phenomena can mimic relapse or spread of disease (metastasis), but PET scanning or biopsy may prove that these are not disease.

Many oncologists who treat lung cancer consider five years of cancer-free survival to be the equivalent of a cure.

Regardless of the schedule of your follow-up visits, new or returning symptoms must be taken seriously and reported to your doctor immediately. Never assume that your doctor will think that you're worrying too much. It's always better to err by communicating too much instead of too little when it comes to aftercare.

Regression of symptoms and side effects

In general, the lingering side effects and delayed effects you may have experienced during treatment should fade away in the months following treatment. Certain side effects may take much longer to regress, though. Difficulty breathing, pain, or weakness may linger for weeks, months, or years. Fatigue often continues for years after treatment. Blood counts can remain low, or low-normal, for months or years after treatment. See Chapter 13, *Adverse Effects of Treatment*.

If you had chemotherapy and lost some or all of your hair, you might notice as it regrows that it's a different color, a different texture, thicker, thinner, curlier, or straighter than it was before treatment. These changes are temporary. If you received radiotherapy to the brain, patches of hair lost might not regrow.

Kathleen Houlihan describes the return of her hair:

> I have had two haircuts recently, one in December and one last week. By mid-December, I had a very thin covering of hair all over my head, but it was messy—all different lengths—some had never fallen out but most had and came back in at different times. So I had a "cut," which took no time at all, but made it look neat and almost intentional. By now, I definitely have hair, even enough to comb and to run my fingers through.
>
> I had another "cut" last week and had it "pixied up," and I have now quit wearing scarves. It's still extremely short, but it doesn't look bad. In fact, I've been getting compliments on it. They've all been from people who know what's going on, but they're still compliments! It remains to be seen whether it will turn curly, as is so often the case, or not. There does seem to be a hint of wave in it even now!

Some time later, Kathleen is pleased about the curls in her hair when it was first growing in:

> A brief update on my hair. It came in curly! Lots of beautiful curls. It's short, so I just wash it, comb it back, put a little gel on it, and it looks great. However, I had it cut last week, and most of the curls are gone. It's reverting back to being straight. All good things must come to an end, I guess. My husband Holt says maybe I should go back for another round of chemotherapy, but I'm not that desperate for curls!

Venous catheter removal

Many people can't wait to have their central venous catheter removed; others prefer to keep it for a while as a talisman against relapse.

Kathleen Houlihan tells of her experience:

> It's gone! I went back to the Cancer Treatment Centers of America for my six-month check-up, six months since the end of chemo, and not only were all the scans clear, but the tumor is gone. It has shrunk down to a scar. In the October and February CT scans, it was stable at 2.5 centimeters, but this time the radiologist says it's not measurable. Neither my husband Holt nor I were expecting this. We both thought I would always have a mass of some size there, and we were just hoping it would be dead scar tissue. But now it's just a scar. It couldn't be better. Of course, it still could come back, but at this point, I'm going to believe I'm cured. The radiologist said it must have been the pilgrimage I made! When pressed about why it continued to shrink after it apparently had leveled off at 2.5 centimeters, he said the radiation can have an effect for quite some time. But I think it was either the pilgrimage or the $200 of MGN-3, a super antioxidant, that I took in February. Those were the only two additions to my program since the February CT scan.
>
> And my port is gone, too. I asked the doctor when he thought I could have it removed. Since the tumor is gone and I'm doing so well, he said I could have it out now. So at about noon the next day (Friday), I had the port removed, in the OR, under local anesthesia. The procedure took sixteen minutes and wasn't bad at all. Holt was shocked when I walked out of the OR to find him in the surgery waiting room.

If your stage and type of lung cancer entail an increased risk of recurrence of disease, it might be wise to consider keeping your catheter, especially if additional surgeries with general anesthesia are required to remove it and reinstall it. Weigh the wisdom of keeping it to avoid extra surgery, should it need to be reimplanted, against the inconvenience of keeping it clean, and the increased risk of infection it may entail.

Emotional responses

Almost everyone looks forward to finishing treatment with feelings of joy, relief, and celebration. Indeed, there are reasons to feel joyous and celebratory. Side effects will diminish, energy will return, expectations of freedom from disease are cherished, and life will begin to return to normal.

Larry Coffman, five-year survivor of SCLC, is ready to live:

> The emotional scars are the worst for cancer patients, in my opinion. The discomfort of the treatment side effects fade rather quickly, but the emotions that one experiences during that period remain for many, many years.
>
> I have never asked "why me?" because it doesn't matter. I enjoy talking to and hugging my kids, watching the flowers bloom in the spring, and the misty rain that falls from time to time. I have adjusted my lifestyle to my condition and am thankful for each and every new day that I see. I concentrate on the positive aspects of my position.

Kathleen Houlihan describes her joy when finishing chemo:

> I'm mostly recovered from my last round of chemo! I spent an extra day there doing all "the scans"—brain MRI, bone scan, and CT scan of the chest and abdomen, as well as a chest x-ray and the usual blood work. Everything looks good! My CEA is still in the normal range at 1.5. The original tumor has shrunk down to 2.5×3 centimeters (from 7×8 centimeters), and is presumably all dead scar tissue by now. The CT scan showed a new spot behind the original one, which scared me, but my doctor thinks it is most likely scar tissue resulting from the radiation treatments, not a new malignancy. "The cancer is gone, for the most part," says he. I gave him a hug, a few tears, and a bouquet of fall flowers to thank him for saving my life.
>
> I am now a former cancer patient, a lung cancer survivor. My hair is starting to grow back, I only have two more Neupogen shots to go, and my white cell count should return to normal in a month or so. Life is good. In the latest issue of Coping with Cancer magazine, Bernie Siegel recommends figuring out what you would want to do if you had only fifteen minutes left to live, and then doing it for the rest of your life. Anyone care to dance?

However, many people also report at least some ambivalence at the end of treatment. Side by side with the expected good feelings can be other, more painful feelings.

The remainder of this section talks about negative feelings that might unexpectedly arise at the end of treatment. These feelings, and all of the feelings described in this chapter, are completely normal. Some of them may not strike you as useful reactions, but they are nonetheless normal reactions for the circumstances surrounding cancer survivorship and should be honored as such. If you decide to join a support group, for example, you'll likely hear many people describing these kinds of reactions and offering very good ways to turn reactions into useful acts.

Keep in mind as well that many lung cancer survivors have long periods of feeling happy, sound, capable, productive, and blessed. For many, the positives outnumber the negatives.

Max Baldwin describes his spiritual evolution since diagnosis:

> I believe that after the initial shock of learning you have cancer, you then adjust your thinking and actually become a bigger and better person. I have an enhanced appreciation of friends, family and increased enjoyment of simple things like rain, green grass, and on and on and on. . . .

Moving on

Everyone who has had lung cancer wants to leave cancer behind and move on to normal living. Some people succeed well with this.

Kathleen Houlihan ruminates on her experience:

> A year ago today was the worst day of my life. I had had the biopsy the day before, on what was probably tied for being the second worst day of my life, the day my mother died, almost twenty years ago now. Then a year ago today, a Wednesday, my husband Holt and I waited all day for the results of the biopsy. When we hadn't heard by about 4:00 PM, we finally called my doctor, who called the pathologist and then called us back. Holt took the call, but I could hear the doctor tell him, "It's an adenocarcinoma."
>
> In talking with friends about my situation, one asked if I had been through hell this past year. I thought for just a minute and said that no, I had been scared as hell, but I really didn't feel like I had been through hell. I sure didn't feel very good for the whole month of April last year,

during the radiation. I was extremely tired all the time from the radiation, and I had pretty bad joint pain, along with some fevers and/or chills from the cancer (who knew fever and pain were symptoms of cancer?!), and those symptoms continued to a lesser degree throughout May, but that certainly wasn't hell. If I had had surgery, the recovery from that would have been hell, I'm sure. But without it, I haven't had very much in the way of physical discomfort.

Now I feel almost as good as I did before. I don't have quite as much energy as before, but otherwise I feel pretty much normal. And even though I am reminiscing about the events of a year ago, I can honestly say that today is one of the best days of my life. We just returned from a wonderful visit with Holt's family in Los Angeles—his four brothers and two sisters and their families, including eight of our nine nieces and nephews out there. We saw my father and brother and his son last month. We're in close touch with our local friends. And long-distance friends continue to visit. The dogs and cats are all doing well. I'm gearing up to plant a garden this year. Life is good!

So today I celebrate being a one-year lung cancer survivor. I intend to continue doing well, having one good day and one good year after another.

Kathleen is also discovering new aspects of life to enjoy:

Speaking of turning to other matters, I've always loved music, but ever since I made a "C" in choir in the seventh grade, I've been resigned to the fact that I can't sing. Not! A couple of years ago, I came across a woman who says she can teach anyone to sing. That's nice, but I knew she couldn't teach me. Well, she can! After the appointment with my psychotherapist in Tulsa last month, I started thinking about what I was passionate about, and music was near the top of my list. So I decided to take singing lessons from Sue. At the first lesson, she had me start by singing scales (just on the vowel "ah") with her and the piano. As soon as I started, I could tell I was singing the right notes, and I started to cry. I sure wasn't expecting that! But Sue says it's not uncommon. I've had four lessons now, and I still cry some, but much less each time. I'm singing songs of my choice, beautiful songs I've always loved (Today, I Could Have Danced All Night, Cabaret, etc.), and it feels so good. I'm still far from perfect, but Sue says I have a "lovely" voice (she's a super cheerleader), and I'm doing so much better than I ever dreamed possible. I think it's the best thing I've ever done for myself.

Many people, however, are able to force this difficult mental shift.

Some people succeed in blocking the experience entirely and immediately submerge themselves in their old life. This is a very healthy and useful form of denial, as long as one doesn't skip follow-up medical appointments. Some people succeed well in readjusting after their course of treatment, but cannot recapture this serenity if disease recurs and they face more treatment—even if their odds of survival after retreatment are promising.

Many people feel almost like their old selves until it's time for their periodic testing, when very strong fears resurface.

Abandonment

Some people fear the end of treatment because they feel that medical intervention and care are all that's standing between them and cancer. Often, people secretly feel abandoned by their surgeon, oncologists, or the medical staff at the end of treatment. To the emotionally charged survivor, the medical personnel's behavior during a normal wrap-up appointment may seem brusque or emotionally flat. Where are the trumpets, the pat on the back, the teary eyes?

If, on the other hand, the staff was loving and helpful throughout treatment and congratulatory at the end, afterward you may miss the all-pull-together camaraderie that was shared and the special kindness you received.

You may fear the absence of regular and close physical scrutiny given by the doctor. The thought of waiting two or three months to the next blood test, scan, or other reassessment may seem like forever.

Karen Parles describes how she felt when treatment ended:

> By far the most difficult time for me emotionally was after treatment stopped. I knew that I was at a high risk of recurrence, and I knew recurrence meant I would die from my disease. I looked well enough, so family and friends were reassured that I would be OK—they called and visited less frequently. Ironically, this is the time I most needed emotional support. One of my lifelines during this post-treatment period, was an in-person lung cancer support group run by Cancer Care. The other survivors in my support group could relate to my anxiety over recurrence and provided comfort through their understanding. I remain vigilant about follow-up visits to my oncologist, but the only thing that truly relieves my worry is the passage of time.

Absence of feeling

Sometimes cancer survivors report feeling nothing at all when their treatment ends and their doctor says their chances are good that their survival will be a long one. This numbness may come about as a protective mechanism or from burnout. Most often, feeling will return with the passing of time.

Fear of relapse

Nobody can guarantee that you won't experience a relapse of lung cancer or develop a second cancer. In spite of many reassurances, it's human to be afraid. Most cancer survivors have fears of relapse that range from occasional to paralytic. Often, the fears can be put to bed for months at time, but they may resurface when it's time for a checkup or when an odd pain emerges.

Kathleen Houlihan describes her intermittent fears:

> I've been kind of nervous lately because I am at the prime time for a recurrence. Most recurrences for lung cancer happen in the first two years, and I'm just short of one and a half years since diagnosis. So every time I have an ache, pain, or bump, or can't remember how to spell a familiar word (I couldn't remember how to spell busy a few months ago— it's called "chemo-brain"), I think I'm having a recurrence, or a metastasis to the bone, or brain, or wherever. I no longer have the "just tough it out, ignore it and it will go away" attitude. I did that for seven months with the pain in my shoulder that turned out to be the lung tumor.
>
> But now that I have the normal results from the AMAS test, I no longer suspect that I may have something "cooking" that could make itself known at any moment. I now think that I am really cancer-free. I know it could still come back, but I'm starting to really believe that it may not. So I intend to start seriously putting this whole cancer episode behind me and moving on.
>
> I do want to put all the supportive information I have on a web site (if I can ever get around to it!), so I can share what worked for me with anyone who is interested, especially newly diagnosed lung cancer patients. But other than that, I don't intend to spend much time on things cancer anymore. As an almost six-year survivor of lung cancer says, "Don't let yesterday take up too much of today."

Fear of relapse is entirely normal. There's no known way to remove this fear entirely, but several ways to diminish these negative feelings might include:

- Learning all you can about your type and stage of lung cancer

- Keeping abreast of improvements in treatment

- Retraining your thinking to focus on the positive

- Maintaining reasonably healthy lifestyle habits

- Attempting to enjoy the small, free joys offered by each new day

- Giving up smoking, if you smoke

Vigilance

Many people experience pronounced, abiding concern about relapse when a new ache or odd body trait is noticed. Fears of relapse are, of course, perfectly normal, and you're to be commended for monitoring your body's reactions and status. You're not a hypochondriac.

Battle fatigue (post-traumatic stress reaction)

Some people experience insomnia; nightmares about their cancer; fear and avoidance of doctors and hospitals; jumpiness or lack of trust during common interactions with medical personnel, such as annual influenza vaccination; or extreme anger or sadness when hearing of someone else with cancer.

Ruminations, doubts

Once the heat of the battle is past, some people may begin to recall survival statistics they've seen. You might become less than happy with what you perceive your odds of surviving to be. You might begin to second-guess whether what you went through was worth it, whether it was the right treatment choice, whether you'll ever be physically adept again, whether anything else in life is worth doing in comparison to battling cancer.

Diminished coping skills

For such a long time, all that was expected of you was to focus on beating cancer. Now it may seem that the rest of the world expects you simply to pick up where you left off with your normal responsibilities. For those who were not able to continue working throughout treatment and who have not retired, the thought of returning to a full workload of regular responsibilities can be overwhelming. If your breathing is not as good as it was, you might feel tired most of the time, even when physical effort is not necessary.

As you attempt to re-enter your wider world, you may notice that things that you used to be able to ignore may annoy you or things that used to annoy you may anger you.

Anger

Now that the time- and energy-consuming process of being treated is behind you, you may find that you're feeling angry about having cancer. You may find that you want to learn all you can about what causes lung cancer or that you want to become politically involved to force legislation that favors cancer research or cleanses the environment of carcinogens.

If you've quit smoking, seeing others smoke might infuriate you.

If you still smoke, you might become very angry if anyone mentions quitting smoking in your presence. You might feel that you've been through enough and you just want to be left alone to enjoy life as you see fit.

Longing for the past

Some people expect and hope that they'll feel and perform exactly as they did before cancer became a problem and are disappointed if they cannot. Sometimes the recovery of physical and intellectual stamina is a slow process. If you need supplemental oxygen support, you may have periods during which you're convinced life will never be the same. At times, you might perceive that all changes or a diminution of performance are cancer-related, when in fact they might be attributable to a number of other things.

Excessive caution

Some people feel that the gods would frown on pride if one celebrates at the end of treatment, so they avoid jinxing themselves by celebrating. They may spend years afraid to enjoy a return of reasonably good health.

Alienation and loneliness

People who haven't had to deal with cancer may strike you now as insensitive or shallow. Those who have had cancer, but not lung cancer, might seem unable to understand the stigma or the prognosis you feel you're facing. The vacuous things others say about your cancer experience or their inappropriate curiosity might leave you astonished or hurt. The everyday topics they want to discuss may bore you. You may find the issues that they view as problematic trivial. You may feel you no longer have anything in common with old friends, nor even with loved ones. You may begin to consider a job change or a divorce.

If you've recently given up smoking, friends who still smoke and know of your illness might be ill at ease around you, or might avoid you—or you them.

Altogether, you may feel out of phase with the rest of the world—until you meet a fellow lung cancer survivor, and a long, intense conversation follows, during which you're impervious to your surroundings, perhaps sharing funny stories about your experiences that healthy people would find morbid. Suddenly, you're aware you're not alone and that cancer support groups may be a good choice for you.

Watchful waiting

Those with slow-growing types of lung cancer that are monitored for long periods, with no treatment but "watchful waiting" and those with ambiguous test results, face special circumstances. Retesting at some future date will be necessary for clarification. The intervening time may be filled with unbearably obsessive worry about the possible failure of treatment, sleeplessness, crying, lack of concentration, and other extremely uncomfortable feelings.

Anxiety and depression

All of the above, combined with the physical toll of treatment, often result in anxiety or depression for many people. Anxiety and depression are discussed more fully in Chapter 15, *Stress and Stress Reduction* and Chapter 16, *Getting Support*. A counselor who specializes in cancer survivorship can help you with these and other problems.

Social and professional aftereffects

You may be quite surprised to discover that those around you who have never had cancer are totally unaware of the mixture of feelings you're experiencing—that, in fact, they may have a very full agenda of their own feelings, both happy and distressing, to sort out. Conversely, you may find that cancer survivors are a tremendous resource to you in this stage of your adjustment.

Reactions of family and friends

Your closest family members and friends who have seen you throughout treatment have probably adjusted to your circumstances, by the time your treatment ends, in a way that benefits all concerned. Nonetheless, you may find that some family members expect that, almost instantly, you'll be just as healthy and active as you were before, particularly if you're a young survivor of lung cancer. They may even become strident on this point, so strongly does human nature yearn for things to return to normal. You need to communicate clearly with them when you're feeling tired and under par, explaining that many cancer survivors experience long-term aftereffects, such as fatigue.

Some family members and loved ones may have feelings of anger, frustration, or impatience that they suppressed during your treatment. They may now allow these feelings to emerge. Candid discussions may defuse these feelings, but if the negative feelings are directed at you, family counseling may be a good choice.

In some cases, a spouse or partner may decide that this is a good time to end the relationship, now that it's "over," and you're "fine." This is more likely in relationships that were experiencing problems before the cancer diagnosis.

Your very young children or grandchildren, lacking adult coping skills, might still remain mired in the distress and terror they experienced during your diagnosis and treatment. They might need long-term therapy or support with social and academic issues.

Getting out socially after treatment among those who know you less well can be entertaining and enriching or exhausting and disappointing. The reactions of coworkers, discussed below, mirror in some ways the responses you're likely to encounter from the rest of society. Unlike coworkers and family members, though, social contacts may not usually have the benefit of seeing you performing and producing, so their reactions may be more skewed and less informed.

It might be wise to be prepared for a variety of reactions that range from loving and positive to very odd, indeed, if you haven't already encountered the entire spectrum of these reactions in the course of being treated. Some lung cancer survivors report, for example, that others don't want the survivor to talk about their experiences at all. Others report that friends who avoided them during treatment relax and reapproach them after treatment ends. Still others find that they are stigmatized by the association of tobacco smoking and lung cancer, whether or not they smoked, and that in some cases others never really forgive them for having smoked.

Larry Coffman describes his life and activities now:

> The doctors won't let me work and I don't think I could handle it anyway, so I am taking a course here and there at the local community college to keep my mind sharp. I have to take my oxygen bottle with me, and you should see the stares I get. I see people putting cigarettes out kind of fast when I approach. At my two youngest's Middle School, I tell the kids that want to know (and some that don't) about the dangers of smoking and allowing our environment to be poisoned. I consider this a privilege and an honor.

You might be able to defuse negative reactions, reinforce your reputation for tenacity and positive thinking, or even be a little audacious if you're in the mood for humor and not concerned about the social consequences. Some of the negative reactions and questions you'll encounter are simply the result of ignorance or a lack of careful thought, or are a front for competitiveness, spite, or sadism. You're under no obligation to go along with agendas that are not in your best interest, nor to waste a lot of emotional energy answering seemingly serious questions that in fact haven't been thought out carefully. See Chapter 16, *Getting Support*, for more information about dealing with the ignorance or unkindness of others.

Reentering the workplace

Resuming the full complement of professional responsibilities or volunteer commitments after cancer treatment has ended can be a wonderful experience, a way to occupy the mind with healthy things, a way to reinforce your belief in yourself and your re-emerging health with productivity and creativity.

Often the feelings your coworkers express are a tremendous reinforcement for your well-being. To know you were needed and missed can be uplifting; to be part of a team again can make you feel you've rejoined the human race. Many cancer survivors report that welcome-back parties are planned to greet them and that coworkers pinch-hit for them if they continue to feel tired.

Kathleen Houlihan is looking forward to returning to work and life:

> We're getting geared up for the holidays. We're going out to dinner with friends for Thanksgiving, my father is coming here for a few days over Christmas, and we're trying to get out to visit Holt's family sometime soon. Then I'll be teaching in the tax class in January, and teaching an intro to linguistics class, and doing income tax as a volunteer in the spring. Life is getting back to normal.

I have a lot to be thankful for this Thanksgiving. I'm thankful for the convoluted set of circumstances that led me to the treatment center I chose, and I'm thankful for all the wonderful doctors, nurses, technicians, and staff there. I'm especially thankful for my recovery and for the love, support, and encouragement I've received from all of my friends!

Occasionally, the return to work is less rewarding. If you have been queried over and over throughout your treatment about when you will return, for example, you may feel that your employer thinks you're just a cog in the machinery rather than a human worthy of her concern. If some coworkers are reluctant to recognize your illness because of their own fears or lack of social skills, they might not refer to it ever, not even to wish you well or to say they're glad you're back. Very rarely, a cancer survivor will experience horrible reactions from coworkers, such as discovering that, in one's absence, one's desk was sprayed with antiseptic "in case the cancer was contagious," but these extreme reactions from coworkers fortunately are rare.

Often the public has misconceptions about lung cancer and how it can be treated. Some coworkers might treat you as if your days are numbered, even if your prognosis is quite good.

But more often, the hurtful reaction will be, "The treatment is over, so now you're fine, right? Ready for a full workload now, right?" If you're still feeling like something Jacques Cousteau would've thrown back, be sure to make it clear that you'll be phasing back in gradually, that you're not feeling up to working a full day or a full week for the first month or two.

Another fairly common reaction among the blissfully healthy is, "Why are you in such a pensive mood? Aren't you glad it's all over?" Your attitude about putting it behind you or not putting it behind you might be worth an explanation, but this explanation might meet with limited success with the less perceptive and empathic of your coworkers. American culture, like some other cultures, has a quick-fix or even a superstitious mentality toward many problems, including health problems.

In general, it's nobody's business how you're coping with the detritus of treatment, but problems can arise if you don't keep your immediate supervisor informed about problems you might still be experiencing. If your supervisor is unaware of your health problems and a dispute arises about your job performance, you might have trouble winning your supervisor as an ally if you inform her of health problems after the fact.

More subtle reactions from coworkers and employers are possible, as well, such as denying a promotion to a person who had cancer several years ago, assuming she will never again be able to meet certain challenges.

Remember that cancer is considered a disability under the Americans with Disabilities Act. You have legal recourse for negative consequences that result in demonstrable harm to you or your livelihood.

Unused drugs or equipment

Often, at the end of treatment you may have drugs and equipment left over. There may be ways to pass these unused drugs along to those who cannot afford them. Although in general federal law prohibits transferring drugs prescribed for one person to anyone else, you might ask your oncologist or veterinarian if there are exceptions to this law.

Nonprescription drugs can be offered to fellow patients and veterinarians.

To donate drugs for use in developing countries with few health resources, contact International Aid Inc. in Spring Lake, Michigan, at (616) 846-7490.

If you have supplies you no longer need, such as a wig or cleaning supplies for a catheter, many groups, such as the American Cancer Society, accept them as tax-deductible donations to help patients who cannot afford to buy their own.

Summary

Earl Weaver, the long-time manager of the Baltimore Orioles baseball team, used to say, "It's not over until it's over." With cancer, sometimes it's not over when it's over. Certain physical, emotional, and social aspects may take longer to realign with the new you.

Many lung cancer survivors gradually see the cup as more than half full and experience increasingly good health and productivity and a goodly measure of happiness. Many have occasional or ongoing fears and concerns that time, professional help, or support groups can alleviate.

Dr. Wendy Schlessel Harpham's book, *After Cancer* (Harperperennial, 1995), is an excellent in-depth guide to meeting the challenges after treatment ends.

CHAPTER 19

Recurrence of Disease

*We do not know what we mean by cure because there is a
great difference between cure and long-term survival.*

—Arthur Holleb

AT TIMES IT IS ALMOST IMPOSSIBLE to think of anything except the possibility that cancer
will return. This fear might be fleeting, or it can be trenchant, obsessive, and compelling, occupying both waking and sleeping thought.

Depending on the stage at which your lung cancer was diagnosed, the type of lung
cancer you had, and what you've learned about it, you might be somewhat prepared
intellectually and emotionally for recurrence, perhaps with a new treatment plan
already selected. On the other hand, you might be emotionally broadsided by the
news, even if you are prepared intellectually.

This chapter begins with a definition of recurrence of disease and then describes who
is likely to experience a recurrence, how recurrence is detected, in what areas of the
body it might emerge, when it's most likely, and why it occurs. A discussion follows
regarding the difficult emotional issues that arise at this time, which often are different from those one encounters at first diagnosis.

There are instances of test results mistakenly being interpreted as recurrence of
disease—and we discuss what findings may constitute equivocal results—but chiefly,
this chapter focuses on true recurrence.

It's possible to mistake some aftereffects of treatment for symptoms of recurrence. It
might relieve you of some anxiety if you review Chapter 13, *Adverse Effects of Treatment*, which describes most of these physical changes.

The definition of recurrence

As defined by Roberta Altman and Michael Sarg in *The Cancer Dictionary* (Checkmark
Books, 1999), relapse or recurrence is the return of disease in a patient who, by the

best measures available, appeared to be disease-free for longer than 30 days after treatment ended. One who has quantifiable evidence of tumors remaining after treatment is said to have had only a partial response to treatment and is very likely to experience a progression of disease. The patient who, after successful treatment, experiences a return of disease within 30 days is said to experience a progression of disease rather than recurrence.

Some lung cancer survivors have tumors that shrink less than 50 percent and then remain the same size for some period of time, a condition called stable disease. Others might have tumors that shrink greatly, but never entirely disappear. This residue might be noncancerous scar tissue.

A very late recurrence might be a new lung tumor, known as a second primary cancer. These tumors should be biopsied to classify them correctly as NSCLC, SCLC, or a mixed type, because shifts between lung cancer types are possible.

True absence of disease after treatment of any kind is very hard to determine with complete certainty. The surgeon's eyes and the specific imaging tools and blood tests used today to detect remaining or recurring disease unfortunately are not foolproof.

How recurrence is detected

Some lung cancer survivors experience old, familiar feelings of malaise in the chest or airways or notice other alarming symptoms, such as blood in sputum, that trigger a visit to their oncologist. Other survivors note entirely new symptoms that they might not think of as related to lung cancer, but somehow they know that things just aren't right. Still others might be feeling fine, yet a routine imaging study indicates a possible return of disease.

If you have worrisome symptoms, contact your doctor immediately. Do not allow concerns about being thought a hypochondriac interfere with getting timely medical care that might save your life. Symptoms of lung cancer are discussed in great detail in Chapter 1, *Symptoms of Lung Cancer*.

It's likely that your oncologist will order one or more tests if either you or he notices anything that hints at a return of disease. Many of these tests, such as imaging scans or blood testing, will be familiar from your experiences during your initial diagnosis and follow-up care. Kathy describes Marty's follow-up:

> Well, we made it to the last chemotherapy treatment on December 27, 1999 (my uncle had died the week before of prostate cancer). The doctor told us he thought it would be a long time before Marty would have to go

back on chemo. We were so excited, a little scared but I was looking forward to trying to be normal for a while—little did I know that we were creating a new normal for ourselves.

Shortly after Marty's January appointment with the oncologist, he started having a pain in the middle of the chest. This was about the same time he went off the MS Contin and got the diarrhea. The doctors all said it couldn't be the cancer; it was too soon. He continued to work with our general practitioner, but constantly complained of a pain in the middle of his chest.

The day before I was to return to work after my hysterectomy, Marty had his three-month CT scan done and he had two exploratory procedures—one for the esophagus and one for the colon. Then we got a call from the oncologist; they wanted to see Marty right away. I knew it was bad news. There were tumors in the lymph nodes.

In April, he started back on chemo: Gemzar and carboplatin. We were devastated.

If suspicious lesions reappear in the lungs or in well-studied sites of lung cancer metastasis, such as bone or brain, treatment might proceed without biopsy. If new lesions appear in unusual places or recurrence occurs years later, however, your doctor might wish to confirm the re-emergence of disease with a second biopsy before proceeding with treatment.

Often these decisions about biopsy depend on the type of lung cancer first found and the stage of the original disease. A person originally diagnosed with extensive stage small cell lung cancer, for instance, is considered likely to experience involvement of many organ systems eventually, whereas a person diagnosed with stage I non-small cell lung cancer has a lower chance of recurrence. Thus, liver lesions appearing on an imaging scan for a stage IV survivor might be interpreted as very likely representing a further spread of disease, whereas a stage I survivor might be questioned, as possible benign scarring, fatty lesions, or a new primary tumor, needing further testing.

Why disease recurs

The most widely accepted theory for recurrence is that not all lung cancer cells were removed or killed by the original treatment.

Recent research has shown that cancer cells can acquire resistance to chemotherapy drugs by turning on genes that block the cellular intake of certain drugs and others related to them, a phenomenon called multiple drug resistance (MDR). This appears to be the case with small cell lung cancer, whereas non-small cell lung cancer might be somewhat resistant to chemotherapy from the very beginning rather than acquiring resistance as treatment proceeds.

Other theories hold that genetic predisposition, widely damaged lung tissue, or continued or repeated exposure to environmental toxins might be responsible for the return of disease, but it can be argued that these latter instances are independent (metachronous) cancers and not recurrence, progression, or spread of the first cancer.

Who experiences recurrence

Very broadly, and only in the context of today's treatments, one can say that those diagnosed in advanced stages of illness or with aggressive tumors are more likely to experience a recurrence than those diagnosed in early stages or with tumors of low malignant potential.

With many new treatments being developed for lung cancer, however, it's not wise, correct, or ethical to adhere to generalities without continually revisiting the progress of research and without noting exceptions. Solitary tumors in the brain or adrenals, for example, might be addressed successfully with radiosurgery or traditional surgery. Chapter 6, *Prognosis*, discusses these exceptions in detail.

Where disease recurs

The return of disease can be classified as local, regional, or distant, and can vary based on the type of lung cancer first found and the type of first-line treatment used.

Locoregional recurrence

Recurrence at or very near the site of the first tumor, known as locoregional recurrence, is common for both NSCLC and SCLC. Recurrence in the same (ipsilateral) lung is possible if any lung tissue remains on that side. Recurrence in the opposite (contralateral) lung is possible, but less likely than same-side recurrence or recurrence in distant organs. Recurrence is possible outside the lung, but within nearby neck or chest structures: mid-chest lymph nodes, the heart or its blood vessels, ribs, chest fluid, larynx, and other chest or neck structures can be invaded by recurrent disease.

Distant recurrence

In Chapter 26 of the first edition of *Lung Cancer: Principles and Practice* (Lippincott, 2000), David Midthun and James Jett say, "There is hardly a body tissue that is immune from the metastatic presence or effects of bronchogenic carcinoma." Distant recurrence of lung cancer is most common in the brain, with 30 to 50 percent being solitary tumors. Adrenal glands, liver, or bone (most often in the spine, ribs, pelvis, or legs) are also common sites of recurrence, although this varies based on the kind of lung cancer one has. Small cell lung cancer is more often diagnosed at late stages with multiple organ involvement than is non-small cell lung cancer, and it reappears more often in distant organs or in rare sites than does non-small cell lung cancer.

Geri Capasso tells of her aunt's unexpected recurrence of disease:

> *In 1988 my aunt, whom I loved very much, had part of her lung removed and had radiation treatments as a follow-up. The doctor said she was cured, but she routinely had chest CT scans. Right before her fifth-year, cancer-free anniversary, she started to get terrible headaches. The lung cancer metastasized. It was not caught soon enough, but she fought with radiation and chemo. She lost the battle within six months.*
>
> *That is when I learned that lung cancer cells commonly hide in the brain. I still cannot understand why they weren't checking her brain. She was 66 years old and ironically had given up cigarettes about one or two years before diagnosis. I remember that she also had clubbed fingers.*
>
> *I think it's important to stay on top of things, and, if need be, to catch it early and not wait for symptoms.*

Gray areas and delays

In the last ten or fifteen years, we have benefited from the tremendous progress made in medical science's ability to detect cancers at much earlier stages. Nevertheless, current sophisticated imaging tools still provide just a glimpse into the body's complex workings. Consequently, blood tests and imaging studies sometimes yield equivocal results that must be qualified with additional testing or a second biopsy.

Following some types of chemotherapy, for example, fatty or scarring lesions can form in the liver. Following lung surgery, scarring (sclerosis) might occur. These benign lesions might appear upon CT scanning as metastases. Positron emission tomography (PET) or MRI can, in some cases, distinguish benign lesions from recurrent lung cancer.

Blood tests that are sometimes used to track possible re-emergence of cancers are not always reliable indicators of recurrence in the absence of other findings. CEA (carcino-embryonic antigen), for instance, can become elevated as a result of other bodily or disease processes or as a result of changes in smoking or alcohol consumption habits. Different laboratories sometimes use different manufacturers' assays to measure blood levels of various substances, and their results can't always be compared with accuracy.

When does risk abate?

In general, the longer you remain disease-free, the less likely you are to experience a recurrence of disease. You might be considered by insurance companies and your oncologist, for example, to be cured of the primary tumor once you have been in remission for five years. Those with bronchial carcinoid tumors, however, might experience a very long disease-free period followed by recurrence.

It is known that those who have had lung cancer face a very high risk for a second lung cancer. Unlike colon or breast cancers, lung tissue cannot be removed in its entirety to ensure that disease will not return. Some researchers believe that the same environmental or genetic aberrations that triggered the first tumor remain to cause a second tumor; that is, a tumor whose development is distinct from a recurrence or metastasis of the first tumor. This means that, for some people, the quest for cure of the original tumor might be only half the battle.

If the survivor has a family history of lung cancers, especially among never-smokers, he should never relax the vigilance of follow-up testing to detect second cancers or recurrence. These genetic disorders might predispose one to multiple cancers of the lung and, in some cases, cancers of other organs.

All lung cancer survivors, with and without hereditary traits, should continue to have periodic tests at intervals determined by their oncologist.

Treatment options

How a recurrence of disease is treated depends on how your first appearance of disease was treated, what type of lung cancer you have, what organs are affected, and how healthy you are overall. Because lung cancer treatments are evolving continually and because patients' medical circumstances differ, attempts to describe very specific treatments your doctor might recommend would be quickly outdated or incorrect for your circumstances. Several general points can be made, however.

Clinical trials

The National Cancer Institute recommends that all lung cancer survivors experiencing a recurrence of disease should consider clinical trials of new substances or techniques. If you didn't familiarize yourself with clinical trials during your first experience with lung cancer, now is a good time to do so. Clinical trials are a good way to gain access to newer, possibly more effective treatments before they are made available to the general public. Having some familiarity with what chemical agents, surgical techniques, and radiologic techniques are being tested will position you to make sound decisions about subsequent treatment. Chapter 20, *Clinical Trials*, Chapter 22, *Researching Your Illness*, and Chapter 23, *The Future of Therapy*, can help guide you through the process of choosing a clinical trial for recurrent disease.

Recurrent NSCLC

Recurrent NSCLC might be found in a single site, such as with several new lung tumors or a solitary brain tumor, or it may recur as widespread disease affecting several organs. A new lung tumor after a substantial disease-free period is evaluated and treated as if it were the first lung tumor.

Treatment options recommended by the NCI and our medical reviewers:

- Radiation therapy to relieve symptoms rather than cure disease
- Chemotherapy:
    - Cisplatin, vinblastine, and mitomycin
    - Cisplatin and vinorelbine
    - Cisplatin and paclitaxel
    - Cisplatin and gemcitabine
    - Carboplatin and paclitaxel
    - One medical reviewer notes that docetaxel is now used, as well
- Surgery or stereotactic radiosurgery to remove an isolated brain tumor, only if no other tumors remain in the lungs or elsewhere
- Surgery to remove a single tumor in a single metastatic site, such as the adrenal gland
- Laser therapy or interstitial radiation therapy for endobronchial lesions to ease breathing, not to cure disease

Recurrent SCLC

Recurrent SCLC might be found in a single site, such as a single brain tumor, but it most often recurs as a distant and widespread disease affecting several organs, including bones such as the ribs, spine, pelvis, or legs. A new lung tumor after a substantial disease-free period should be evaluated and treated as if it were the first lung tumor, and it should be rebiopsied for SCLC versus NSCLC.

Treatment options recommended by the NCI and our medical reviewers:

- Radiation therapy to relieve symptoms, not to cure.

- Second chemotherapy attempts, which might provide some relief from pain or uncomfortable symptoms for patients who were previously sensitive to earlier chemotherapy. NCI says, "While no single chemotherapy regimen should be considered standard, those that have shown activity as second line treatment include:

  - Oral etoposide

  - Etoposide/cisplatin

  - Cyclophosphamide/doxorubicin/vincristine (CAV)

  - Lomustine/methotrexate

  - Paclitaxel

  - Topotecan"

- Endobronchial laser therapy, endobronchial stents, or brachytherapy to relieve symptoms of airway obstruction.

- Trials of new chemotherapy agents.

Drug resistance

If chemotherapy is planned and you have received chemotherapy previously, your oncologist might assume that the drugs you were given at first, at least at their initial doses, would not be the best choice for treating recurrence. The thinking is threefold:

- If these drugs were very effective, your disease would not have recurred.

- Certain lung cancers can become resistant to drugs.

- Some drugs are toxic to various organs; their lifetime dose must be limited.

This means that, for subsequent chemotherapies, it's usually the case that a second drug or series of drugs will be attempted.

Emotional issues

Clearly, recurrence is an emotional lowland for almost anyone affected by lung cancer, including the survivor, family, friends, and the oncologist.

The emotional issues faced at recurrence are different in quality and scope from those encountered at first diagnosis and endured during treatment. What follows are some of the reactions that many lung cancer survivors describe having.

Fear and terror

Feelings of fear or raw terror might overcome you, even if your odds for long-term survival look good. A sense that your options are narrowing might grow stronger, even if you are aware that, by medicine's best assessment, they are not. Thoughts of death that you might have been able to put aside during and after treatment crowd back in, even if you know that there are still treatment options open to you. Fear of different, stronger, more damaging treatments might emerge.

Loneliness and abandonment

Facing cancer is almost always a lonely experience. Facing a recurrence of cancer is even more so. Lung cancer, in particular, has great potential to alienate others because of public awareness of the link between smoking and lung cancer. This abandonment, real or implied, is particularly bitter if you have never smoked or if you quit smoking many years ago.

You might find that those who were supportive until now begin to withdraw. Even if they remain supportive, you might find yourself fearful that they will very soon withdraw support. You might find that cancer survivors in your support group are made uncomfortable by the proximity of someone who is facing a recurrence.

Unfairness

There might be a sense that you fought the good fight, and now you deserve peace, contentment, and normalcy. Not only are you not getting these just rewards, you're getting something that could hardly be worse. You might wonder why unethical, unkind humans go about happy and healthy. You might find yourself wishing that certain particularly unpleasant people would get cancer, too.

Anger

Anger over these terrible circumstances, perhaps kept in check or rationalized during initial treatment, might now emerge and cause you and those around you much discomfort. What psychological adjustments you might have made to your illness might go out the window, seeming to be a waste of time. Anger might manifest as rage, irritation, cynicism, or depression.

Grief

Many people grieve from the moment of diagnosis. They grieve for lost health, energy, and diminished opportunities of many kinds—from career opportunities they had to forego to have treatment, to loss of sexuality, loss of bodily integrity, ruptured relationships, or the possible loss of life.

Not surprisingly, an expanded sense of grief might emerge upon recurrence. Some people can't help but remember having heard that, for many cancers, failure of first-line treatment entails a poor prognosis. Although you might know that this generality does not apply to all lung cancer survivors, it's still a frightening thought that makes some people grieve for the life they might lose.

Despair

The initial diagnosis of lung cancer and its first-line treatment often are addressed with a can-do attitude that might be difficult to sustain at recurrence, even if your chances of long-term survival are good. There's something about facing the battle all over again that might make you weary at the very thought of it. You might feel that the difficult treatment you've already endured was a waste of time. You might question the quality of your life. You might contemplate suicide.

Loss of trust

You might lose trust in the medical system in general or in your oncologist in particular. If a strong faith sustained you during diagnosis and first-line treatment, you might find yourself questioning this faith now. You might lose confidence in your own ability to meet physical and emotional challenges.

Acceptance

Many lung cancer survivors marshal their emotional resources to start additional treatment or search for clinical trials. Others begin to consider the process of dying and ways to approach death with serenity.

Family and friends

The reactions of friends and family might be completely supportive, positive, and loving, or particularly inept. Unless they're kept well informed about your illness and its likely patterns, they might give up on being supportive, instead treating you as if you have one foot in the grave. They might mourn prematurely; they might practice living without you emotionally.

Employers might begin to lose patience with you at the prospect of yet more absenteeism. Your young children or your grandchildren might once again exhibit earlier, less adaptive behaviors that they had outgrown, such as clinging, aggression, bedwetting, or temper tantrums.

Getting help

If you are facing a recurrence of lung cancer, you should consider clinical trials of new substances and techniques. Contact the NCI at *http://cancernet.nci.nih.gov/ trialsrch.shtml* or by phone at (800) 4-CANCER for information on clinical trials.

Cancer counselors have a considerable amount of experience with those who are dealing with cancer as a chronic, recurrent illness and sometimes are cancer survivors themselves. You can locate a cancer counselor by contacting your hospital's social worker, the local Wellness Community, or the local office of the American Cancer Society for referrals.

Support groups are an inestimable resource for regaining emotional footing and a balanced outlook. If you didn't examine options for finding support during your first experience with lung cancer, it would be wise to do so now. It's not an overstatement to say that you'll be overwhelmed by feelings of hope and energy when you discover how many other people have gone through what you're experiencing and came through it in good shape.

Many forms of support are available for cancer survivors in general and lung cancer survivors in particular. Chapter 16, *Getting Support*, details these options.

Summary

Recurrence of lung cancer is an extremely difficult time for most people. Fear, hopelessness, anger, and overwhelming sadness are common feelings.

Recurrence is not a death sentence. There are good options available for retreatment, and many people report feeling much better after they familiarize themselves with the options available.

Key points to remember:

- You should tell your doctor immediately about any suspicious or worrisome symptoms you experience. Do not concern yourself with fears that others will think you're a hypochondriac.

- Re-emergence of disease is not an automatic death sentence. Certain tumors that recur or spread can be treated in some instances.

- For clinical trials of new treatments, visit the NCI's web site *http://cancernet.nci. nih.gov/trialsrch.shtml* or call them at (800) 4-CANCER.

CHAPTER 20

Clinical Trials

"Come to the edge," he said. They said: "We are afraid."
"Come to the edge," he said. They came.
He pushed them ... and they flew.

—Gillaume Apollinaire

WHY WOULD ANYONE CHOOSE an experimental therapy over standard lung cancer treatments that have well-known risks? Aren't clinical trials of new treatments dangerous? Aren't these experimental treatments just for people who have no other choices left? And why are they called clinical trials?

Lung cancer is the subject of a great deal of very promising research. These new and possibly better treatments are available to lung cancer survivors in carefully controlled settings called clinical trials.

Many of the treatments now in the pipeline are of very low toxicity, unlike some traditional, standard chemotherapeutic agents. Many experimental treatments, such as monoclonal antibodies, use natural cancer-fighting body products that are amplified outside the body and then reinserted. Others, such as idiotype vaccines, use your own white blood cells that are retrained to attack tumors. Other treatments aim for and destroy the parts of the cancer cell's chromosomes that make cancer cells immortal.

In this chapter, we discuss the structure of clinical trials, how they're run, their advantages and disadvantages, safeguards for the patient, and your rights as a patient. We show you why it's often to your advantage to do your own searching, instead of relying on trials your doctor may recommend, and how to evaluate different trials. We explain what to expect and what to do when you're finally enrolled in a trial.

This chapter focuses on finding and evaluating clinical trials for treatment, not for support, prevention, or detection. For the sake of readability, we will use the word "substance" throughout this chapter, with the understanding that either new substances or new methods can be the objects of testing.

For more information on clinical trials, see Robert Finn's book, *Cancer Clinical Trials* (O'Reilly, 1999).

Who should examine clinical trials?

The National Cancer Institute recommends that if you have any stage of small cell lung cancer, or non-small cell lung cancer at a stage beyond IA, examination of clinical trials may be very much worth your while. The factors that contribute to this statement are discussed at length in Chapter 6, *Prognosis*.

All lung cancer survivors should become familiar with methods for finding clinical trials and with the general structure and function of trials. If you wait until you need a trial to attempt to learn these things, you may run out of time.

Geri Capasso, whose brother Anthony participated in a clinical trial, reinforces this need for preparedness:

> *No matter which treatment you're on, find out how they are measuring the results and, as soon as it's not working, be ready with a second line of treatment. We sent my brother's tumor cells to the Weisenthal lab in California for chemosensitivity testing, and he is now on weekly Taxol with daily thalidomide. There have been a few articles about some work with low-dose, more frequent chemo, which seems to lessen the adverse side effects and seems more effective. Don't hesitate to speak to the oncologist about symptoms.*

What are clinical trials?

Clinical trials are the tests by which new treatments are evaluated to see if they offer more benefit than existing treatments. Success of a new treatment in the highly structured, controlled environment of a clinical trial is required by the US Food and Drug Administration (FDA) before treatment can be approved for wider use by doctors and patients in less controlled settings. When clinical trials show that a new treatment is better than older, standard care and these results are verified by objective third parties, the treatment that was used in the clinical trial becomes the new standard for care.

Clinical trials are tests run in the clinic, or, more clearly stated, on humans. The word "clinical" distinguishes these trials from tests done on tumor samples or on animals. Clinical trials are not started on humans until a substance has shown promise when tested first on human tumor samples and then on animals, usually mice.

There are many kinds of clinical trials. The ones that usually interest most lung cancer survivors are the ones that focus on treatment, but trials also exist to improve cancer support, detection, and prevention. A clinical trial can test either a new substance, a new combination of substances, a new surgical technique, or a new method for administering treatment.

Clinical trials are designed and structured so that the results can withstand the minute and critical scientific scrutiny necessary to determine if a new treatment is effective. Three study designs that aid in ensuring that the results of treatment are attributable to the new agent and not to chance or confounding factors include randomization, blinding, and double-blinding. Blinded and double-blinded trials are rare in the testing of new cancer therapies, but an explanation of these concepts is included here so that you will be well informed should you be asked to participate in a blinded trial:

- A randomized trial is one in which a large number of patients with the same disease are assigned via computer to receive either the new treatment or existing, standard treatment. This means that you might not receive the new substance at all. Randomization is used to demonstrate as clearly as possible that a group of similar patients did either better or worse, and that only the treatment given explains the difference in outcome. The ideal randomized clinical trial would treat only patients that are alike in every respect except for the treatment given. This would ensure that the only difference that accounted for success or failure is the treatment used. In reality, this regimentation is not possible because patients are human beings who might differ in many respects.

- In a blinded trial, not only are patients randomized, they also are unaware of which treatment they're receiving. This is considered necessary to rule out the placebo effect, defined as the ability of the human body to respond differently to treatment in measurable, physical ways, based on complex psychological and motivational factors experienced by the patient. Some patients might respond better to a treatment, for example, simply if they know they're getting a new treatment as opposed to an older one. Passive, compliant patients might report responses that they think will please the doctor and staff. The placebo effect is the subject of some controversy, with some researchers maintaining it's truly measurable, and others believing that its supposed effects can be attributed to other phenomena, such as inaccurate metrics or patient subjectivity.

- A double-blinded trial is one in which the patients and some of the medical staff are unaware which substance is received by whom. For example, the patient, the nurse who measures vital signs, and the pathologist who examines tissue samples might be unaware of which substance is received. The doctor writing orders as outlined by the trial's protocol is aware, though, because she must be prepared to deal with side effects that arise. Double-blinding is used to eliminate the possibility that the patient might sense subtle factors, such as motivation and mood on the part of the nursing staff. These could account for differences seen in the progress of the group receiving the new treatment compared to those receiving the old—see the placebo effect, described in the preceding paragraph.

- A case-control study is one in which patients are matched on as many characteristics as possible, then one group is given a particular treatment and the other group is not. For cancer clinical trials, the characteristics on which patients are matched are disease characteristics. Very few case-control studies are designed for cancer treatment, although they are for cancer prevention.

Here are examples of cancer trials both randomized and double-blinded currently in the NCI's clinical trials database:

- Phase III randomized, double-blind study of warfarin versus placebo for chemo-prevention of thrombosis in central venous access catheters in cancer patients

- Phase III randomized, double-blind study of megestrol versus dronabinol versus both drugs in patients with cancer-related anorexia and cachexia

Because of their trilevel structure, peer-reviewed design, and enforced controls, clinical trials differ from less rigorous tests designed and administered by doctors and researchers working independently on new substances in for-profit cancer clinics. These researchers—some of whom are well respected by the broader medical community, some of whom are not—often lack complete records and consistent evidence that can be verified by impartial observers. Often, their patients are not subjected to the necessary long-term evaluation of five years or more that determines whether the new treatment truly made a sustained difference in patient survival.

In general, if trials are run by a university, an NCI-designated regional cancer center, or a pharmaceutical company adhering to NCI and FDA guidelines, the chances are very good that safeguards for the patient are part of the design and that the substance being tested has been reviewed and approved for use by a committee of responsible and knowledgeable researchers. Therapies offered by independent researchers in their own for-profit clinics, especially those that involve ingesting or injecting an untested substance, should be avoided or, at the very least, approached with extreme caution.

Why use clinical trials?

Aside from the altruistic aspect of participating in a trial in order to benefit others—an aspect that may or may not motivate you—clinical trials offer you a good chance to receive more effective treatment, and perhaps a cure, years before it's available to the general public.

Steve Dunn is a nine-year survivor of metastasized kidney cancer. In CancerGuide, he tells of his difficult experience with this cancer, which, prior to the availability of inter-leukin-2 therapy developed at the NCI, had five-year survival statistics in the 2 to 3 percent range. Like most people facing cancer treatment decisions, Steve started at ground zero with no medical background or insider information to assist his search.

Steve's story is available at the CancerGuide web site, *http://www.cancerguide.org*, one of the best cancer sites on the Internet. His personal story alone is probably enough to convince most people of the benefits of finding the best clinical trial for their circumstances. Moreover, his advice to patients for locating, examining, and choosing a clinical trial is unparalleled in the scientific and lay literature.

Won't I be just a guinea pig?

In the US, the long and not altogether honorable history of the clinical trial process has resulted in laws, procedures, and methods that safeguard the patient. For example, each clinical trial has a lengthy plan, called a protocol, that will be given to you if you ask for it. The protocol describes what will be done and when, and what action will be taken if certain undesirable effects occur. You should always ask for, and read thoroughly, a copy of the full protocol.

Informing the prospective patient and obtaining consent from the patient are time-consuming and repetitive processes done to ensure that all risks and benefits are made clear. For example, the patient should be made aware that she can drop out of the study at any time and that care cannot be denied her if she does so.

Unfortunately, sometimes patients are pressured to sign clinical trial consent forms without full information, or at the last minute, without time to consider other options. Remember that very few lung cancers progress fast enough to require a same-day decision.

- Always ask that the consent forms and the protocol be sent to you well in advance of your scheduled visit.

- Do not sign a consent form until you have received and read a copy of the full protocol and have considered all other clinical trials for which you might be eligible.

Only institutions funded by the federal government or governed by pertinent local laws are required to abide by consent guidelines. If you're in a for-profit hospital that receives no government support, it's possible for you to be treated in a study without your knowledge or consent, thinking that you're getting standard treatment. Ask your doctor if your treatment represents state-of-the-art treatment as defined by the NCI or if you're being treated in a study. In addition, phone your state health department to determine if your state has its own laws regarding consent issues.

Placebos

For cancer clinical trials, true placebos are almost never used. A true placebo is a drug or treatment that has been made to look exactly like the active substance or the effective procedure, but has no effect. In clinical trials of antihistamines, for instance, the placebo used most often is a sugar pill.

For randomized cancer treatment trials—usually phase III trials, of which more is said later in the chapter—the new treatment is compared to existing, accepted treatment, not to a placebo. Exceptions to this ethical policy are new treatments for which no corresponding previous treatment exists, such as trials of the earliest efforts to purge bone marrow of cancerous cells prior to bone marrow transplantation. In that instance, standard care was represented by reinfusion of unpurged marrow, and the test treatment involved reinfusion of marrow that was purged using an experimental technique.

How are clinical trials run?

Clinical trials are organized into three stages: phase I, phase II, and phase III. Each phase attempts to address different and increasingly complex issues concerning the success of the new treatment. Some drugs are tested in trials that are a combination of two phases, such as phase I/II or phase II/III. Usually this is done if some knowledge of the new treatment's effect in humans is already known so that its development and testing can be expedited.

There may be clinical trials in which you can participate locally on an outpatient basis, but many require travel and inpatient stays.

Phase I clinical trials

The primary purpose of a phase I clinical trial is to measure the safety and toxicity of different doses of a new substance in the human body. Some phase I studies may also assess tumor response, therapeutic effectiveness, the amount of drug that accumulates in the body, and a substance's general behavior (pharmacokinetics) in the body.

Phase I trials are preceded by animal studies that measure toxicity, so an estimated safe human dose is already known. Rigorous controls are enforced to be sure that no patient suffers adverse effects. For example, blood or urine values of certain body substances may be measured several times a day to ensure that the liver and kidneys are not compromised. Doses that are found to be unacceptably toxic are lowered.

Phase I trials usually enroll just a few patients, perhaps ten to thirty. Often these patients have a variety of different cancers. Sometimes one cohort of patients will receive only a low dose of the drug, and a different group will receive higher doses; but in other studies, the same patients who initially receive a low dose may be given a higher dose later if toxicity is not too profound.

The advantages of a phase I trial are:

- You may receive a treatment that may be better than anything else currently approved by the FDA years before it becomes available to the general public.

- If this drug is already in use for other illnesses, its toxic effects might not be completely unknown.

- Candidate substances for cancer treatment are not approved for phase I trials unless the substance has shown reasonably acceptable toxicity, as well as activity against cancer, in cultured tumor cell lines and in animal studies. Of every five thousand substances tested in animals, only five enter phase I trials.

- Doses found to cause unacceptable toxicity are lowered.

The disadvantages of a phase I trial are:

- For every 100 drugs tested in phase I trials, only 70 will prove successful or safe enough to carry forward into phase II trials.

- Because phase I trials are chiefly concerned with discovering dose-limiting toxicity, they are brief compared to phase II and III trials. You may receive too few doses of the test substance to destroy all of your cancerous cells.

- Phase I trials usually test one substance alone, yet experience has shown that, at least for the chemotherapeutic agents commonly used today, combined drug regimens often are more effective against most cancers than single-drug regimens.

- The substance, although it may be an approved drug for other illnesses or even for other cancers, most likely has never before been used in humans for your illness. Although it has been tested in cultured tumor cell lines and in animals implanted with tumors, it may not be effective against your tumor, or it may be no better than existing treatments.

- The substance, although it may be an approved drug for other illnesses or even for other cancers, may be administered to you at a much higher, more toxic dose.

- The dosage will be varied among those enrolled, thus its effects on your tumor may not be directly comparable to the effects on the tumors of others enrolled in the trial . . . and patients do talk among themselves.

- The use of patients with different tumor types makes it difficult for you to compare your progress to that of other patients.

- Toxicity may cause substantial discomfort, illness, or permanent damage, in spite of the safeguards designed to prevent damage.

- Often phase I trials are run by one principal investigator at one institution. You may have to travel to participate in a phase I trial.

Here are the titles of a few phase I trials for lung cancer selected from the NCI clinical trials database. These trials illustrate the broad variety of cancers being studied simultaneously in phase I trials. Note that the titles state the phase number and, at this phase, make no reference to randomization or blinding. Don't be distracted by the overly technical verbiage in these titles. You'll become more familiar with the terminology as you read more about your illness:

- Phase I/II study of Lepirudin in patients with recurrent or extensive stage small cell lung cancer

- Phase I study of Bryostatin 1 in patients with advanced cancer

- Phase I pilot study of vaccine therapy with tumor-specific mutated ras peptides in advanced cancer

Phase II clinical trials

Phase II trials measure the effectiveness of new treatments against cancer after phase I trials have demonstrated the maximum safe dose. Some phase II trials also attempt to measure how best to deliver the drug to the tumor—orally, by infusion, and so on—and how often the dose should be given.

Phase II trials enroll many more patients than phase I trials, perhaps fifteen to eighty, so that the substance will receive a more thorough test and the statistics collected will be more meaningful.

Sometimes, but not always, phase II clinical trials are divided into arms, with one arm getting one version of the experimental treatment and a second arm getting another—perhaps the same experimental agent combined with an established, FDA-approved cancer-killing drug; or delivered by another route; or on a different dose schedule.

Because some phase I trials seek preliminary evidence of efficacy against disease,[1] a clearer idea might exist regarding what cancers will benefit most from this treatment when it's used in a phase II trial. Nonetheless, the researchers designing the trial usually determine the types of cancers that will be addressed in a phase II trial. Sometimes parallel phase II trials for different cancers will be designed and funded.

Phase II trials take more time than phase I trials because, unlike phase I trials, more of the new agent is administered for a longer time in an attempt to cause tumor regression.

The advantages of a phase II trial are:

- Candidate substances for cancer treatment are not approved for phase II trials unless phase I trials have shown that the substance is safe at a given dose and, in some trials, that the substance has some activity against cancer in humans.

- You'll be receiving a treatment that may well be better than anything else currently approved by the FDA several years before it becomes available to the general public.

- Only doses of acceptable toxicity, determined during phase I testing, are utilized.

- Randomizing and blinding usually are not used in phase II trials. Therefore, you are assured of receiving the experimental treatment.

The disadvantages of a phase II trial are:

- More than half of the drugs used in phase II trials will be found ineffective against cancer or too problematic for use. Of the original 100 drugs that entered phase I trials, of which 70 survived to pass to phase II, only 33 will survive phase II testing.

- The substance, although it may be an approved drug for other illnesses or even for other cancers, may not prove to be better than existing treatments for your illness.

- Although its toxicity was determined in the phase I trial of this substance, the substance is still an evolving treatment with the potential for unexpected side effects.

- More of your time will be needed for a phase II trial than for a phase I trial.

- You might have to travel to participate in a phase II trial.

Here are a few examples of phase II trials for lung cancer selected from the NCI clinical trials database. Note the occasional use of randomization and that fewer cancer types are eligible:

- Phase II study of intensive chemotherapy with peripheral blood stem cell support in patients with small cell lung cancer

- Phase II randomized study of autologous tumor cell vaccine in patients with advanced cancer

- Phase II study of vasopressin receptor type I-A antagonist SR49059 in patients with refractory small cell lung cancer

Phase III clinical trials

Phase III clinical trials test a new substance's efficacy compared to existing standard treatments.

Phase III trials are much larger than phase II trials and are almost always multi-center trials; that is, trials run in many sites simultaneously. They run for years, including multiyear follow-up of the patient's cancer status and overall health.

The large number of patients in a phase III trial tends to flatten any aberrant statistics that result from patient differences that would lessen the usefulness of statistical data collected in a smaller trial. For this reason, patients in a phase III randomized trial can be of various ages and both sexes, for example, as long as they're all stage III NSCLC patients or all SCLC patients with limited disease, and so on.

Phase III trials are almost always randomized (case-control studies are not), but are not always blinded or double-blinded. When blinding is used, patients might discover which treatment they're receiving based on side effects, comparisons in conversations with other patients, or other overt or subtle phenomena.

The advantages of a phase III trial are:

- A substance that has survived the scrutiny of phases I and II is very likely to be better than current treatments: either more efficacious, or equally effective but less toxic.

- You'll be receiving a treatment that may be better than anything else currently approved by the FDA a year or two before it becomes available to the general public.

- If, during the trial, a new treatment shows itself to be profoundly superior to existing treatment, those receiving the existing treatment are switched to the arm of the study utilizing the new substance.

- If a new treatment shows itself to be clearly or dangerously inferior to existing treatment, those receiving the new treatment are switched to the standard treatment regimen.

The disadvantages of a phase III trial are:

- Of the 33 drugs that survived phase II testing, only about 25 will be found effective in phase III trials.

- Randomizing and blinding may not appeal to those who are determined to receive only the new treatment, not the contrasting current treatment.

- The new substance may prove to be just as effective as, but no better than, the existing treatment.

Here are a few examples of phase III trials for lung cancer selected from the NCI clinical trials database:

- Phase III randomized study of Matrix Metalloprotease Inhibitor AG3340 in combination with paclitaxel and carboplatin in patients with recurrent or metastatic non-small cell lung cancer

- Phase III randomized study of Gadolinium Texaphyrin as a radiosensitizer in patients with brain metastases receiving whole brain radiotherapy

Which phase is best?

This chapter cannot offer you absolute advice about which type of clinical trial is best for you. Only you and your treatment team should make this decision. Several aspects can be considered, though:

- A phase III trial that offers randomization to either standard therapy or a new therapy might be the choice that's right for you. The relative safety of receiving a known regimen might be reassuring to those who discover that they have not been randomized to the new treatment arm.

- A phase III trial in which all patients receive the new drug and only an ancillary feature of treatment (such as one antibiotic against another to control infection) is randomized might be as good a choice as a phase II trial of a less well-known substance.

- A phase II trial of a very promising substance might appeal to patients who find phase I trials too risky and phase III trials too controlled.

- A phase I trial of a drug with a long, safe history of use for another illness might be a reasonable choice for you if animal studies have shown that the agent is active against lung cancer and if you have tried other treatments without success.

Where are clinical trials run?

Clinical trials are found most often at NCI-designated Comprehensive Cancer Centers, Clinical Cancer Centers, and at other university medical hospitals that receive federal funding and cooperate with the NCI on clinical trials. Your community oncologist may participate through association with the NCI's community clinical oncology programs. See Chapter 3, *Finding the Right Treatment Team,* for more information on NCI-designated cancer care centers.

Finding trials for lung cancer

If you're an adult with lung cancer, you must take an active role in finding the best care for your disease. Adults with cancer are seldom asked to join a trial unless they are being treated in a regional cancer care center. (The approach needed by adults is different from that for children with cancer, whose families are commonly approached regarding enrollment in clinical trials, and 75 percent of whom eventually are enrolled in clinical trials.) The NCI estimates that less than 5 percent of adults eligible for clinical trials enroll and that minorities are underrepresented in the clinical trial process.

Geri Capasso tells of her brother Anthony's participation in one clinical trial and their search for others:

> It has been a difficult week for my brother. Two weeks ago when he went for his Gemzar treatment, his oncologist said he had bronchitis and sent him home with antibiotics. He was very fatigued, and by last weekend he could hardly breathe. He went to the ER last Sunday and is still in the hospital. On Monday, they drained 1.5 liters of fluid from his lung area. The biopsy of the fluid was cancer. His oncologist said that his CT scan showed significant growth, and consequently discontinued the Gemzar/cisplatin chemo treatment. He is still taking a double-blinded trial drug AG3340.
>
> On Wednesday, he got a port and began Taxotere. His breathing was still labored, and his oncologist saw growth in the heart area, so he had an echocardiogram and was put into the cardiac care unit. Early Thursday, a heart surgeon drained the fluid around his heart. His oncologist has suggested talc to stop the fluid leakage. We are praying that the Taxotere works, and we sent fluid to the Weisenthal chemosensitivity lab in California for testing with different chemos. We are considering Thalidomide and looking into new trials. My brother is still full of fight, for which I'm thankful, but I just hope that we can find the right treatment.
>
> The following Tuesday, my brother Anthony had a talc procedure to scar the lining of the lungs to stop fluid leakage. He finally didn't need the oxygen by Friday, when he began Thalidomide, and we discontinued his participation in the double-blinded Phase III clinical trial of AG3340 (I really don't think he was getting the real drug).
>
> Meanwhile, he had CT scans and a brain MRI, and a "speck" showed up, so yesterday he had a spinal tap; the fluid was replaced with a chemotherapy agent. We sent the MRI film to Staten Island Hospital for review. Today he started Taxol.
>
> Based on the chemosensitivity report, Taxol was active with his cancer cells. He is still taking Thalidomide. We had a stain test to see if he expressed Epithelial Growth Factor (EFG) and it came back positive.

We are looking into experimental drugs Iressa and ZD1839. Today he got out of the hospital, and he looks great and is breathing fine. He is physically and mentally ready to continue this fight. I'm so glad for that!

Several weeks later she says:

I'm very excited and have my fingers crossed. My brother began a clinical trial for the anti-EGF drug that Pfizer makes. It's similar to Iressa and ImClone's C225. We had previously been turned down by the FDA in requesting C225 on a compassionate plea. He has tested positive for overexpression of EGF, and I hope that he gets the same good results as others have. He is hanging in there, only using his O^2 sparingly, the second talc treatment seems to be holding against pleural effusion. He hasn't had any more problems with blood clots, and the Aredia seems to be holding the bone metastases at bay. According to the latest CT scan, his liver has about 70 percent functioning capacity, and as his oncologist nicely put it, "you can function with 30 percent." So there are rays of sunshine here and there.

You can use several methods to find clinical trials:

- Ask your oncologist which trials would suit your medical circumstances. This has its advantages and disadvantages, one advantage being that you need to do very little except trust. The disadvantages are described in the next section, "Why research trials on your own?"

- Call the National Cancer Institute at (800) 4-CANCER and ask about trials for your subtype of lung cancer, being sure to ask for the full document, not the summary, and to specify whether you're willing to travel—otherwise they'll send you local trials only. Be warned that if you call often with this request, which is not an unreasonable thing to do, because new trials are added every month, eventually they may decline to send you any more listings. This has been the experience of some cancer survivors who've used this service, which is provided by various regional cancer care centers under the auspices of the NCI.

- Research US and international clinical trials on your own at the NCI's web site, *http://cancernet.nci.nih.gov/prot/protsrch.shtml*. This, in conjunction with learning to use Medline, is by far the most comprehensive way to check on new treatments being tested. This service alone may be worth the cost of a personal computer and the time spent learning to use it. At one time, Medline was available only to those who subscribed to the NCI's Information Associates' program for an annual fee, but now the NCI provides this tool free of charge on the Internet. Note that you should examine all trials available for lung cancer, not just those in your area.

- Contact pharmaceutical companies or visit their web sites to see what trials they offer. You can also see a list of pharmaceutical web sites at Karen Parles' *http://lungcanceronline.org*.

- Use CenterWatch (*http://www.centerwatch.com*) to track new cancer treatment trials. CenterWatch has improved their service greatly in the last few months, adding new information that shows what agent is being tested and at what center the trial is being held, instead of only a general trial title and city. (This additional information is imperative if you're searching for trials at a top-notch cancer center in a large urban area.) The listings are still by state, however, forcing you to review some of the same information over and over for each state if you're willing to travel and want to be familiar with all trials available.

- Use the services of commercial Internet service providers, such as America Online (AOL), to receive email press releases from pharmaceutical companies concerning new products in development. Be aware, though, that press releases often will simply echo in less detail the medical information that you may already have found elsewhere. Furthermore, press releases typically are written to attract or reassure investors, rather than to impart fully accurate information to cancer survivors.

Why research trials on your own?

Some people who have depended only on their oncologists for comprehensive and up-to-date information on clinical trials have been disappointed. In many cases, oncologists in clinical practice—and that means most oncologists—are aware only of the high-priority trials that receive emphasis in such publications as *Oncology Times* or those that are offered nearby. Some still do not use a computer to search the NCI's database for all applicable trials. Perhaps they haven't the time to do so: remember that most oncologists in the trenches must track information on every cancer known, whereas you have the opportunity to focus intensely on your own cancer, subtype, and stage.

At the other end of the lung cancer oncologist spectrum is the oncologist associated with a university medical school or cancer research center. You can usually expect very good to excellent treatment from such a specialist, but often, when consideration of clinical trials is appropriate, they are biased toward their own research or toward trials run by colleagues at their own institution.

The following story is an all too common example of our need to educate ourselves about clinical trials:

> Several months ago, I had a phone call from a friend who now has a second cancer, a lymphoma, following treatment as a child for bone cancer. She thanked me for sending her information on the FDA's approval of a new monoclonal antibody treatment for lymphoma.
>
> She was originally enrolled in an antiviral trial at a prestigious east-coast cancer center, but the trial was halted following concerns about safety. When she showed her doctors the information on the new monoclonal antibody, they immediately put her on it. "They had never heard of it," she said.

The ideal oncologist is one somewhere in the middle: educated about most trials, able to find information quickly on new trials, aware of what's a good fit for you, but not biased toward her own work or that of colleagues.

Life doesn't often approach the ideal, so it's a good idea to learn to search for clinical trials on your own and to repeat your search every month, because new trials are constantly opening.

At the time of this writing, there are 105 trials for non-small cell lung cancer and 40 for small cell lung cancer. Once you have found a trial for which you believe you qualify, you should bring it to your doctor's attention. Suppose you find several trials that seem to admit patients with your profile? How can you tell which trial would be best for you? Clearly this is one of the most important questions that will arise in your experience with lung cancer.

At this point, you need to acquire skills for searching Medline and reading the studies that result from your searches. The substances used in each clinical trial may have results published regarding their previous use in animals or in humans. These studies should be found, evaluated, and compared, by you and your doctor, to single out the substance most likely to benefit you. Detailed techniques for searching Medline are discussed in Chapter 22, *Researching Your Illness*.

If your oncologist is unwilling to help you, is negative, or is at best ho-hum about your proactive attitude toward searching for trials, find a new doctor, because you'll need a doctor's recommendation to get admitted to a trial.

Getting admitted to a trial

Once you have found one or more clinical trials that you think you're eligible for, you must ask your oncologist to consult with and refer you to the treatment center running the trial for an evaluation to be admitted. If your doctor is unwilling to do so, seek a second opinion. You might try phoning the principal investigator listed in the trial description. Many principal investigators are willing to speak directly with prospective patients about the details of the trial and the patient's medical history. The names and phone numbers of the principal investigator and participating doctors can be found at the end of the document that describes the clinical trial.

You and your medical records will be scrutinized closely by your doctor, the doctors at the institution offering the trial, and perhaps your insurance company, to see if you're truly a candidate. Various physical parameters, such as the condition of your lungs and liver, may be factors. The kind of tumor you have, how large it is, or whether your disease is progressing must be considered.

One of the chief considerations in evaluating patients for most clinical trials is how much previous treatment they've had and what kind. Some trials want only those who have been heavily pretreated; others require patients who have not had any treatment resembling that proposed for the trial. Still others seek patients who have had no treatment at all.

You should read all of the entry criteria listed for the clinical trial and become very familiar with the results of your various tests so you'll have a good idea whether you're eligible before you approach your doctor for a referral. Questions that many other cancer survivors feel overwhelmed by—such as how long the trial will run, where it is located, and what the side effects are—will not be a problem for you because the description of the study will have answered many of these questions for you.

In order for you to be accepted, there may need to be a great deal of rapid cross-communication among you; your medical care providers; your insurance company, which will almost certainly insist on pre-approval; the oncology nurse in charge of administering the trial at the center you've targeted; the social worker; the housing assistant (if you must travel for this care); and the principal investigator (an MD) running the trial. You may need to make one or more trips to the cancer center for an evaluation. You may be pleasantly surprised by how kindly you're treated—some doctors phone personally, for instance—or you may be dismayed by lost records, lack of communication, and red tape. Other patients experience heartache and anger when, after passing all the benchmarks, a reviewing MD employed by their insurance company denies payment for the treatment after finding some discrepancy. More on this topic is discussed later in the section "About payment."

The evaluation process is the time to ask for your own copy of the full protocol. The protocol is the lengthy, fully detailed document that describes what will be done, when, and what action will be taken if certain undesirable effects occur. You should always ask for, and read thoroughly, a copy of the full protocol.

Do not sign a consent form until you have received and read a copy of the full protocol and have considered all other clinical trials for which you might be eligible.

You can expect to feel conflicting emotions at this time. The excitement of finding a treatment that may be more effective than current treatments, the fear that the treatment might have unknown effects, concerns about being away from home, nagging worries about financial considerations, and the thrill of empowerment on finding the best care may suddenly emerge as overwhelming feelings after months of relatively calm feelings about coping with your illness.

No doubt the very detailed information that is part of the full protocol will answer many of your questions and will trigger several others. In addition, consider these less-than-obvious questions, which are adapted from Nancy Keene's book, *Working With Your Doctor* (O'Reilly, 1998):

- Who reviews this study, and how often?
- Who monitors patient safety?
- Why do you believe that this treatment is better than standard treatment?
- What are the potential short- and long-term side effects of this treatment?
- Will participation in the study mean that I have to change oncologists?
- Must I be hospitalized to participate?
- What will be my costs, and what will my health insurance pay?
- Does the study follow patients for the long term?
- Who pays for any care I'll need if the treatment has negative effects?

Once you're enrolled

Detailing exactly what to expect after you're enrolled in a clinical trial is not possible in this or any book because each trial is quite different; but, in general, most people find they feel well cared for in a trial setting. It might be wise, however, to expect the unexpected. One cancer survivor, for example, traveled a great distance to take part in a clinical trial, only to be told upon arrival that the trial had been closed because of safety concerns. Others meet delays because the paperwork necessary was never forwarded by those who promised to do so, especially insurance company pre-approvals for payment.

Once treatment is underway, some people are surprised that the extensive and detailed protocol outlining the treatment really is just a guideline. Although a great deal of homage is paid to adhering to the protocol for the sake of science, the truth is that the protocol can be changed if you're suffering adverse effects. This is particularly true in a phase I trial that's measuring toxicity.

If at all possible, have a friend or relative with you during treatment to verify what medications are given, to provide emotional support, and to be an advocate if you need one. This is especially important if you have traveled some distance for care or are using morphine, for example, to control side effects.

Remember that you have the right to withdraw at any time from a clinical trial, to read your medical records, and to ask that deviations from the protocol be made if you're experiencing very bad side effects.

Experimental drugs outside clinical trials

There are several ways, other than clinical trials, to obtain drugs that are still in testing phases. See the FDA web site (*http://www.fda.gov/cder/cancer/access.htm*) for information about their regulations: "If the eligibility criteria in a study protocol are not suitable for a particular patient, it may still be possible to be treated according to the study protocol as a special exception (sometimes called compassionate exemption).... Another alternative is for a physician to file a single patient or emergency IND directly with the FDA."

Investigational new drugs (IND)

Gaining early access to drugs still being tested is possible under the FDA's treatment Investigational New Drug (IND) program, sometimes called the compassionate use program. This access is reserved for those with life-threatening diseases that have no other satisfactory treatment. According to FDA statistics, since 1987 more than 20,000 patients with cancer have received treatment under a treatment IND. For more information, contact your doctor, the drug manufacturer, or the FDA at (800) 532-4440.

Paralleling a trial

Once the FDA approves a drug for a given condition (commonly referred to as its indication), a doctor is free to prescribe this drug for any illness. This is called off-label use and demonstrates the FDA's faith in the medical community's integrity and knowledge.

If a clinical trial is testing drugs or radiation therapy techniques that are already approved by the FDA, but in new combinations or at new dose levels, your doctor might be willing to administer these to you as they would have been given within the trial. Contact your oncologist for more information.

Importation of a foreign drug

If an illness has no cure using drugs currently approved by the FDA, drugs made in foreign countries might be imported. Only those drugs meeting strict FDA regulations, though, are permitted. Among other requirements, the manufacturer must file an investigational new drug application with the FDA, and a letter justifying importation must accompany the request. For more information, contact your doctor and contact the FDA CDER division at (888) 463-6332.

About payment

Many people have found that they have difficulty getting their insurance companies to approve payment for care administered under the auspices of a clinical trial or for an investigational new drug.

One might surmise that, because cancer is a very expensive chronic disease, it would be to the financial benefit of insurance companies if better treatments were found. Nonetheless, individual companies often are unwilling to assume the costs of these studies. The trend, however, is that more companies are paying for trials than in the past or can be convinced to make exceptions for those who need treatment in trials.

The federal government has set a good example by ruling that federally insured employees will be covered for their treatment within NCI-sponsored clinical trials. Rhode Island has passed a law requiring insurance companies to pay for cancer clinical trials. The State of Maryland has passed similar legislation that will require payment of fees for treatment given as part of a clinical trial for any illness, as long as the trial is NIH-approved. Contact your state health commissioner to determine if your state has enacted similar laws.

Some cancer survivors have had success getting insurance payment approval by having their doctors supply evidence that previous tests of the new treatment showed some superiority over existing treatments, or by writing "letters of necessity" demonstrating that this experimental treatment is the only good choice available. Others have luck when their employers intervene, especially if the employer is self-insured. Still others use the news media to generate publicity that is embarrassing for the insurance company. Some cancer facilities offering clinical trials make provisions for those who want to participate but cannot pay.

IND programs may offer drugs at a reduced price.

Importation of foreign drugs for single-patient use under the FDA's strict guidelines will almost certainly be an expense you'll have to bear on your own, but do check with your health insurance company, because policies vary widely.

An excellent source of additional information on negotiating for payment of treatment is Nancy Keene's book, *Working With Your Doctor* (O'Reilly, 1998).

Free treatment

The National Cancer Institute in Bethesda, Maryland, offers free treatment for those who qualify for their trials. This is a top-notch scientific institution run by the federal government, and has some of the best cancer researchers in the country. Those who have used their services sometimes say, though, that they were very aware that they were in a research setting, as opposed to a setting oriented toward patient care and comfort. Call (800) 4-CANCER.

Non-US citizens are also admitted to trials at the NCI at the discretion of the principal investigator. Criteria that are weighed in making this decision include whether a US citizen would be denied treatment if a non-US citizen were enrolled and whether treating this particular individual's illness would benefit medical progress.

Summary

The NCI recommends that clinical trials, a means of testing new therapies in order to improve cancer treatment, can be a good choice for those with small cell lung cancer or non-small cell lung cancer at stages beyond IA. It is most wise to become familiar with clinical trials before you think you'll need one because the effort involved might require time and energy.

Clinical trials are organized into three phases that evaluate increasingly complex aspects of treatment success. Each phase has its advantages and disadvantages. A careful assessment of all clinical trials is necessary to choose the one that's best for your circumstances.

Patient rights and safeguards are carefully observed in the clinical trial setting. You are free to withdraw at any time, and you cannot be denied care if you do so.

You can find information on clinical trials by asking your oncologist, calling the NCI at (800) 4-CANCER, or searching for trials on your own. See Chapter 22 for more information on searching for trials.

Being admitted to a trial may be preceded by a flurry of administrivia surrounding your evaluation that may thrill you with its cut-to-the-chase aspect or may disappoint you with delays and miscommunications. The administrative offices of certain cancer care centers can be quite disorganized in spite of the institution's fine reputation for practicing excellent medicine.

Plan to have a friend or loved one act as an advocate for you during your treatment. It can be difficult to resolve certain problems, especially if you're far from home or using morphine, for example, to control side effects. Your emotional reactions might be surprising and conflicting, but overall you can probably expect to be confident that you've made a good choice.

CHAPTER 21

If All Treatments Have Failed

Death, the refuge, the solace, the best and kindliest
and most prized friend...

—Mark Twain (Samuel L. Clemens)

NOT SURPRISINGLY, THE PERSON who has had lung cancer, or indeed any cancer, sometimes feels compelled to consider what experiences he faces if his treatments do not succeed, and likely will do so with more clarity, urgency, and fear than the person who perceives himself to be reasonably healthy.

This chapter discusses what dying appears to be like. It assumes that your treatment options either have been exhausted or are potentially too uncomfortable or damaging to continue. Before reading further, please consider carefully whether reading this chapter will be bad for you emotionally if you still have options remaining.

Speaking to and for the patient—not for family and friends—is our chief goal, because this chapter must communicate a great deal in limited space, and many books already exist for those who will grieve. This chapter offers information about dying as an incipient event rather than addressing the problems of living well with lung cancer. We discuss the physical and emotional aspects, but not the philosophical, religious, or financial aspects of approaching death.

In the last twenty years, and especially in the last few years, many good books have become available on the topics of dying and dying well. Some, such as several by Elisabeth Kubler-Ross, tend to address those nearest the dying rather than speaking directly to the dying person. Others by Kubler-Ross, as well as such books as *How We Die* by Sherwin Nuland (Vintage Books, 1995), *The Art of Dying* by Patricia Weenolsen (St. Martin's Press, 1997), *The Dying Time* by Joan Furman and David McNabb (Random House, 1997), and *A Graceful Exit* by Lofty Basta (Xlibris, 2000), speak directly to the dying person. Please see the *Notes* for these and other books.

Preparing emotionally for death

There are probably as many emotions about dying as there are human beings, and there is no one "correct" way to die. If death is somewhat expected and not too rapid, the emotions of loss that we experience are likely to mirror those one felt at first diagnosis of lung cancer. In fact, the evolving feelings associated with loss that were described in Chapter 2, *Diagnosis and Staging*, were first described by Elisabeth Kubler-Ross following her observations of the dying. They are common to many people in the time approaching death:

- Denial that death is approaching

- Anger that you're being taken too soon or unfairly

- Bargaining with God, or with others, for more time or less pain

- Depression and sadness that death is inevitable when bargaining fails

- Acceptance that death will occur

Not everyone goes through all of these stages, evolves through them in the same order, or lingers in these stages for the same amount of time. The person experiencing great pain, for instance, is likely to long for and accept death's approach quickly rather than be angry about its approach.

These stages are not necessarily sequential and discrete: you don't necessarily feel anger until it's spent, and only then move on to bargaining, for instance. The stages often are overlapping or concurrent.

Larry Coffman has given thought to these issues:

> *How one handles the finality of death is a personal issue. The end of life is as much a part of life as the beginning, and its approach is different for each of us. My own belief is that "I'll be okay, either way."*
>
> *The stresses we face are manifest in different ways for different people. When I get really stressed out, they are manifest physically; with my wife, it is emotional and physical. You should find your own peace with what you may or may not need to face in the coming months, be it mediation, prayer, or conversation with another caregiver who has been there. Hospice is a great place to start.*
>
> *Most people have a definite problem when it comes to discussing death, but we have only two choices to apply our energies, and those are living or dying.*

I recently told my sister (diagnosed with mesothelioma recently) that she needed to make her choice. I put it this way, "Sis, are you going to continue to feel sorry for yourself, or begin the process of living, or apply your energies to dying?" I think and hope that she has chosen to live, even though the prognosis is serious.

Having faced my mortality, I have a tendency to be reality-oriented, and that makes some of those around me uncomfortable. It seems that I can discuss death as easily as I can discuss life. My family and friends don't want to discuss it either. I just force the issue at times. Besides, when it is my turn, I want to "live" until the very end and know that I'll be okay either way.

Asking for honesty

You might not be able to prepare to die as you would like if those around you are not willing to admit it's imminent. At the very least, you can expect and ask for honesty from doctors, even if family members continue to deny your approaching death in order to protect themselves a little longer.

If you have trouble getting honest answers from those around you, you might try pointing out how much it means to you to make sense of this final experience, to be ready for it, and to be as comfortable as possible. If you are convinced that death will occur soon, you might also attempt to tell those you love, because often the patient is more aware than others—sometimes even more aware than medical personnel—that the end is quite near.

Difficult family issues

Unfortunately, at this very difficult time one often needs to deal not only with one's own feelings, but with those of loved ones. This may be made even more difficult if their experiences with loss and grief are out of phase with your own. A relative's denial that you are dying is not the only issue that may sadden your final days. They may grieve earlier than you do, anticipating your death before you yourself have accepted it—or indeed, perhaps before you're dying at all. They may lag behind you in the stages of acceptance, continuing to bargain with medical personnel for life-support measures when you're ready to let go. Or perhaps your family will express anger toward you for asking questions about dying, a railing against any sign that you've given up.

You might be able to ease your family's acceptance of your death by reassuring them that they will be taken care of, by telling them that you love them, that you're weary of the battle and you welcome death, and by saying good-bye in loving ways, either openly or symbolically.

What to say to children

Dependent children and grandchildren need unique reassurances that they will be loved and well cared for after you're no longer available to love and help them. Of course, if you have dependent children, by now you've most likely done your best to arrange loving care for them, and they probably know of these arrangements.

Fortunately, there are many good books you can use to help your child or grandchild understand death in general: see Appendix A, *Resources*, and the *Notes* (in particular *I'm With You Now* by M. Catherine Ray). In general, it's considered wise to give children as much honest and literal information as possible, in terms that are appropriate for their age. For instance, it may be upsetting for your child to hear you say that you're in pain and are taking medicine for pain, but it's likely to be much more damaging if he sees you suffering, wasn't prepared to see this, and thinks your suffering can't be relieved.

Make it clear to your children and grandchildren that your circumstances were not caused by anything they did. Children are egocentric and must be reassured repeatedly that their thoughts and actions did not cause this illness.

Make it clear as well that your spouse and the child's siblings and parents are not to blame. Expect that young children will be openly or secretly angry with you for leaving them: spurts of this anger are natural and inevitable. At the same time, they may understand that it's not acceptable to blame you for dying. This doesn't leave the anger anywhere to go. Thus, the path that the young psyche may take—if they cannot blame you, and the burden of anger and self-blame is too great to carry alone—is to blame the surviving grandparent, parent, or a sibling. Make it as clear as possible that nobody is to blame and that everybody is feeling sad and sorry about your dying.

Tell them over and over that you love them and that you would not leave them if you had a choice.

There are specific points to be avoided, though, when talking to a child about dying. In her book, *The Art of Dying* (St. Martin's Press, 1997), Patricia Weenolsen suggests you avoid saying the following:

- Do not say you're simply going to sleep for a long time. Children may develop a fear of falling asleep if it's compared to dying, this phenomenon that is making all the grown-ups act so sad. If your faith includes a belief in an afterlife during which one awakes and is reunited with loved ones, try to explain that by using an analogy that does not parallel the child's normal daily actions.

- Don't tell them you're going on a long trip. They may never accept that you've died, and they may never again trust others to return. Using allegorical detail with children who are too young to do other than take what you say literally might be unwise.

- Be cautious about suggesting that your spiritual presence will remain nearby. If your children believe in and act fearful of ghosts, they may become fearful of haunting after you've died.

Forgiveness and other emotional closures

Some religions emphasize that, before one dies, certain spiritual life tasks must be completed, such as forgiving those who have harmed you, forgiving yourself, and admitting your wrongdoings.

Only you need to be satisfied with the state of your inner being as you prepare to die. You may choose to adhere closely to religious beliefs or you may decide they're not your cup of tea, that you wish to die peacefully without trying to contact everyone you've wronged, for example.

Anger about smoking

If you or your family believe that your lung cancer is related to smoking tobacco or to inhaling other carcinogens, it is to be expected that you or they will be angry with the tobacco industry or with other political or industrial groups as your death approaches. It is hoped that the anger can be channeled to useful causes, but it is possible that you or other loved ones might become the target of each other's anger.

Detachment

Just as one may have withdrawn quite naturally from healthy, unaware friends after diagnosis, cleaving instead to other cancer survivors, as death approaches, you may find yourself wanting and needing to withdraw from the living. This is a natural process, partly physical as one weakens and perhaps suffers physical pain, but it might also be a shift in the spiritual or emotional needs of the nonphysical self.

You may sense that people who have died are trying to communicate with you; you may dream about those who have died or of places distinctly not of Earth's confining dimensions. Although it's beyond the scope of this book to speculate on the meaning or veracity of such events, we can share with you that others who are dying have reported such happenings and appear to be much comforted by them. Often, these dreams and perceptions occur in the last week or so of life.

The outside observer sometimes is appalled by the sight of the family sitting in the dying person's room, talking among themselves as if the patient had already died. Although ignoring the dying person's need to communicate does sometimes happen, at other times it's a reflection of the family's tacit understanding that the dying person is withdrawing from the living.

Permission to die: the last gift of love

Many reports of the experiences of the dying tell us that some people need permission from their loved ones to let go. If you are blessed with time, you might discuss this in advance with your family. Particularly if you are in pain, try to make it clear to them that they give you a great gift when they give you permission to die.

At times, even among those who have had this discussion, a final gesture of letting go by the family, verbally or by touch, appears to be necessary in one's final moments to allow death to occur.

Physical aspects of dying

Many lung cancer survivors and their families ask what dying will be like.

How will we die?

Dying from lung cancer can occur in several ways, depending on which organs are most affected by disease. Life-threatening symptoms usually will be related to the failure of organs invaded by or near a tumor mass. Lung cancer widespread in the lungs may gradually reduce available oxygen or cause the heart to fail. Lung tumors metastasized to the brain may suppress the brain center that controls breathing or may cause seizures. Lung cancer spread to the liver or kidney may cause toxins to accumulate in the bloodstream that, in turn, cause coma.

Because lung cancer can manifest in several ways, your oncologist is the best person to prepare you for the physical symptoms you are most likely to face and what level of pain, if any, you may need to counter with medication.

Even a death preceded by great pain and discomfort sometimes is, in its very last stage, peaceful and illuminated by a brief cognizance.

When will it occur?

No human knows the answer to this question: not for lung cancer or for any other form death may take. There are well-known physical signs associated with the very last stage of life, yet some people have revived after all signs of life are extinguished. Many people have rallied for months or years after feeling so ill they wished for and surrendered to death, or after their doctors had given up all hope for survival. We can know only that our death will occur in our lifetime.

The final moments of life

Most people at this stage of death seem not to be aware of what is happening to their body or they seem to drift in and out of awareness. The perception of family members looking on at this stage is that the patient is in great discomfort, but those who have had near-death experiences do not report remembering great distress at this stage. The truth is unknown.

The visible physical signs seen most often just before death comprise the "agonal" stage and might include muscle spasm, one or more large gasps for breath, breathing that starts and stops, heaving of chest or shoulders, a single deep exhalation, clear or unclear vocalizations, or noisy breathing. All muscles relax, including bowel and bladder sphincter muscles. This might not release any body waste, though, if no food was taken recently.

These signs may be visible for just an instant or may last for several minutes.

Geri Capasso describes her brother Anthony's final hours:

> The evening my brother passed away, the interventional radiologist spoke to him about putting screens in his veins for blood clots. (He had been off blood thinners that week because of blood in the pleural effusion.) The radiologist told my brother that the pulmonologist wanted Anthony on a respirator, but he wanted to try without it, and if the stress was too much during the procedure he would be ready to hook him up. My brother said, "Go for it." I remember looking out of the window by my brother's bed. It was pouring rain, and I thought to myself that the angels were crying.
>
> A surgeon stopped by and spoke to my brother about doing another talc procedure to stop pleural effusion (it would have been his third), or a video-assisted thoracoscopy (VAT) early the next week. I helped transport Anthony's bed down to the operating room for the screen procedure. He was a bit anxious; his pulmonary doctor stayed throughout, although he didn't have to.
>
> During the procedure we heard an emergency code come from his room, and they had to put him on the respirator. It was quite tense for all of us waiting right outside (my sister-in-law, her mom, my mom, my sister, three couples who are very close to Anthony and his wife, my sister's boyfriend, and the faith healer who had a session with Anthony earlier). Anthony always said that he felt bad for anyone going through this without support, saying it would be almost impossible. It used to break my heart when he would thank me for the littlest things.
>
> I helped transport Anthony back up to ICC. My sister and I were going to spend the night (Anthony's wife spent the previous night and needed rest). Everyone was getting ready to leave. The interventional radiologist told us that they were stabilizing Anthony, and he said he was sorry about the respirator, that they would try to wean him off of it. He said he would see us tomorrow and left. Because Anthony was in ICC, the nurse didn't want us there and had us wait in the lounge area. My sister and I took turns to monitor his room, and the numbers (his vital signs) looked fine. The pulmonologist then told us that they were having a hard time stabilizing him, and that the numbers were chemically induced.
>
> My sister and I pleaded with the nurse to let Anthony's wife in, and she refused. My sister and I kept monitoring, and when it looked bad, we got

my sister-in-law into the room (I don't know where that nurse was). I took my Mom to the room. There were so many doctors. I was right outside the curtain with my Mom. Anne held Anthony's hand and told him how lucky she and the kids were to have him and how much everyone loved him. She told him, "It's okay. You can go. It's okay. It's okay." That was when his vital signs bottomed. The doctors asked her if they should try to resuscitate, and she said, "Try only once."

My Mom told us that she saw Jesus standing at Anthony's bedside when the doctors were trying to stabilize him. He was taller than everyone, and he laid his hand on Anthony's head. She thought Jesus was there to heal Anthony, not to take him. I asked her what Jesus was wearing, and she said a tunic in earth colors.

Even though we lost Anthony, I still believe in fighting this battle.

Finding the ACOR lung cancer discussion list was truly a blessing for me, and still is. I have often wondered about how people not on the Internet get information, how a publication could serve as a great benefit for them and for lung cancer awareness in general. Anthony's lung cancer was a part of his life and we are not ashamed of it (maybe because he never smoked); we are only proud of how he fought to stay here with his kids and loved ones. and I truly believe that if we keep our memories alive and often think of Anthony, then he will never be gone.

How medical staff define death

Currently, brain death is the criterion used to ascertain that death is irrefutable because other classic signs of death, such as cessation of heartbeat or breathing, can be misleading or can be reversed using twenty-first century medical technology.

Signs of brain death include loss of all reflexes, such as the blink reflex or the pupil's response to light; failure to respond physically or verbally to urgent or painful stimuli; and the absence of electrical activity within the brain, as measured by an electroencephalogram (EEG).

If a lung cancer patient dies in a hospital or under hospice care, though, medical workers are very likely simply to check for pulse and breath as death approaches. Under these circumstances, an EEG would most likely be unwarranted.

Can we make dying easier?

Easing death can take several forms: receiving physical and emotional comfort, finalizing affairs, or perhaps forgiving one's self and others for old grudges and sins. Some of these topics are addressed in other chapters; spiritual comfort and philosophical adaptation are addressed in many fine books. The following sections discuss the topics of pain control, hospice settings, and euthanasia.

It's wise to plan in advance on having a say in the comfort of your death. If you have the luxury of choices and the time to make them, draft a living will or advance directives, or both, and plan to die at home or in hospice care instead of within the hospital. Studies of care administered in hospitals show that advance directives expressing wishes against extraordinary life support measures often are ignored by doctors when care is administered in the hospital. Hospice care or care by loved ones is more likely to assure your comfort than life-saving hospital measures are. See the NCI's information on advance directives at *http://cancernet.nci.nih.gov* under "Support issues."

Pain control

The most pressing concern for many people with terminal lung cancer is the control of pain. In the past, several studies have shown that dying cancer patients did not receive adequate medication to control pain because of misconceptions on the part of medical doctors about addiction or accidental overdose. In the time since these studies have been published, however, many physicians have become better informed about pain control for the dying cancer patient. They're doing a better job of providing palliative care, but patients and especially caregivers must remain vigilant about insisting on adequate pain medication.

Hospice and hospice home care

One of the most useful resources for the comfort of the dying person and his family is hospice care, a comfort-centered concept that emerged in Europe and migrated to the United States following many years of the failure of medical technology to provide comfort for the dying. Hospice care is devoted only to making one comfortable and loved in his dying days, not to prolonging life. A peaceful and less expensive variation of hospice care is hospice home care, now quite common in the US.

Hospice nurses are on call for you twenty-four hours a day. They might visit one or more times daily if needed, or perhaps once a week or less if your needs are minimal. They are able to administer pain medication; provide skilled nursing care, such as monitoring vital signs; and train family members to provide care. They are trained to recognize the signs of impending death, and they can help the family with the arrangements that are necessary just after a death has occurred in the home. Their focus includes the physical and emotional comfort of the patient and the well-being of the surviving family members after death.

Under many hospice programs, home health aides also are available to help caregivers with some household chores and certain kinds of patient care, such as bathing.

Some hospice services charge little or nothing for those who cannot afford the service; others provide free hospice care regardless of one's financial status.

To qualify for hospice Medicare benefits and for many private insurance companies' benefits, a doctor's statement is necessary stating that the patient has less than six months to live.

The Association of Cancer Online Resources (ACOR) offers a support group, Cancer-Hospice, for patients and families under hospice care. See *listserv.acor.org*.

Euthanasia

Unfortunately, there can be painful preludes to death for which no amount of medication is adequate. In some cases, the dying and their loved ones are willing, indeed almost compelled by horrific suffering, to end life earlier than the disease would end it.

Euthanasia, the hastening of the end of life by active intervention, has been much discussed in the US recently. Groups such as the Hemlock Society and the American Medical Association have expressed divergent points of view. The American Medical Association states that doctor-assisted suicide violates their standards. The Hemlock Society publishes literature on dying and the right to die, including the 1997 book *Final Exit*.

In his book *How We Die* (Vintage Books, 1995), Dr. Sherwin Nuland, a surgeon, says:

> *In my medical practice, I have always assured my dying patients that I would do everything possible to give them an easy death, but I have too often seen even that hope dashed in spite of everything I try. At a hospice too, where the only goal is tranquil comfort, there are failures.*

Some doctors will privately state that they have broken assisted suicide laws to ease a patient's going. A personal friend who is a physician stated that, among his fellow medical doctors, about half will help a patient of their own to die when medicine and technology cannot relieve suffering.

Planning your own memorial ceremony

It's an odd fact that many people who cannot bear to think of the dying process, who cannot even conceive of their mortality, are quite happy to plan their own memorial ceremony and burial. As death becomes a certainty, many people find comfort in planning how others will remember them and celebrate their life.

Some of the things you might want to consider are:

- Whether you would like to be buried or cremated
- Where and how you would like your remains to be preserved or honored
- What memories of your life you'd like retold at your service
- If there are special songs or poems you want read or sung
- Whether the ceremony will be a religious one
- If your burial or the scattering of your ashes will be private

Summary

Dying cannot be described accurately by the living, much less by the well. Nonetheless, we have tried to listen to those preparing for death, to learn from what they say and from those nearest them, and to share these insights with you.

It is a blessing to be living during a renaissance of interest in society about dying and death and to benefit from cultural considerations of how to die well. You will find many books available to make the journey called dying as peaceful as possible.

Key points to remember:

- Adequate control of pain is often possible and should be discussed in advance with your doctor.

- Hospice care is an excellent choice for those facing death, because they provide extraordinary physical and emotional support for the dying person and his family.

- If you have time, prepare wills, living wills, and advance directives so that your wishes about dying will be known and honored.

- Communicate with your loved ones about dying. The last days or weeks of life can be beautiful and peaceful if you have the support, acceptance, and love of those around you.

CHAPTER 22

Researching Your Illness

Chance favors the prepared mind.

—Louis Pasteur

THIS CHAPTER WILL OFFER YOU ways to find information about lung cancer, outside of simply relying on your doctor. First we cover a few generalities about one's approach to learning, then we discuss the National Cancer Institute's Internet, phone, fax, and clinical trials services; using medical libraries and research journals; and hiring a search firm to do the legwork for you. We also offer methods for checking drug side effects, verifying your chemotherapy dosage, finding support groups, interpreting test results, and evaluating unproven remedies.

For each type of information, ways to access the source with and without a computer are outlined when it is possible to do so. For instance, the *Merck Manual* section on laboratory results is available both on paper and on the Internet. Certain unique resources, however, are found only on the Internet.

Reasons to research

Cancer survivors and their loved ones choose to search for information for many reasons. Many feel a compelling need to learn all they can as quickly as possible about what they'll be facing, or they feel that they must do something to contribute to their recovery. Some just like to verify that the doctor is relaying accurate and up-to-date information, even when the care they've received has been very good. Others are faced with having to assume a greater responsibility for their health care because of living in areas with few doctors or perhaps because of having had a bad experience with a doctor's lack of knowledge. HMO policies that might deny the best care in order to keep expenses down are a driving force for many. Loved ones of cancer survivors sometimes need to feel they're doing something to help, and finding information might satisfy that need.

Larry Coffman describes his reasons for doing his own library research:

> *I happen to think that any physician who would let his or her patient suffer needs to review the Hippocratic oath. Avoiding unnecessary pain is another good reason why patients, especially cancer patients, need to empower themselves with as much knowledge of their particular disease and possible treatments as they can. It's funny how different an oncologist will react when you express an understanding of what is going on. As with real estate's slogan, "location, location, location," the cancer patient's slogan should be "knowledge, knowledge, knowledge." A good source of material (albeit somewhat out of date) is the public library. The Alliance for Lung Cancer Awareness, Support and Education (ALCASE at http://www.alcase.com) and various other web sites are excellent. One needs to take extreme care and not believe everything on the Web, though. There are a lot of well-meaning people with inaccurate information. Try sticking to the "accredited" sites: ACS, ALCASE, CANCERCARE, and so on.*

The decision to research your illness is the beginning of an empowerment that will do more than just serve you in good stead for making decisions. Research on stress and cancer hints that a proactive attitude might contribute to long survival. The more you learn, the more control you have over how events unfold, not only because you'll be making better health and treatment choices, but because you can take back some of the control that is lost in the clutter of automation that now accompanies cancer diagnosis and treatment.

Max Baldwin expresses his dismay about communication with his doctor:

> *Getting information from my oncologist was like pulling teeth. Very seldom would he give a definite answer about anything. The Internet provided the best info I could find. However, a word of caution! Be sure it is a legitimate medical web site as opposed to either personal opinions or someone wanting to sell something. Many questionable sites seem to encourage megadoses of many different vitamins and other things. Remember, if it hasn't been professionally tested, it could be dangerous.*

Prerequisites and perspectives

Before you start, you need to know a few specific facts about your diagnosis to make searching more fruitful. You also will benefit by knowing what to avoid and what to insulate yourself against.

Prerequisites

You'll need three things before you start: the exact name of your lung cancer sub-type, its stage, and a medical dictionary.

If you don't know your precise diagnosis, you'll waste a lot of time and precious energy reading the wrong material. You might even frighten yourself unnecessarily by finding distressing, but wrong, information, not realizing that it doesn't pertain to you.

Your doctor's staff can read you the exact name of your lung cancer subtype from your pathology report. Better yet, ask them to send you a photocopy of this and of all your medical records.

Purchase a medical dictionary for between five and twenty dollars to help you with the terminology you will encounter, which becomes increasingly easy to understand with greater exposure. Several reasonably priced medical dictionaries are listed in Appendix A, *Resources*. One of the most useful is *The Cancer Dictionary*, by Roberta Altman and Michael Sarg (Checkmark Books, 1999).

Perspectives

The following perspectives are helpful to keep in mind while researching your condition:

- **Persistence.** Please don't feel intimidated by the volume of information on lung cancer or its seeming complexity. As with any other task of assimilation, small steps ultimately will yield great gains. If you're wary of trying to search for information because medicine seems like an alien frontier to you, it might be helpful to know a few interesting facts:

  - Academic success does not account for all that much of success in life. Success also is a result of being flexible and adaptable, developing social skills, having luck, being persistent, having patience, and so forth.

  - If one person can understand something, generally so can another person, and if the second person doesn't understand, it might be because the first person isn't explaining it very well.

  - Contrary to popular mythology that kids are computer whizzes and older people are not, the fastest growing group of Internet users is the group consisting of those over age 65.

In short, if you're persistent in asking about, searching for, and trying to absorb medical information and in turning away from doctors who are condescending, seeking instead those who respect you, you'll succeed. You won't need a degree in medicine or an abnormally high IQ to understand what you find, just a medical dictionary and the motivation to acquire new skills. It might take you twenty minutes longer to understand a certain medical concept than it takes an MD, but it's worthwhile if that twenty minutes makes the difference of a lifetime.

- **Clarity.** When asking for help, be specific about what you need. If you ask friends for help or hire a search firm to do a medical search, the same considerations about clarity and intent apply.

  Educate yourself first as to what options are available. We suggest you ask for full information, rather than edited versions that might exist. For example, when communicating with the National Cancer Institute (NCI), consider requesting the information for physicians, not for patients, if you already are somewhat familiar with lung cancer. The PDQ patient information statement is quite basic, and, although it might be useful to you initially, soon it will seem less than edifying. If you find that this is the case, it's time to request the physicians' version of PDQ information.

  Likewise, ask for the full information on clinical trails, not the summaries. Specify a national search, unless you want to limit yourself to only those trials in your area.

- **Humility.** Don't forget that you should always verify what you find with your oncologist. It's imperative that you focus on correct, current information and that you understand what it means regarding your specific circumstances. At times people simply are not equipped to evaluate what they've found, but it's almost a certainty that your doctor has a good frame of reference for doing this evaluation.

- **Courtesy.** Good manners dictate that you make an appointment to discuss lengthy topics with your doctor or other health professional or that you offer to pay for a telephone consultation. See Nancy Keene's book, *Working With Your Doctor* (O'Reilly, 1998), for a good discussion of improving patient/doctor relationships.

- **Diplomacy.** Some doctors react badly to the idea that their patients find information on the Internet because the information available on the Net ranges from abysmal to superb. If you use the Internet to research your illness, avoid using the word Internet when discussing your findings with your oncologist. Instead, use terminology that credits the original sources on which your Internet findings are based: Medline, the PDQ database of the NCI, CancerLit, certain reputable medical journals, and so on.

- **Self-respect.** If your doctor is not interested in what you find or seems threatened by your efforts, consider discussing this attitude with him or consider changing doctors.

- **Serenity.** When you have started researching your illness, you might find some information that's upsetting, such as survival statistics. Keep in mind that statistics always describe composite results of studies involving numbers of people and cannot be applied to the progress and circumstances of a single individual. For example, when a researcher averages the survival times of 80 patients treated with drug X whose survival ranges from 2 months to 212 months, she might calculate that the average survival following treatment is 13 months. An individual has no idea where to place herself on this continuum, however, unless she knows intimately the health factors of all 80 people and can match herself to at least one of them. The average will tell the researcher whether the treatment is worth further development; but for the individual, statistical averages are just data, not information.

Ways to find information

Here's a summary of ways that you can obtain information about lung cancer. The sections that follow describe these methods in detail.

The Internet

If you have a computer, you can find an almost limitless amount written about lung cancer on the Internet, some of which is highly accurate, some of which is of lesser quality:

- The highly reliable information at the National Cancer Institute's site *http://cancernet.nci.nih.gov* should be your starting point, and the latest medical research papers should become and remain an ongoing source of information.

- If you have siblings, children, or grandchildren with a computer and you don't feel like starting from scratch using a computer amidst your worries about cancer—and who would blame you?—ask them to do Internet searches for you. Make sure you tell them the specifics of your diagnosis, and what you're looking for: treatment options, complementary therapies, stories of other patients, clinical trials, and so on.

Cancer organizations

Several nonprofits and government agencies can help you find accurate, current information:

- Alliance for Lung Cancer Advocacy, Support, and Education (ALCASE): (800) 298-2436; *http://www.alcase.org*

- The American Cancer Society: (800) ACS-2345; *http://www.cancer.org*

- The National Cancer Institute: (800) 4-CANCER, or ask for instructions for using their CancerFax service

Hospital resources

Hospitals and medical schools can be good sources of information:

- If you're friends with a doctor, nurse, or librarian, ask them to do searches of various resources, such as the National Library of Medicine's Medline database and NCI's Physician's Data Query (PDQ).

- The local hospital should have a library of patient-oriented resources. This is now a requirement for accreditation by JHACO.

- Visit an academic or medical library to research the medical journals in the periodicals section and their medical texts.

- Ask your doctor for help getting copies of research papers from medical journals, but offer to pay for any photocopying that's needed.

Commercial search services

Pay a commercial firm that specializes in this activity to do a search for you, but check their credentials first because some are more reputable than others.

How to obtain the NCI's information

The information on cancer amassed and maintained by the NCI, a division of the NIH, is the granddaddy of all cancer databases and should be your starting point for learning the basics about lung cancer. It's accurate and current. You can access this information in several ways.

By phone

You can call the NCI at (800) 4-CANCER and request that information on lung cancer be sent to you by mail free of charge. Remember that the information geared to physicians is much more useful and detailed than that written for patients. If you feel uncomfortable asking for physician information, you can give some justification. For example, you could say that your doctor asked you to request this information. One patient said that she was writing a newspaper article that required in-depth material. You might want to ask as well for literature that describes all of the NCI publications that one might order, such as tracts that describe dealing with fatigue or depression.

By fax

The information available by phone request is also available by fax. You can call (800) 4-CANCER and ask for instructions for faxing.

By personal computer

If you have a computer, you can read the NCI's state-of-the-art lung cancer treatment statements for physicians, as well as an immense collection of other literature, at their web site *http://www.cancernet.nci.nih.gov*. Note that there are separate statements for non-small cell and small cell lung cancers.

Alternately, you can retrieve the NCI physician's statements on lung cancer via email by keying "help" into the message area; be sure not to include any other information, such as your signature, in the message area. Send this email to *cancernet@icicc.nci.nih.gov*.

How to obtain medical research papers

Reviewing the research papers published in medical journals is the best way to get the most current information about your illness. Textbooks are out of date almost as soon as they're printed because of the time delays of production. NCI PDQ information is a good foundation, but doesn't reflect every emerging trend still in the test phase—just state-of-the-art standards for care.

Journals that publish many papers on lung cancer include *Lung Cancer*, *Chest*, and *Thorax*. Several other cancer journals that are not specific for lung cancer or pulmonary disease, such as the *Journal of the National Cancer Institute*, also publish top-notch research on lung cancer.

Many medical and scientific journals are now on the Web, including *Science, The Journal of the American Medical Association,* and *The Journal of the National Cancer Institute.* Many of these cannot be viewed online in their entirety unless you're a subscriber to the standard paper edition, but a few, such as the *British Medical Journal* and *Blood,* provide full text free of charge.

Reading medical research papers is arguably the most difficult part of learning about progress against lung cancer, as well as the best way to keep abreast of progress. A medical dictionary will serve you well in this effort, and you should ask your doctor about any parts that are not clear. Often the abstract—a long summary of the paper—will suffice, because abstracts of cancer research studies normally contain conclusions, but obtaining the full text of a paper will be necessary if you intend to base treatment decisions on these studies. Certain details regarding patients in these studies and how they might differ from you, such as the characteristics of their disease, can be determined only from the full text of a research paper. Moreover, abstracts can contain errors because often they are written not by the coauthors of the paper, but by a technical writer not necessarily familiar with the study.

When you use the full text of a paper, don't try to understand the whole thing at first. Just read the introduction, the conclusions, and the discussion. The middle sections deal with scientific methodology that's important in verifying that the research was performed to strict scientific standards, but this part has been peer-reviewed by other scientists and the editors of the journal. This material is usually, but not always, less important to a patient trying to find good prospects for care. As you become better acquainted with research papers and their terminology, you might want to read the remaining sections occasionally, as well.

By subscription

Subscription costs for some journals such as these usually start at about one hundred dollars per year, and can go much higher. The disadvantage of subscribing to individual journals, besides the accumulation of hard-to-index paper copy, is that good research articles on lung cancer will be spread among several of these, and subscribing to several journals becomes prohibitively expensive.

By using Medline

Medline, a database maintained by the US National Library of Medicine (NLM), is an indispensable resource—some say the most important resource—for library research on medical issues. Medline contains pointers to more than eleven million medical research papers in the National Library of Medicine. Medline is indexed by hierarchical categories called MeSH terms, which are described in more detail below.

If you don't have a computer, ask a friend or relative to do a search for you. Alternately, a nurse, a medical librarian, or someone affiliated with a hospital or library may have Medline access.

NLM's PubMed

Various Medline search engines exist on the Internet, but the one offered by the NLM, PubMed, is described in this chapter.

The NLM's PubMed web address is *http://www.ncbi.nlm.nih.gov/entrez/query.fcgi?db=PubMed*. If you need help with PubMed, you can call the NLM at (800) 272-4787 or (301) 496-6308, or see the PubMed help page at *http://www.ncbi.nlm.nih.gov/entrez/query/static/help/pmhelp.html*.

Searching with PubMed

The PubMed site offers a search engine that accepts keywords and returns titles of studies that match your keywords. For example, if you key the terms, "lung cancer treatment gemcitabine" and click "Go," you'll receive in return more than 300 titles of studies regarding treating lung cancer with gemcitabine. You will almost certainly want to narrow this search to fewer studies, and this process is described below.

Note that placing quotes around search terms causes the search engine to treat these words as a single search term. Take care not to enter too many keywords because this will result in too few or no results.

The latest studies are displayed first. In some cases, even though a search has returned many results, you might be interested in only the latest studies because they might represent the most recent progress in cancer care. Here are some tips for searching with PubMed:

- Clicking on a single title will cause an abstract of the study's results to display on your screen.

- Clicking on the box to the left of the title flags the information for later retrieval. Normally, this box is used when you want to see the abstracts of several studies at once. You choose the level of detail at the top of the screen next to the "Display" box. Choose "abstract" for a summary of the paper and then click "Display."

Don't be discouraged by the medical terminology you see in these abstracts. After you've read a few, the terminology will become more familiar.

Narrow the search

Several options are available to narrow the number of studies returned to a smaller number for a more incisive review.

You can use the "Limits" option just beneath the keyword box. Once selected, the limit screen allows you to specify a specific age group, gender, or human or animal studies. The "Limits" option also allows you to restrict to articles published in a specific language and to specific types of articles, such as review articles. You can limit results to certain publication dates. You might choose, for instance, to limit your results to papers published in the last five years.

You can also create a more incisive list of results by repeating the search using additional keywords you found while browsing. For example, adding the additional keywords "NSCLC" and "vindesine" to our original search: "lung cancer treatment Gemcitabine NSCLC vindesine" returns only eleven studies.

Take care when using this winnowing technique that you do not accidentally omit a study that's worth seeing. It's better to err on the side of producing too many results and spending additional time browsing titles than to over-specify search terms and miss information that might be pivotal in your decision making.

Reviews

A good way to get background information on any medical topic is to find review articles for that topic in Medline. Review articles attempt to cover medical progress to date on a given topic and often are geared to those who are not medical super-specialists. Including the word "review" with your search terms or choosing it as an option from the "Limits" page will retrieve abstracts of review articles appearing in more generalized publications, such as *Family Practitioner* or *Nature*; these articles contain more explanatory material and make fewer assumptions.

Suppose, for instance, that you have fluid accumulating in your chest and your surgeon has suggested a procedure called pleurodesis to create scar tissue that will stop fluid accumulation. You can read reviews about the pros and cons of pleurodesis discovered over time by searching for the keywords "pleurodesis lung cancer review," which returns eight review papers, as opposed to 32 studies when the word "review" is omitted.

If a clinical trial of vaccine therapy is being recommended to you, you might want to search for review papers by keying "lung cancer vaccine review," which returns 25 review papers, as opposed to the 174 studies that discuss lung cancer and vaccines, but might not be reviews of all past research.

If you've been told your non-small cell lung tumor exhibits neuroendocrine characteristics more often found in small cell lung cancer, you can search for "NSCLC neuroendocrine review," which returns five research abstracts, instead of 53 studies that might or might not be reviews.

Advanced PubMed features

PubMed offers many other ways to refine and limit searches for optimal results, such as Boolean operators (AND, OR, NOT), Preview/Index, History, and Clipboard. For more detail, see the PubMed help page, which can be accessed on the left sidebar of the main PubMed page.

MeSH terms

Almost all of the web-based Medline search engines use an organizational hierarchy called Medical Subject Headings (MeSH). MeSH terms group references by category so that you'll get more specific research papers returned for your searching efforts, even if you're not familiar with the right medical terms or if you misspell a word slightly. Some Medline search tools invoke MeSH terms behind the scenes when you enter a keyword; others will prompt you to pick a MeSH term from a list that is associated with the keyword you entered. Still others have advanced searches you can invoke using MeSH terms explicitly.

You don't need to know MeSH terms to search Medline, however. Many people find that searching by keyword comes more naturally to them.

Obtaining full text

If the Medline abstracts you read are more tantalizing than edifying, you can order the full text of any research paper from companies that specialize in this service. Some of these companies, such as InfoTrieve, are web-based; others can be found by calling a medical school library and getting recommendations from a librarian. Unfortunately, at the time of this writing, the National Library of Medicine's service does not offer full text retrieval to those not associated with an academic library. Those who are, however, can use the Loansome Doc service to order full text of papers.

On the Internet, the Medline service providers HealthGate, Medscape, Helix, PhyNet, PDRnet.Com, SilverPlatter, Ovid On Call, Infotrieve, PaperChase, and others offer full-text services for a fee.

By using medical libraries

Another way to find articles in medical journals is to visit a medical or university library and examine their journals, borrowing or photocopying what you find most useful. US copyright law permits photocopying one copy of a journal article if it's for your own immediate use.

Note that some university and medical libraries restrict entry to those affiliated with the institution in some way.

Your local hospital might have a medical library. Recent upgrades in standards for hospital accreditation require that hospitals build and maintain patient libraries.

You can find the nearest medical library open to the public by calling the National Network of Libraries of Medicine at (800) 338-7657.

To find articles in medical journals, ask the main information desk where periodicals are stored and how to search them by subject. There's some variety in how different libraries store, search, and retrieve journal articles. Some academic libraries have all periodicals stored on CD-ROM, for example, but others are still stored as paper copy in the stacks. Regardless of these differences, there's always a way to search by subject, and this should be your starting point. The library you visit might also have access to Medline.

Often the periodicals section of a medical or academic library will have staff devoted to helping you. All should have material you can read at your leisure describing how to search their collection.

Don't be shy about asking for help. Most librarians are proud of their ability to root out obscure references and are in that career because they want to connect people to information.

Arrive prepared to pay for photocopy fees and with coins for photocopy machines.

By hiring a search firm

Before hiring a commercial firm to do a search of the medical literature, you might want to call the National Library of Medicine's Management Desk at (800) 638-8480 and ask for whatever help they can provide.

You might choose to pay a search fee to one of a number of companies who provide this service. Tell them what topic you're interested in, but keep in mind that the more specific you can be, the better: treatments for stage III non-small cell lung cancer for those under age 50, rather than just "lung cancer," for instance, will yield more useful material on this topic. The search firm will locate and mail copies of articles from medical journals.

It would be wise to check the credentials of such firms before deciding to use one because some are more reliable than others.

Here's a partial list of such companies. Their being included here does not imply an endorsement of their service:

* The Health Resource, Inc.: (501) 329-5272

* Can Help: (360) 437-2291

* Schine On-Line Services: (800) FIND-CURE

How to obtain medical textbooks

Texts on cancer genetics, immunology, and lung cancer can provide you with the foundation for understanding more timely sources, such as the papers published in medical journals. In general, the more recent the text, the better.

A source of background information might be an oncology text aimed at premed college students or first-year medical students. The terminology might be a notch higher than many people are comfortable with, but not nearly as difficult as that found in medical journals, and it's definitely geared to providing broad, fundamental information.

Using the list of books in Appendix A as a guide to reliable texts, visit your local public or academic library.

You can also buy textbooks. They'll probably range in price from $40 to $200. Some of the largest well-known bookstore chains carry hard-to-find textbooks, or they can order them for you. Several bookstores have web sites that greatly facilitate ordering books, especially if you're not feeling well enough to drive, park, browse, and lug heavy texts home.

It's fairly easy to get used copies of textbooks at college and university bookstores. Medical bookstores usually are found near medical schools.

Because of the high cost of textbooks, borrowing texts is an attractive alternative for most people.

If you haven't used a public library lately to search for holdings, you might be pleasantly surprised to find that, in many cases, the old card catalogs are gone, replaced by fast and easy-to-use computer workstations. Their databases can tell you within a few minutes how many copies of a book are in their system, which branches of the library own the book, whether another borrower has charged it, and when it's due back.

If your public library is in a large urban area, the materials you need might be readily accessible; if not, your library system may be able to borrow the materials you need even if they're not in their holdings. As with searching for medical research papers, it pays to ask for help. You might have to wait longer for an interlibrary loan, but it can save you the cost of an expensive text.

How to find clinical trials

New and possibly better treatments are available to lung cancer patients in carefully controlled settings called clinical trials, which are described in depth in Chapter 20, *Clinical Trials*. You should become familiar with the trials that are available before you need one, for frequently trials are needed when events have reached crisis level and time is running low.

We strongly suggest that you examine all trials available for lung cancer, not just those in your area.

In order to choose the best from among several clinical trials, it's necessary to be familiar with the track record, if any, of the treatments being used in each trial. Each of the drug names or surgical techniques appearing in a trial's title can be used as a keyword to search medical journals for any previous research studies published, as described in the earlier section "How to obtain medical research papers." This can be a daunting task: do not expect to finish it in one sitting or even in a few days. Once it's done, though, you only need to search for new treatments as they first appear in the clinical trials database or among your other sources of information.

You can use several methods to find clinical trials: asking your oncologist, calling the NCI, hiring a search firm, or searching on a computer.

By asking your oncologist

You can ask your oncologist which trials would suit your medical circumstances. This has its advantages and disadvantages; one advantage being that you need do very little except trust. A full discussion of advantages and disadvantages of relying only on your oncologist for trial information can be found in Chapter 20, but patients should not be deterred by a negative or apathetic oncologist from seeking out trials on their own.

Note that your entry into a clinical trial must be coordinated between your oncologist and the investigators running the trial, so you will need her cooperation.

By calling the National Cancer Institute

Call the NCI at (800) 4-CANCER and ask about trials for lung cancer. Be sure to specify whether you're willing to travel—otherwise they'll send you local trials only—and be sure to ask for the full document, not the summary. Be warned that if you call often with this request (which is not an unreasonable thing to do, because new trials are added every month), eventually they may decline to send you any more listings. This has been the experience of some cancer survivors who've used this service, which is provided by various regional cancer care centers under the auspices of the NCI.

If you have a personal computer, you can use the NCI's search engine for clinical trials: *http://cnetdb.nci.nih.gov/trialsrch.shtml*.

By hiring a search firm

Commercial firms that can do a medical literature search for you also exist. A partial list of such companies appeared earlier under the topic "How to obtain medical research papers."

By personal computer

You can use a computer and the Internet to research US and international clinical trials at the NCI's web site, listed at the end of this paragraph. This, in conjunction with learning to use Medline, is by far the most comprehensive way to check on new treatments being tested. Once available only to those who subscribed to the NCI's Information Associates' program for $100 per year, this tool is now provided free of charge by the NCI on the Internet at *http://cnetdb.nci.nih.gov/trialsrch.shtml*.

When you visit this site, you'll be presented with a menu of choices for finding trials by cancer type, location of trial, kind of trial, and so on. Use the down arrow next to "Type of cancer" to expand the list of cancers, then scroll down and click on one of these:

- Lung cancer, small cell

- Lung cancer, non-small cell

- Lung cancer, pulmonary carcinoid tumor

- Metastatic cancer

- Solid tumor, unspecified, adult

If you're using this search engine for the first time, it's a good idea to view all lung cancer treatment trials that are available for your type. Use the down arrow next to "Type of trial" to select the word "treatment," then click the search button, leaving the other fields with their default values. The result will be a very large list of all trials for lung cancer that focus on treatment. You will be asked to either view these or narrow the search. The first time through, quickly browse all the titles to gain a broad familiarity with the trials available.

Then repeat the search using these delimiters, selecting one or more of these fields for an increasingly narrow list of results:

- "City" and "State" to see trials only in your own area, if you're unable to travel

- "Stage of cancer" set to I, II, III, or IV

- "Phase of trial" to see only phase I, phase II, or phase III trials, which are explained in Chapter 20

- "Modality" to select trials using a specific technology, such as monoclonal antibodies, which are categorized as antibody therapy

- "Drug" to search for a specific drug name

- "Clinical trials added to PDQ this month" to repeat your search every 30 days for only the newest trials

Other means of finding clinical trials include:

- CenterWatch's site on the Internet to track new cancer treatment trials: *http://www.centerwatch.com.*

- Commercial Internet service providers, such as America Online (AOL), to receive email press releases from pharmaceutical companies concerning new products in development.

- Drug manufacturer web sites to locate privately funded pharmaceutical trials. Karen Parles' Lung Cancer Online, *http://www.lungcanceronline.org*, contains links to a great deal of useful information including links to pharmaceutical companies that run clinical trials of their own investigative substances. Karen is a lung cancer survivor and a medical librarian who was kind enough to review this chapter. Visit the site *http://www.lungcanceronline.org/websites.htm#pharmcos*.

How to find support groups

Local hospitals, a local branch of the national Wellness Community, the American Cancer Society, ALCASE, and the Internet offer solid information, as well as access to others who have been through it, too. Their help and comfort are beyond estimation. The American Cancer Society can be reached at (800) ACS-2345; ask for their *I Can Cope* program. The Wellness Community in your area is listed in the phone book. ALCASE can be reached at (800) 298-2436 or at *http://www.alcase.org*.

If you have Internet access, the Association of Cancer Online Resources (ACOR) has pointers to all of the Internet cancer email discussion groups. Highly recommended are the lung cancer lists for emotional support and medical information. For this and other Internet discussion groups, ACOR offers a handy automatic subscription feature. See *listserv.acor.org*.

How to verify drug information

Pharmaceutical information tools are useful for finding drug side effects, mode of action, and marketing names. Your pharmacist, your library or bookstore, your computer, and the FDA can be sources of information.

You can call your pharmacist for information about drugs or ask for the foldout paper of small print that comes from the drug manufacturer, but is seldom included with your prescription unless you ask for it.

The Physician's Desk Reference (PDR), a compendium of information about drugs, is now reprinted in versions that are easier for the general public to understand. In addition to PDR, many other drug encyclopedias are available for the general public.

The Food and Drug Administration is a good means for verifying drug information. Call (888) 332-4543 or (800) 532-4440, or visit *http://www.fda.gov*. You can report adverse effects of drugs to the FDA, or use their MedWatch web site: *http://www.fda. gov/medwatch/how.htm*.

If you have a computer, the following sites have search engines requiring only the drug name:

- Clinical Pharmacology Online (free, but requires registration): *http://www.cponline.gsm.com*

- Rxmed: *http://www.rxmed.com*

- DrugInfoNet: *http://www.druginfonet.com*

- HealthTouch: *http://www.healthtouch.com/level1/p_dri.htm*

- Mythos Pharmacy Online: *http://www.mythos.com/pharmacy*

How to verify your chemotherapy dose

For most drugs, you can use a general formula for calculating dosages of your chemotherapy drugs and can compare it to the amount that is recommended for you in your medical records. Keep in mind, though, that your doctor might be using a different dose for very good reasons or that your regimen might include drugs that are not given based on body surface area, but instead on renal function, for example.

Glaxo's DoseCalc site (*http://www.meds.com/DChome.html*) deserves special mention as a user-friendly research site because it's a great way to verify your chemotherapy dosage. Enter your height, weight, and a drug name. Behind the scenes, it calculates your square feet per meter (yes, square, not cubic, feet per meter—the basis for most chemotherapy dosages) and gives you the standard dose administered for a person your size.

You can also do this calculation using your body surface area and the standard recommended dose for your body surface area by using one of the following web sites to calculate your body surface area:

- Cornell University: *http://www-users.med.cornell.edu/~spon/picu/bsacalc.htm*

- Medical College of Wisconsin: *http://www.intmed.mcw.edu/clincalc/body.html*

- Martindale's HS Guide: *http://www-sci.lib.uci.edu/HSG/Pharmacy.html*

Or, try a web search on the phrase "body surface area." Note that some of these sites use slightly different formulae, and so the results will differ slightly.

For the truly dedicated, calculation of body surface area can be done by hand. One formula for calculating your body's surface area in square meters is the DuBois & DuBois formula:

$$(kg^{.425}) \times (cm^{.725}) \times 0.007184$$

or:

(your weight in kilograms raised to power 0.425)
times (your height in centimeters raised to power 0.725)
times 0.007184

How to interpret test results

There are several ways to find the normal values of tests that you can compare to your own test results. Please note that a value outside of the normal range does not always indicate a problem. Your doctor is generally the best person to tell you how to interpret test results, but for your own edification, there are several references available for comparing your test results to normal values.

Appendix C, *Test Results*, lists the normal adult values for a variety of blood, urine, and pulmonary function tests.

The *Merck Manual*, either the paper version or at their web site, has a section devoted to laboratory pathology. Many public libraries have a copy of the *Merck Manual* in their noncirculating reference section. At Merck's web site, just enter the test name and click on the search button. *http://www.merck.com/pubs/mmanual* is the page from which you can find the search facility.

Each of the following web sites has a search engine for finding the normal values of various test results:

* The University of Michigan Pathology Laboratories Handbook. Enter the test name and click search: *http://po.path.med.umich.edu/handbook*.

* The Lupus Lab Tests web site has tests commonly done for Lupus, but many of these are also done for various cancers, such as lung cancer: *http://www.mtio.com/mclfa/lfalt1.htm*.

Results of pulmonary function tests (PFTs) vary by age, weight, and height. For norms, see:

- Johns Hopkins University Pulmonary Function Lab results calculator: *http://www. med.jhu.edu/pftlab/pfthome.html*

- Virtual Hospital for pulmonary function tests: *http://www.vh.org/Providers/ClinRef/ FPHandbook/Chapter03/06-3.html*

How to assess unproven remedies

If your treatment isn't giving you good results, you might become vulnerable to claims for a quick cure made by certain practitioners. Although some of these treatments might have merit, others are simply the means by which charlatans realize financial gain. How can you separate treatments that might have unrecognized medical potential from those that have been tried and discarded by reputable researchers and those that are, or were, the focus of legal action?

- QuackWatch on the Internet gives the medical scientist's evaluation of those unusual remedies you've been hearing about and provides pointers to reliable sources of information. Visit them at *http://www.quackwatch.com.*

- The National Cancer Institute publishes a great deal of information on untested remedies. Call (800) 4-CANCER.

- The American Cancer Society has a list of questions you should ask before becoming involved with unusual remedies. Call (800) ACS-2345 or visit their web site at *http://www.cancer.org.*

- The Consumer Health Information Research Institute provides an integrity index—a credibility of publication index, including one that rates cancer books. You can contact them at 300 E. Pinkhill Road, Independence, MO 64050; (816) 228-4595.

Unique web resources

If you don't have a computer yet, or if your spouse or kids won't let you near it, this section might convince you how easily and quickly you can get the answers you've been looking for.

Please note that web sites might be inaccessible on occasional days because of data reorganization or maintenance and that web site addresses can change:

- The American Medical Association has a doctor locator and other useful features: *http://www.ama-assn.org*.

- Steve Dunn's CancerGuide is an excellent source of information on clinical trials and researching your illness: *http://cancerguide.org*.

- Oncolink, sponsored by the University of Pennsylvania, is a highly reliable source of cancer information: *http://www.oncolink.upenn.edu*.

- The *Merck Manuals* online are an indispensable source of medical information: *http://www.merck.com/pubs/mmanual*.

- Cancer News has links to several sites containing press releases: *http://www.cancernews.com*.

- Mid-South Therapeutics, Inc. hosts a web site with information for patients about radiologic tests and procedures: *http://www.msit.com/patients.htm*.

- HealthAnswers offers a web site with a search engine that can supply information about how to prepare for tests, and so on: *http://www.healthanswers.com*.

- The Thrive Health Library is a good general site for questions and answers: *http://www.thriveonline.com*.

- WebMD is another good site with a wide variety of information: *http://www.webmd.com*.

What next?

Think of researching your condition as a cyclical activity. Although you can accumulate and absorb the basic facts about lung cancer in a burst of initial activity, certain parts of the literature search process should be repeated about once a month in order to stay in touch with improvements in care. Three areas in particular should be revisited on a regular schedule:

- The NCI updates the physician's state-of-the-art treatment statements as standards of care change. If the treatises on lung cancers are modified, the NCI can notify you via email, you can check the web site's last changed date (*http://cancernet.nci.nih.gov*), or you can call the NCI at (800) 4-CANCER each month and ask them to check the date of last update on the lung cancer physician's statement.

The NCI classifies changes to these documents as either substantial or editorial. (Editorial changes are usually considered minor and might include replacing one citation with a better one.)

- Every month, new research papers on lung cancer are published in many medical journals, and their abstracts are collected in Medline and in Cancerlit, which is a subset of Medline consisting of cancer literature only.

- New clinical trials for treatment are added to the NCI database every month.

Summary

This chapter describes three critical techniques: tapping NCI information repositories, accessing medical research papers, and locating clinical trials. It also discusses supplementary resources, such as finding medical textbooks, verifying test results, locating information on drug side effects, and locating support groups.

Your approach to learning can make a difference, and the learning experience is a continuous one. It's best to keep an open mind and to repeat your search efforts from time to time.

Key points to remember:

- The National Library of Medicine's online Medline database contains more than eleven million medical research papers, accessible at *http://www.ncbi.nlm.nih.gov/entrez/query.fcgi?db=PubMed*. For assistance, call (800) 272-4787.

- The National Cancer Institute offers a search engine for clinical trials. Visit *http://cnetdb.nci.nih.gov/trialsrch.shtml* or call (800) 4-CANCER.

- The National Cancer Institute maintains state-of-the-art treatment information for all cancers. Call (800) 4-CANCER or visit *http://cancernet.nci.nih.gov*.

CHAPTER 23

The Future of Therapy

Every great advance in science has issued from a new audacity of imagination.

—John Dewey

THIS CHAPTER IS AN OVERVIEW of lung cancer treatment research being conducted by the mainstream oncology community.

Cancer treatments are being improved constantly. This chapter represents merely a snapshot of new therapies at the time this book was written and is subject to change as research progresses. You should review new therapies periodically by calling the National Cancer Institute at (800) 4-CANCER or visiting their clinical trials web site at *http://cnetdb.nci.nih.gov/trialsrch.shtml*.

The first section discusses broad trends in research. Next is an encyclopedic list of treatments now in trials, organized by mode of action. Finally, we discuss therapies we're likely to see in the more distant future, consisting of substances and approaches, such as tissue regeneration, that are not being tested against lung cancer at this time. Because space is limited, we do not discuss clinical trials aimed at preventing or detecting lung cancer.

None of the descriptions that follow should be construed as a recommendation for treatment. Oncology experts should carefully evaluate any treatment that you find here or elsewhere before your treatment decisions are made. You can gain access to new treatments that are still in clinical trials if you and your doctor decide it would be advantageous to do so. See Chapter 20, *Clinical Trials*, for more information.

The sources of information for this chapter are the National Cancer Institute's clinical trials database (*http://cnetdb.nci.nih.gov/trialsrch.shtml*) and research papers accessible through the National Library of Medicine's Medline, a collection of more than eleven million published medical papers.

Cancer cell genes

Cancer is an illness resulting from damaged genes. The descriptions of new treatments that follow will be easier to understand if you are somewhat familiar with the genetic basis of cancer. This topic is covered in detail in Chapter 5, *What Is Lung Cancer?*

An overview of research trends

The spirit of cooperative academic endeavor, a coalescence of insights from multiple medical disciplines, governmental prioritization, a highly developed research infrastructure, and the uninterrupted scientific focus of nations at peace have given us promising new cancer therapies.

Over the last twenty years, broad trends in cancer research have taken several concurrent paths:

- A much more targeted approach to identifying and testing potentially useful anticancer substances, enabled by our improved understanding of the genetic origin, development, and metabolic milieu of tumors.

- An effort to fight cancer with substances our own bodies make, instead of using external plant-based or manmade substances.

- Interdisciplinary cooperation that yields coordinated treatments with better results.

- An emphasis, at the request of many patients, to design drugs and procedures for supportive care—drugs that do not destroy cancer, but instead contribute significantly to survival by eliminating the secondary effects and illnesses related to treatment. The drugs that control coughing or nausea or stimulate growth of new blood cells after chemotherapy, for example, fall into this category.

- An interest in preventing cancer and examining its causes.

- Development of exquisite imaging tools and tests that reveal the smallest of tumors and metastases.

- Refinements in surgical technique that permit sparing of healthy tissue and more thorough removal of tumors.

- Refinements in radiotherapy that permit more careful targeting of cancerous tissue, sparing healthy tissue.

- The combination of surgery, chemotherapy, and radiotherapy for optimal results.

Substance identification and testing

For many years, anticancer drugs were discovered by testing many natural and man-made substances wholesale—often in excess of 5,000 per year—against tumor samples that were kept alive in laboratories. Substances that worked in this setting were then tested in mice; those that worked in mice were tested in humans. Those that worked better in humans than existing drugs became part of standard treatment—all without understanding the drug's mode of action until afterward, if ever.

Although this approach is still often used, a trend toward understanding a drug's mode of action before its use has emerged because of great advances in biochemistry, genetics, molecular biology, and many related fields of science, such as engineering and computer science. You'll see this trend reflected in almost every drug category discussed later in this chapter—indeed, the fact that they can be categorized at all reflects this new understanding.

For instance, one problem that often emerges in cancer therapy is the inability to deliver a high dose of toxin directly to the tumor, either because it's encapsulated within or entwined with healthy tissue, is many cell layers thick, or has high internal pressure that makes penetration difficult. Many of the newer approaches to cancer therapy target specific barriers such as these, rather than just a wholesale killing of the tumor by unknown mechanisms.

This refined testing relies on our greatly improved understanding of the genetic causes and biologic pathways of cancer. Using this understanding, a researcher might be able to identify the portion of a molecule that's responsible for the specific anticancer activity the researcher is hoping to accomplish. Often, this design and simulation are computerized, atom by atom, including animation that shows how the molecule will interact with the binding site of the tumor or other bodily substance that aids cancer growth. This isolation of design is followed by a computerized search of a database of millions of substances, retrieving all that match this characteristic. Sometimes among the substances that match will be a tried and true drug for another illness; sometimes it will be a drug tried for other purposes, but abandoned, such as thalidomide. Sometimes it will be a new, plant-based biological compound found during a pharmaceutical company's last foray into the rainforest or ocean to collect samples of all flora.

Some researchers take this understanding several steps further and attempt to build from scratch custom-made drugs that have a lock-and-key fit to the tumor cell type or to some biological mechanism that supports tumor growth. This approach is called rational drug design.

Biological anticancer substances

Almost any anticancer substance could by definition be called biological because it has an effect on the body, but in this book, the term includes only those substances made by the body to fight intruders. These substances have accumulated a tremendous following among many patients and some researchers as potential cures for cancer. As a distinct class of drugs, they are appealing for many reasons. One fairly overt reason is the popular contemporary cachet of "natural substances" and their alleged low toxicity. Another less obvious reason is the sense of balance provided by the theory that cancer is an internal process run amok and that a corresponding internal substance may correct it. The third and best reason is that they may work, as have interleukin-2 and interferon-alfa-2B, against some kidney cancers and melanomas.

Five biological anticancer substance types are in clinical trials for use against lung cancer at the time of this writing. Each type is discussed in detail in the following sections:

- Monoclonal antibodies
- Growth factors
- Tumor vaccines
- Leukocyte therapy
- Cytokines

Much work remains to be done in the area of biological substances because the concept is very promising and has hardly been tapped. Combining monoclonal antibodies with toxic substances, such as radioisotopes that will target only the tumor instead of healthy tissue, is being pursued hotly. Growth factors that support tumor growth or the growth of blood vessels to feed a tumor are now well studied and make promising targets for therapy.

It's useful to keep in mind, though, that some substances that have long been used against cancer also are "natural." Mitomycin, for example, is derived from a fungus, and paclitaxel is based on a highly toxic substance found in yews. In other words, natural substances are not always harmless and magically effective, just as steroids—including such substances as estrogen, vitamin D, and cholesterol—are not necessarily rage-producing, dangerous, and illegal.

A subcategory of drugs considered to be biological therapy is the biological response modifiers, another somewhat ambiguous name, because any substance that modifies a bodily response might in theory fit this category. In this instance, though, we include only substances made by the body and replicated in the lab, such as:

- Cytokines, such as the interleukins and interferons that are part of a normal immune response

- Colony-stimulating factors for red and white blood cells and platelets, discussed under "Supportive care"

Interdisciplinary cooperation

Cancer survivors sometimes report that a medical oncologist's assessment of their condition includes a recommendation for chemotherapy, while a radiation oncologist's assessment suggests that radiotherapy is the best choice.

Although this unenviable dilemma still arises for some cancer survivors, now more than ever, the surgeon, medical oncologist, and radiation oncologist work as a team, often with computerized technology. New treatment combinations, sometimes called adjuvant therapies when combined with surgery, are the subjects of ongoing study for lung cancer and many other cancers. Several clinical trials now underway test combinations of treatment.

Supportive care

Although this chapter does not discuss investigative drugs used for supportive care simply because space is limited, they should not be underestimated. Many of the gains made in lengthening life or curing cancer have come about because of drugs for supportive care, such as Zofran for controlling nausea, Neupogen for reestablishing infection-fighting white blood cells, and epoietin (Epogen, Procrit) for reestablishing adequate levels of red blood cells.

Cancer prevention

Years ago, cancer epidemiology consisted of asking those already diagnosed with cancer to recall incidents and lifestyle habits from many years ago. Their answers were examined for patterns that might correlate to the incidence of cancer in a population.

Today, we're seeing different kinds of detection and prevention trials, such as those designed to examine lifestyles, diet, and environmental factors as they're occurring and to tally and track all cases of cancer in these groups as they develop. This is a more accurate way of assessing risk and correlation than asking patients in a highly stressful setting to recall, for example, dietary habits from thirty years ago.

Other trials include asking participants to adhere to a specific diet for a number of years, and then recording the incidence of cancers in this group as opposed to the incidence among those who had no dietary restrictions.

Still others may involve participants who are taking vitamin supplements, exercising on a schedule, using estrogen supplements, or losing weight. These groups are followed for many years, and any cases of cancer that occur are recorded and followed.

Imaging tools and tests

The ability to visualize body organs and to delineate the status of disease without invasive procedures truly is one of the great gifts of 21st-century medicine. X radiation, computed tomography (CT), magnetic resonance imaging (MRI), positron emission tomography (PET), scintigraphy, needle biopsy, fluorescence endoscopy, and ultrasound (US) give us better information than ever about the health and disease status of individual organs.

The use of such tools has shown us, though, that even better tools are needed. Computed tomography, for instance, does not clearly display soft tissue, but MRI does; and although one or the other may delineate an unusual internal mass, they may be unable to determine if it's a cancerous or a harmless lesion. Positron emission tomography, on the other hand, can distinguish the metabolic rate of glucose in tissue, and by this measure may identify a mass as cancerous or benign. Endoscopy generally sees best only those tumors nearest the airways.

For lung cancer, a new form of CT called spiral or helical scanning has, in some studies, found very early lung cancers, and a test of body fluids such as urine is being developed at Johns Hopkins that can detect mitochondrial DNA uniquely changed by lung cancer. Each of these techniques promises earlier detection and a better chance for cure.

Surgical technique

The surgeon operating today has many new advantages to offer you. Some are aimed at improving the removal of all tumors; others aid healing; others extend the surgeon's ability to perform less invasive surgery:

* Bloodless surgery
* Camera-guided microsurgery
* Computer-enhanced imaging tools
* Nerve-sparing surgery
* Radioimmunoisotopes to highlight hidden cancerous cells for removal
* Imaging dyes to track cancer's spread to specific lymph nodes
* Stereotactic radiologic surgical tools for brain metastases
* Tools that access and repair areas not reachable with human hands
* Manmade materials to replace diseased organs

Refinement of radiotherapeutic technique

Newer types of radiotherapy afford protection to healthy tissue while maximizing destruction of cancerous tissue.

Three-dimensional conformal radiotherapy incorporates computerization to sculpt radiation beams that exactly match the tumor and can be changed dynamically without resimulation. Beams can be preprogrammed for delivery from many more angles than conventional external beam radiotherapy, allowing delivery of a maximal dose of radiation to cancerous tissue while minimizing exposure of healthy tissue.

Fractionated stereotactic radiosurgery, similar to the gamma knife, uses a CT scanner to pinpoint cancerous tissue with high accuracy. By fractionating the dose over many days, a safer, more effective dose is delivered.

Recombinations of treatments

Although recombining existing treatments might not seem exciting or intuitively effective, some of the most successful treatments devised for other types of cancer have involved this technique. The tremendous success in treating the most common type of childhood leukemia, for instance, which is now cured in over 90 percent of cases, involves combining eight or more drugs for a period of two years or more. Certain types of lymphoma also are treated this way.

This approach is being attempted for both SCLC and NSCLC. These trials are not discussed specifically in this chapter because the drugs involved usually are already approved by the FDA. Your oncologist can discuss with you the advantages and disadvantages of various combinations of chemotherapy, radiotherapy, surgical techniques, and variations in their schedules.

Current trials of new drugs and techniques

Currently, there are over 111 clinical trials of treatment for non-small cell lung cancer and 44 trials for small cell lung cancer. Some are trials of treatments already approved by the FDA, but with restructured timing or dosage for better results; some are trials of entirely new substances, techniques, or devices. In some cases a trial admits patients with NSCLC or SCLC.

Note that the substances and techniques listed here were in trials at the time this book was written. For the most current information on substances in clinical trials, use the NCI's clinical trials search engine at *http://cnetdb.nci.nih.gov/trialsrch.shtml*.

Treatments are grouped by category, but some substances or techniques fit more than one category.

3D Conformal Radiotherapy

This radiation therapy technique involves computerized imaging to shape a beam of radiation to match the tumor. Often, the beam is directed at the tumor from several angles to maximize the dose of radiation given to the tumor and to minimize the exposure of healthy tissue.

See also "Stereotactic radiotherapy."

Adjuvant therapies, combination therapies

Many new combinations of surgery, radiotherapy, and chemotherapy are being tested for lung cancers. Sometimes these combinations involve drugs already approved by the FDA, but on a different schedule. Including a full list here would be too lengthy and quickly outdated. For a comprehensive list of all adjuvant therapies being tested for NSCLC, contact the NCI at (800) 4-CANCER or visit the NCI clinical trials web site at *http://cnetdb.nci.nih.gov/trialsrch.shtml*.

Antiangiogenesis therapy

Most tumors trigger growth of many new blood vessels to support the increased metabolic needs of the tumor. This growth of new blood vessels is called angiogenesis. Antiangiogenic agents interrupt the ability of the body to grow new blood vessels, causing tumors to shrink.

Some of the substances being studied now to reduce the blood supply to starve tumors, an approach called antiangiogenesis, cause concern because they also are likely to reduce the blood supply to normal tissues. The normal tissues of concern are found near wound healing and, for example, in the uterus of a menstruating woman. Refined methods of curtailing a tumor's blood supply are being examined, and include triggering clots only in tumor blood vessels by preferentially binding clotting substances to proteins found only on tumor cells.

Some antiangiogenesis drugs now in clinical trials for either NSCLC or SCLC are thalidomide, low molecular weight heparin, marimastat, carboxyamidotriazole, BMS-275291, AE-941 (shark cartilage extract), and prinomastat (AG3340).

Antibody therapy

Antibodies are substances (proteins) secreted by white blood cells called B cells. They attach to foreign material and pathogens so the invaders can be destroyed by other white blood cells called T cells and macrophages.

Antibodies engineered in the lab to attach to only one cell surface receptor—monoclonal antibodies—have long been used in research and cancer diagnosis to tag cancer cells for visibility and quantification. Now, they're beginning to be used to treat cancers.

Monoclonal antibodies (moabs) being tested include:

- ABX-EGF against endothelial growth factor for NSCLC
- LMB-9 for NSCLC tumors that express the Lewis Y antigen
- R115777 and Trastuzumab (Herceptin) for both NSCLC and SCLC
- Trastuzumab alone for NSCLC

Anticytokine therapy

This is a broad category of anticancer drugs that contains some agents in other categories.

By definition, cytokines are proteins our bodies manufacture to trigger activity in other cells (cyto, meaning cell, and kine, meaning activity). Using this definition, almost any protein or enzyme is a cytokine, but for cancer and inflammatory processes, special cytokines are in play. All of the interleukins and interferons are cytokines, as are tumor necrosis factor and the colony stimulating factors.

Some cytokines appear to cause cancer growth under certain circumstances, such as interleukin-6 (IL-6) in myeloma studies. Some cytokines work in opposition to each other, such as interleukin-10 and -12 .

The substances being tested as anticytokines for either SCLC or NSCLC are low molecular weight heparin (Dalteparin), thalidomide, marimastat, and prinomastat (AG3340).

Antifolate therapy, folate antagonists

Folate is needed to make the building blocks of DNA, purines and thymidylates. Absent these, new copies of DNA cannot be made. Because cancer cells divide more rapidly than most normal cells, and because they commandeer major supplies of the body's nutrients, treatments such as folate antagonists are expected to affect cancer cells more strongly than most healthy cells.

The antifolates pemetrexed disodium (LY231514) and 10-Propargyl-10-Deazaaminopterin are being tested against NSCLC.

Anti-growth factor therapy

This therapy targets any one of many growth factor receptors identified for SCLC or NSCLC. Drugs that are able to inhibit growth of various types of tissue surrounding cancer cells show promise against cancer. Epidermal growth factors (EGF) and vascular endothelial growth factors are two such substances that aid tumor growth and might be successfully inhibited in cancer therapy.

At this time, an antiepidermal growth factor (EGF) substance known as Iressa (ZD 1839) is in Phase III clinical trials. The manufacturer, AstraZeneca (*http://www. astrazeneca-us.com*), is making the drug available to those in and outside clinical trials in accordance with the FDA's Investigational New Drug program.

Antisense therapy (antisense oligonucleotides)

DNA wants to exist in paired strands, except when a cell is dividing. Because cancer cells are known to have one or more faulty genes somewhere along the length of their DNA, some researchers are experimenting with delivering to the tumor short pieces of DNA or RNA that will match the faulty genes and couple with single strands of the cancer cell's DNA. In theory, these short pieces of DNA or RNA might interfere with a cancer cell's division and replication in a variety of ways.

An antisense drug being tested for SCLC is BCL-2 antisense oligodeoxynucleotide G3139.

Bone marrow transplantation

See "High-dose chemotherapy with stem cell or marrow support."

Chemosensitization/potentiation

Research has shown that some drugs, although having no direct ability to kill cancer cells, appear to heighten the cancer cell's vulnerability to other drugs, perhaps by suppressing the MDR (multiple drug resistance) gene that cancer cells appear able to activate.

The chemosensitizers Biricodar (VX-710; Incel) and G3139 are being tested against SCLC.

Chemoprotectants

These agents are used to offset dangerous effects of chemotherapy by shielding healthy cells from damage or by promoting their regrowth.

A substance being tested for both SCLC and NSCLC is Amifostine (Ethyol), which protects bone marrow, the central nervous system, and the kidneys.

Colony-stimulating factor therapy

Some treatments, particularly those that target the immune system, may work better if red or white blood cells or platelets are abundant when the substance is administered.

Trials for lung cancer exploiting this theory include granulocyte-macrophage colony stimulating factor (Sargramostim) and granulocyte colony stimulating factor (Filgrastim):

- Phase II Randomized Study of Amifostine in Patients with Hematologic Malignancies and Solid Tumors Receiving Cyclophosphamide, Etoposide, and Cisplatin Chemotherapy

- Phase II Study of High Dose Paclitaxel, Carboplatin, and Topotecan with Peripheral Blood Stem Cell Support

- Phase II Study of Intensive Chemotherapy with Peripheral Blood Stem Cell Support

- Phase II Study of Interleukin-11 with Filgrastim (G-CSF) in the Mobilization of Peripheral Blood Stem Cells

- Phase II Study of Oral Topotecan and Paclitaxel with Filgrastim (G-CSF) Support

- Phase II Study of Paclitaxel, Carboplatin, Topotecan, and Filgrastim (G-CSF)

Continuous infusion

See "Prolonged (chronic) infusion therapy."

Cytokine therapy

Cytokines, as discussed under "Anticytokine therapy," are proteins our bodies manufacture to trigger activity in other cells, such as the release of prostaglandins at the site of injury or the growth of new white blood cells. All of the interleukins and interferons are cytokines, as are tumor necrosis factor and the colony stimulating factors. Cytokines such as G-CSF are used in clinical trials in conjunction with other substances to boost an immune response or to support patient recovery.

Manmade cytokines tested for use against either NSCLC or SCLC include:

- Granulocyte-macrophage colony stimulating factor
- Interleukin-2
- Interleukin-11
- Interferon-alfa
- Thalidomide
- Low molecular weight heparin
- Marimastat
- Prinomastat (AG3340)

Note that some of the above are also categorized as antiangiogenesis agents or anticytokines.

Dendritic cell vaccines

Dendritic cells are accessory cells of the immune system. They can be educated to stimulate other white blood cells to kill tumors.

A phase II adjuvant study of immunotherapy with mutant p53 peptide pulsed autologous dendritic cells following standard therapy is underway for those with locally advanced NSCLC.

For SCLC expressing carcinoembryonic antigen (CEA), a phase I study of an active immunotherapy with CEA RNA-pulsed patient's cultured dendritic cells is underway.

Differentiation therapy

Cell differentiation into distinct functional types is part of the normal cell's maturation process. When cancer cells are continually dividing, however, they are not maturing and differentiating into the adult, functioning form of the tissue in which they arose. The result is a large group of cells that not only fail to carry out the function the organ was designed to do, but also crowd out other cells and commandeer a disproportionate share of the body's resources.

Some substances can force cancer cells to mature as normal cells do, stopping the cycle of uncontrollable cell division that characterizes cancer cells. Bryostatin 1 and tretinoin are possible differentiators being tested for NSCLC.

13-cis-retinoic acid (13-CRA) is also being tested as a differentiator for squamous cell NSCLC, although its exact mechanism might vary from differentiator to immune-modulator under some circumstances.

DNA crosslink disruptors

Some chemotherapies work by breaking DNA's ladder-like bonds; others work by creating new, erroneous bonds between DNA strands. A novel substance, glufosfamide (Beta-D-glucosyl-ifosfamide mustard or D 19575, glc-IPM), appears to work by inhibiting repair of DNA cross-links, although this new drug's mechanism is not fully understood at this time.

Demethylation, hypomethylation

In the healthy cell, genes that are covered with methyl compounds are not transcribed into proteins, and genes that are demethylated can in some cases initiate or control desirable orderly cell death. Demethylation of DNA is being tested to activate genes that might promote tumor death.

For SCLC and NSCLC, decitabine is being tested to demethylate DNA.

See also "Methylation."

Drug resistance inhibition

Some chemotherapies cause certain cancer cells to turn on genes that halt the ability of that chemotherapy to work against cancer. Drug resistance inhibitors attempt to undo this effect. Although drug resistance inhibitors generally have no ability on their own to kill cancer cells, it is hoped that they can enable other drugs to continue doing so.

Drugs in this category being tested against NSCLC include hydroxyurea.

Endoscopic surgery

Various surgical techniques aimed at making surgery less invasive, but as effective as traditional chest surgery, are being tested.

Epidermal growth factor (EGF) receptor inhibitor

See "Anti-growth factor therapy."

Farnesyl protein transferase (FPTase) inhibitors

In lung cancers and several other cancers, a gene called ras (which, along with other genes, is responsible for orderly cell division) is mutated. Certain substances can inhibit the growth of cancerous cells that contain a mutated copy of ras, while leaving normal cells unaffected.

R115777 is being tested for both SCLC and NSCLC.

Gene therapy

In its broadest sense, gene therapy is a name applied to several kinds of cancer treatment that involve modifying genes, such as triggering the body's white cells to attack tumors. Conforming to the strictest definition of gene therapy are experiments to reinsert genes into cancer cells that lack properly functioning copies of these genes or to insert a manmade suicide gene into the tumor cell that will make the cell more susceptible to the toxic effects of certain drugs.

Modification of white blood cells to attack a tumor can occur, for example, if a weakened virus, modified genetically to contain a piece of the tumor's DNA, is inserted into the cancer cell. When this weakened virus is unleashed in the body, our white blood cells recognize it as an enemy and destroy it. Because the virus also is expressing part of the tumor's DNA, white blood cells become sensitized to this tumor protein as well, and attack it wherever they find it; that is, either on the virus coat or on the tumor.

Currently, the following gene therapy trials are underway:

- Inserting a working copy of the p53 tumor suppressor and cell death (apoptosis) gene into lung tumors, using one of the common cold viruses (adenovirus) as a carrier.

- For patients with SCLC or NSCLC adenocarcinomas expressing carcinoembryonic antigen (CEA), the patient's white blood cells called T cells are activated outside the body with combined anti-CEA immunoglobulin T cell receptors and then reinfused into a vein.

Graft versus tumor induction

Successful treatments for lymphoma and leukemia have, in some cases, involved using components of another person's immune system to fight the patient's cancer. This principle is being studied for SCLC and NSCLC. The technique involves transferring blood components from a highly specific donor into the patient's vein:

- Phase II Study of Nonmyeloblative Allogeneic Peripheral Blood Stem Cell and Donor Lymphocyte Infusions in Patients with Refractory Metastatic Solid Tumors

High-dose chemotherapy with stem cell or marrow support

Some researchers believe that very high doses of chemotherapy or radiotherapy will kill cancer, but the dose that can be given has in the past been limited to the amount that will not kill bone marrow. Bone marrow furnishes all of our blood cells; without marrow, we will die. High dose therapy with stem cell support is a means of bypassing this limitation by resupplying bone marrow with new stem cells.

Some trials in this genre use the patient's stem cells; some use donor marrow. Some do not use doses of chemotherapy high enough to destroy all of the patient's marrow.

Trials of this type are being conducted for both SCLC and NSCLC, as well as other solid tumors at the National Institutes of Health and certain other research centers:

- Phase II Study of High Dose Paclitaxel, Carboplatin, and Topotecan with Peripheral Blood Stem Cell Support in Patients with Metastatic Small Cell Cancer

- Phase II Study of Intensive Chemotherapy with Peripheral Blood Stem Cell Support in Patients with Small Cell Lung Cancer

- Phase II Study of Nonmyeloblative Allogeneic (donor) Peripheral Blood Stem Cell and Donor Lymphocyte Infusions in Patients with Refractory Metastatic Solid Tumors

High-dose prophylactic cranial radiotherapy

To date, irradiating the brain to prevent the spread of SCLC has been only somewhat successful. Some researchers believe that higher doses of radiotherapy will improve results. This idea is being tested in clinical trials.

Hyperfractionated accelerated radiotherapy

Some researchers have found that smaller, but more frequent, doses of radiotherapy are more effective against some tumors. Small doses several times a day are being studied for their possible superiority against NSCLC.

Hyperthermia

High temperatures sometimes have a fatal effect on cancer cells. One such study is currently underway for lung cancer, a study of isolated lung perfusion with paclitaxel and moderate hyperthermia in patients with inoperable malignancies.

Hypoxic cell toxins

Often, both cancerous and healthy cells die if deprived of oxygen. An agent in this class being tested against lung cancer is tirapazamine.

Inhaled drugs

Some clinical trials are using standard injectable drugs effective against other cancers as inhaled agents.

For both SCLC and NSCLC, doxorubicin is being tested in this manner.

Interferon therapy

See "Cytokine therapy."

Interleukin therapy

See "Cytokine therapy."

Isolated perfusion

Almost since the inception of cancer chemotherapy, it has been recognized that targeting only the tumor and sparing healthy tissue would be ideal. Isolated perfusion is an attempt to treat only the tumor, or only the organ that contains the tumor, rather than exposing the entire body to toxic drugs.

Currently, one trial is underway that isolates perfusion of paclitaxel into the lung for either NSCLC or SCLC.

Leukocyte therapy

This approach uses white blood cells to challenge a tumor. The patient's blood cells are extracted from a vein, resensitized to the tumor, and reinserted.

The following trials using leukocyte therapy are underway:

- T cells, which are white blood cells that can be pretreated to recognize carcinoembryonic antigen (CEA). They are reinserted into the body to attack tumor cells that express CEA.

- Injection of a tumor-specific vaccine containing either the cell-death p53 gene, or ras, a growth signaling gene, with or without cellular immunotherapy with peptide-activated lymphocytes plus interleukin-2.

- Infusion of donor stem cell and lymphocytes.

See also "Gene therapy" and "Graft versus tumor induction."

Methylation

Genes that are coated with a carbon substance—methylated—cannot be translated into the proteins that carry out the work of genes. Methylating substances are being tested to cover tumor-promoting genes in cancer cells, genes that normally control cell death and other normal cell functions. Researchers think that, by covering these genes with methyl compounds and thus deactivating them, they can force cancerous cells to rest or die as normal cells do.

Temozolomide is being tested as a methylating substance for NSCLC.

Monoclonal antibodies

See "Antibody therapy."

Nonspecific immune-modulator therapy

Nonspecific immune modulators are substances that aid in redirecting, suppressing, or boosting the immune system in ways that are either somewhat general or, perhaps, poorly understood. Vaccines often contain aluminum or small pieces of protein, for instance, that are not related to the vaccine material, but are known to elicit a stronger immune response.

KRN7000, an alpha-galactosylceramide that activates natural killer T cells, thus helping to generate strong antitumor activity, is being tested as a nonspecific immune stimulant against NSCLC.

Prolonged (chronic) infusion therapy

Several trials are underway to exploit the observation that some drugs may be more effective against lung tumors and appear to operate biochemically in different ways if administered slowly over long periods, instead of injected all at once during a brief office visit:

- Topotecan is being tested for NSCLC using low doses and prolonged infusion.

- Aminocamptothecin is being tested for NSCLC as a colloidal dispersion as a 120-hour infusion.

- Paclitaxel is being tested for SCLC.

Peripheral blood lymphocyte therapy

See "Leukocyte therapy."

Phosphoprotein inhibition

The drug CI-994 (N-acetyldinaline) appears to act against cancer in a way not observed in the past and might represent an entirely new way to treat cancer.[1] Tumor cells treated in the laboratory with CI-994 lose a specific protein and stop dividing.

CI-994 is being tested against NSCLC.

Radiosensitization

Certain drugs can make tumors more sensitive to damage by radiotherapy.

Gadolinium texaphyrin, or RSR13, used prior to or during radiotherapy appears to make NSCLC cells more sensitive to radiotherapy.

Stereotactic radiotherapy

Stereotactic surgery is surgery guided by a 3D image of the tumor and by multiple targeting criteria that allow precisely aimed microsurgeries. Stereotactic radiosurgery is the aiming of one or more small, precise beams of radiation at cancerous tissue using these stereotactic guiding systems.

Clinical trials of fractionated stereotactic radiotherapy for brain metastases are being conducted to determine the efficacy of this method.

Topoisomerase inhibitor therapy

Topoisomerases are enzymes that our cells use to break DNA bonds before copying and to repair the breaks after copying. Topoisomerase inhibitors interfere with DNA repair, causing the cancer cell to die because damaged DNA cannot be translated into the proteins, such as transport and digestive proteins, that each cell needs to breathe or eat.

New topoisomerase inhibitors being tested against NSCLC include colloidal aminocamptothecin (9-AC), nitrocamptothecin, acridine carboxamide, DX-8951f, pyrazoloacridine, and irinotecan.

Topoisomerase inhibitors being tested against SCLC include topotecan, irinotecan, and epirubicin.

Thoracoscopic surgery.

See "Endoscopic surgery."

Vaccine therapy

Vaccines against cancer can be made with or without tumor cells as a basis and with or without recombination with other anticancer substances. The following vaccines are being tested:

- Phase I Pilot Study of Ras Peptide Cancer Vaccine and Sargramostim (GM-CSF) in Patients with Stage IB-IV Non-Small Cell Lung Cancer

- For NSCLC, Phase I Pilot Study of Vaccine Therapy with Tumor-Specific Mutated ras Peptides in Adjuvant Setting of Colon, Pancreatic, and Lung Cancer

- Phase I Study of Active Immunotherapy with Carcinoembryonic Antigen (CEA) RNA-Pulsed Autologous Human Cultured Dendritic Cells in Patients with Metastatic Malignancies Expressing CEA

- Phase I Study of HER-2/neu Peptide-Based Vaccine with Sargramostim (GM-CSF) as an Adjuvant in Patients with Stage III or IV HER-2/neu Expressing Cancers

- Phase II Adjuvant Study of Immunotherapy with Mutant p53 Peptide Pulsed Autologous Dendritic Cells Following Standard Therapy in Patients with Locally Advanced Non-Small Cell Lung Cancer

- For both SCLC and NSCLC, Phase II Pilot Study of Tumor-Specific p53 or ras Vaccines with or without Cellular Immunotherapy with Peptide-Activated Lymphocytes plus Interleukin-2

- For SCLC, a Phase II Study of Immunization with Polysialic Acid Keyhole Limpet Hemocyanin (PSA-KLH) Conjugate or N-Propionylated PSA-KLH Hemocyanin Conjugate plus Immunological Adjuvant QS21

Future trials

The following strategies are being discussed with vigor among scientists, and some are being tested against other cancers, but they are not yet ready for human trials against lung cancer. Some may prove suitable for treating lung cancer; others may not.

Death receptors

Normal cells, cells being transformed into cancerous cells, and fully cancerous cells have on their surface certain proteins that act as binding regions for a protein called TRAIL (also called Apo2L), which triggers orderly cell death. Cells being transformed into cancerous cells can be destroyed by TRAIL, but normal cells protect themselves from this destruction using "decoy" receptors: they bind TRAIL, but do not transport it inside the cell, thus seeming to render it ineffective. Cancerous cells also appear to have many ways to avoid cell death. Future cancer therapies will examine these differences in behavior among normal, cancerous, and soon-to-be-cancerous cells.

In vitro sensitivity-directed chemotherapy

This approach requires a sample of one's tumor, against which a variety of anticancer compounds are tested to see which works best. In practice, there are problems with this approach because tumor cells that respond well in a test tube may be inaccessible to the apparently useful drug when the same scenario is attempted within the body, and because substances that appear to be inactive in the test tube may become active in the body after biochemical interaction with various substances.

In other words, this technique cannot be used with accuracy to determine agents to which the tumor will respond.

Some clinicians offer this service now, but its use is not widespread.

Mitochondrial DNA

Science and medicine have focused primarily on the activity of genes within the cell's nucleus, but DNA also exists within the mitochondria of each cell.

Mitochondria are small organs (organelles) within each cell that burn oxygen to accomplish cellular tasks. It's theorized that mitochondria are bacteria that were enslaved by the cells of larger species many millions of years ago, because each mitochondrium contains its own DNA and resembles a bacterium in certain other ways. All cells of all higher species contain mitochondria; cells requiring higher levels of oxygen consumption, such as muscle cells, contain more mitochondria than do others.

Mitochondrial DNA can only be inherited from the female. Ova—being fully functioning cells—contain mitochondria, but spermatozoa do not.

These facts are meaningful for cancer research for at least three reasons:

*   Mitochondrial DNA may play a role in diseases that are linked to lung cancer and found in both males and females, but found consistently only on the mother's side of the family.

*   Mitochondrial DNA sometimes exhibits damage that is known to cause cancer, as does the much more closely studied nuclear DNA.

*   Mitochondria appear to respond to chemotherapy and radiation therapy, and mitochondrial DNA can be modified to improve cancer treatment.

*   Mitochondrial DNA can be detected in urine, offering promise for an inexpensive means to detect lung cancer in very early stages.

Molecular oncology

A tumor may arise because a gene is being transcribed incorrectly into an aberrant protein; is not transcribed at all; is overexpressed or expressed at the wrong time; because two erroneously spliced genes are being transcribed into a hybrid protein that is impotent or oncogenic; or because of a combination of any of these. Molecular oncology attempts to substitute the correct or missing gene product for a faulty or missing gene.

Proto-oncogenes, oncogenes, and tumor-suppressor genes

As with many areas of cancer research, this is a well-studied but not yet fully understood area of genetics.

In normal cells, DNA contains oncogenes and precursor genes called proto-oncogenes. Both can trigger growth, but these genes normally are tightly regulated, sometimes kept quite literally under wraps with methylation, so they cannot be transcribed into proteins that would trigger growth until it's time for the cell to divide.

In contrast, and for biological balance, there are about nine known tumor-suppressor genes (of which p53 is the best known) that are sensitive to the activity of the dividing cell, which signal when to demethylate and transcribe growth genes, when to arrest growth, and when to initiate cell death, if irreparable errors are found in the cell's DNA.

Errors in or near any of these genes can cause a cell to become cancerous.

Some studies are examining ways to regain control of oncogenes that have run amok or to substitute for the products of tumor suppressor genes that have been damaged.

Telomerase inhibitors

At the end of each chromosome is a long string of repeating, non-translated genetic material called a telomere. Not too long ago, it was discovered that, as a normal cell ages, the telomere, or tail, shortens. When it is entirely gone, the cell dies in an orderly, shrinking, dissolving way (apoptosis).

The telomeres of many cancer cells, however, never shorten.

Some researchers believe that an enzyme called telomerase is faulty in certain cancer cells and that, by manipulating this enzyme, they can force the cancer cell to age normally and eventually die.

Tissue engineering

Currently, tissue engineering is in limited use to regrow skin damaged by burns and to repair damaged cartilage within joints. Artificial kidneys that are half human tissue, half mechanical device are being tested in animals. Although tissue engineering is not used yet following cancer therapy, it's conceivable that someday new vocal chords, breast, or lung tissue might be regrown in the laboratory and implanted into a cancer survivor weeks or months after laryngectomy, mastectomy, or lobectomy.

The obstacles to this approach are several: the first being that usually a small piece of the patient's own tissue is required to grow the much larger quantity on a base consisting of anchor material and nutrients. For cancer survivors, the risk exists that microscopic cancer growths that might be included in this sample would survive, thrive, and subsequently be reimplanted. The second problem is that even seemingly simple tissues can be quite complex. Cartilage, for instance, is composed of several layers, each having a separate function. Results of cartilage implantation are too new to be certain that the tissue functions as it should for many years later. Although multilayered skin has been regrown and used successfully in burn therapy and is FDA-approved, it's not known at this time whether all tissues, in all their complexities, can be regrown. A third obstacle is expense. One square inch of nutrient matrix for regrowing skin costs several thousand dollars. Tissue engineering for a very complex organ might be beyond reach simply because of expense.

Triplex molecules

In some cases, the antisense molecules, described in an earlier section, that bind to single strands of dividing DNA or RNA also can bind with double-strand DNA that is not in the process of dividing. When antisense molecules do bind to double strands, they form a triplex molecule. Some researchers are pursuing this strategy as a means of cross-binding DNA so it cannot even begin replication, thus causing the cancer cell to become static or to die.

Summary

Many new concepts and treatments are evolving for cancer in general and lung cancer in particular. This chapter has addressed the treatments now in clinical trials.

Key points to remember:

- It's wise to keep in touch with new treatments being developed for lung cancer by consulting your doctor, by browsing the NCI clinical trials database, or by calling the NCI and asking for a list of trials for lung cancer. Chapter 20 and Chapter 22, *Researching Your Illness*, contain information regarding evaluating clinical trials.

- The NCI web site for searching for clinical trials is *http://cnetdb.nci.nih.gov/trialsrch.shtml*.

- The NCI telephone number for getting help finding clinical trials is (800) 4-CANCER.

Resources

THE LISTS THAT FOLLOW reiterate the various groups, publications, services, and web tools discussed throughout this book, and include additional resources that might serve your needs.

Lung cancer resources

This first category includes resources you're likely to use most often: those that are the richest sources of specific lung cancer information.

Organizations

Various organizations support lung cancer patients and their loved ones.

Alliance for Lung Cancer Advocacy, Support, and Education (ALCASE)
1601 Lincoln Avenue
P.O. Box 849
Vancouver, WA 98666
(800) 298-2436
http://www.alcase.org

The Alliance for Lung Cancer Advocacy, Support, and Education (ALCASE), is the only national group for lung cancer issues and is an excellent centralized, comprehensive resource. Be sure to see their Lung Cancer Manual, downloadable from their web site or sent via US mail for a $20 donation. If you cannot afford the donation, they will make arrangements with you to receive a copy for a lower amount.

The National Familial Lung Cancer Registry
Johns Hopkins University School of Hygiene and Public Health
615 North Wolfe Street, Room 6309
Baltimore, MD 21205
(410) 614-1910
fax (410) 955-0863
mmccullo@jhsph.edu
http://www.path.jhu.edu/nfltr.html

The National Familial Lung Cancer Registry at Johns Hopkins seeks families with two or more people diagnosed with lung cancer. Family members and patients can refer themselves to the National Familial Lung Cancer Registry. Their goals are to further the understanding of the causes of lung cancer (beyond smoking) and to provide educational material for those at risk for lung cancer.

Quitnet
Boston University
121 Bay State Road
Boston, MA 02215
(617) 353-2000
http://www.quitnet.org

Quitnet, sponsored by Boston University, is a 24-hour Internet support group and information center for those who wish to quit smoking.

Support groups

Support groups can provide a wealth of information and emotional sustenance.

Alliance for Lung Cancer Advocacy, Support, and Education (ALCASE)
1601 Lincoln Avenue
P.O. Box 849
Vancouver, WA 98666
(800) 298-2436
http://www.alcase.org

ALCASE maintains a comprehensive list of in-person support groups and phone buddies. See their web site at *http://www.alcase.org/support/suprtgrps.html*.

Association of Cancer Online Resources, Inc. (ACOR)
173 Duane Street, Third Floor
New York, NY 10013-3334
(212) 226-5525
http://www.acor.org

ACOR is a nonprofit organization created, funded, and operated by Gilles Frydman, spouse of a breast cancer survivor, to provide Internet-based cancer information free of charge to cancer patients. ACOR offers access to over 100 Internet mailing lists and a variety of unique web sites. The mailing lists provide information and support to over 50,000 patients, caregivers, and those looking for answers about cancer and related disorders. The number of members given is approximate at the time of writing and will vary over time. A handy automatic subscription feature is available for ACOR Internet discussion groups at ACOR's site *listserv.acor.org*

- LUNG-ONC is an ACOR group offering medical discussion and emotional support for all lung cancer patients, survivors, and their loved ones. About 460 members.
- LUNG-BAC is an ACOR discussion group for those diagnosed with bronchioloalveolar carcinoma. Fifty-nine members.
- LUNG-NSCLC is an ACOR discussion group for those diagnosed with non-small cell lung cancer. One hundred and ninety-nine members.
- LUNG-SCLC is an ACOR discussion group for those diagnosed with small cell lung cancer. One hundred ten members.
- Cancer-Pain (249 members), Cancer-Sexuality (160 members), Cancer-Fertility (83 members), Cancer-Fatigue (210 members), and Cancer-Depression (107 members) are ACOR discussion groups for those with cancer-related adverse effects.

Reading and reference material

This section includes books, medical journals, and NCI literature.

Reference material

National Library of Medicine
National Institutes of Health
Bethesda, MD 20892
(800) 272-4787
http://www.ncbi.nlm.nih.gov/entrez/query.fcgi?db=PubMed

The National Library of Medicine's Medline database is the best place to find the published results of studies on cancer treatment and care. It houses more than eleven million research papers. If you need help with searching, you can call the National Library of Medicine at (800) 272-4787 or (301) 496-6308.

National Cancer Institute (NCI)
Bethesda, MD 20892
(800) 4-CANCER
http://cancernet.nci.nih.gov

The US National Cancer Institute, a division of the National Institutes of Health, has a hotline to help cancer survivors with a variety of issues, such as physician referrals; an enormous web site; and numerous tracts, statements, booklets, and books about cancer treatment and care. Many of the statements about cancer come in two versions: one for patients and one for physicians. You might prefer to start with the patients' version, but it's likely that, as you learn more, the physicians' statements will provide better, more detailed answers to your questions. The physicians' information is often part of the Physician Data Query (PDQ).

Lung Cancer Online
http://www.lungcanceronline.org

Created by Karen Parles, Lung Cancer Online contains links to a great deal of useful information for every aspect of diagnosis, treatment, and recovery, including links to pharmaceutical companies that run clinical trials of their own investigative substances. Karen is a lung cancer survivor and a medical librarian.

Texts

Pass, Harvey I., ed., and others. *Lung Cancer: Principles and Practice.* Philadelphia: Lippincott Williams & Wilkins Publishers, 2000. This 1,177-page text is an excellent resource both for medical personnel and for a subset of patients because it assumes the reader knows nothing about certain basics, such as molecular genetics. It also provides up-to-date information about all aspects of lung cancer diagnosis and treatment. Very readable.

Roth, Jack A., ed., and others. *Lung Cancer.* 2nd edition. Malden, MA: Blackwell Science, 1998. This 400-page text is less comprehensive than the Pass text, but it offers a different perspective on information found in the first text. Many high-quality photographs and diagrams are included.

Turrisi, Andrew, ed. *Lung Cancer: An Evidence-Based Guide for the Practicing Clinician*. Oxford, England: Isis Medical Media, 2000.

Detterbeck, Frank, ed. *Diagnosis and Treatment of Lung Cancer*. Orlando, FL: WB Saunders Co., 2000.

Ginsberg, Robert, ed. *Lung Cancer*. Hamilton, Ontario: BC Decker, 2000.

Patient's guides

Alliance for Lung Cancer Advocacy, Support, and Education. *The Lung Cancer Manual*. Vancouver, WA: ALCASE, 1999. This manual is downloadable free from ALCASE's web site at *http://www.alcase.org* or as spiral-bound printed copy sent via US mail for a $20 donation.

Cox, Barbara, et al. *Living With Lung Cancer: A Guide for Patients and Their Families*. 4th edition. Gainesville, FL: Triad Publishing, 1998. This guide is a good basic primer describing what to expect during diagnosis and treatment.

Ruckdeschel, John. *Myths & Facts about Lung Cancer: What You Need to Know*. Melville, NY: PRR, 1999. This very brief guide, although not offering the detailed information many lung cancer patients hunger for, is a good restorative after the shock of diagnosis.

Scott, Walter. *Lung Cancer: A Guide to Diagnosis and Treatment*. Omaha, NE: Addicus Books, 2000. Covers topics from diagnosis to death in 156 pages. A good foundation book, but lacks significant detail.

General cancer resources

These resources are not specifically targeted to lung cancer patients, survivors, and their loved ones, but nonetheless offer an enormous variety of information and services.

Organizations

Many organizations exist to help cancer patients and survivors.

Agency for Health Care Research and Quality
Office of Health Care Information
2101 East Jefferson Street
Executive Office Center, Suite 501
Rockville, MD 20852
(800) 358-9295 (for ordering publications)
(301) 594-1364 (all other calls)
fax (301) 594-2800
info@ahrq.gov
http://www.ahcpr.gov

The Agency for Health Care Research and Quality, a division of the US government's Department of Health and Human Services, "provides evidence-based information on health care outcomes; quality; and cost, use, and access."

American Cancer Society National Office
1599 Clifton Road NE
Atlanta, GA 30329-4251
(800) ACS-2345
http://www.cancer.org

The American Cancer Society has many national and local programs to help cancer survivors with such problems as travel, lodging, and emotional support. ACS publishes an excellent book, *Informed Decisions—The Complete Book of Cancer Diagnosis, Treatment and Recovery.* This hefty book is a comprehensive guide to care and treatment for all aspects of all cancers. ACS also offers a 24-hour support line for both English- and Spanish-speaking cancer survivors. Check your local phone directory for the office nearest you, or call (800) ACS-2345.

American Red Cross
430 17th Street NW
Washington, DC 20006
(202) 737-8300
http://www.redcross.org

The American Red Cross sponsors the Armed Forces Emergency Services program, which provides communication services and money for transport, burial, food, or shelter costs for active military personnel.

Cancer Care Counseling (National Cancer Care Foundation)
1180 Avenue of the Americas
New York, NY 10036
(212) 382-2078 or (800) 813-HOPE
http://www.cancercare.org

Cancer Care Counseling provides free professional help in the form of emotional support, information, referrals, and practical help to people with cancer and their loved ones. They offer a toll-free counseling line and teleconference programs.

Cancer Research Institute
681 Fifth Avenue
New York, NY 10022
(800) 99-CANCER
http://www.cancerresearch.org

The Cancer Research Institute, dedicated to mobilizing the immune system against cancer, offers such services as PDQ searches for clinical trials and free literature on cancer.

Cancervive
6500 Wilshire Boulevard, Suite 500
Los Angeles, CA 90048
(213) 655-3758
http://www.cancervive.org

A nonprofit organization founded in 1985 by childhood cancer survivor Susan Nessim, Cancervive is dedicated to improving the quality of life for cancer survivors by providing emotional support, education, and advocacy. Cancervive offers one-on-one and telephone counseling nationally.

Center for Medical Consumers
237 Thompson Street
New York, NY 10012
(212) 674-7105
medconsumers@earthlink.net
http://www.medicalconsumers.org

The Center for Medical Consumers, a nonprofit organization established in 1976, acts as an independent source of information to assist consumers in evaluating medical information. It publishes a newsletter and maintains a free medical and health reference library designed for consumers that contains more than 1,200 books and periodicals.

Consumer Health Information Research Institute
300 East Pink Hill Road
Independence, MO 64057
(816) 228-4595

The Consumer Health Information Research Institute provides an integrity index and a credibility of publication index, including one that rates cancer books.

Hereditary Cancer Institute
Creighton University School of Medicine
Department of Preventive Medicine
2500 California Plaza
Omaha, NE 68178
(800) 648-8133
http://medicine.creighton.edu/medschool/PrevMed/hc.html

The Hereditary Cancer Institute evaluates families for risk and furnishes educational material and recommendations for surveillance to families with hereditary cancers. Their goal is to save lives through the evaluation and identification of families at high risk of hereditary cancer. Henry Lynch, who first described the Lynch Syndromes of hereditary colon cancer, is a key member of the HCI.

Mautamar Project for Lesbians with Cancer
1707 L Street NW, Suite 1060
Washington, DC 20036
(202) 332-5536

The Mautamar Project for Lesbians with Cancer offers support to lesbians and their families.

National Coalition for Cancer Research
426 C Street NE
Washington, DC 20002
(202) 544-1880
http://www.capweb.net/nccr

The National Coalition for Cancer Research is an activist group that monitors government spending on cancer.

National Coalition for Cancer Survivorship
1010 Wayne Avenue, Fifth Floor
Silver Spring, MD 20910
(301) 650-8868
http://www.cansearch.org

The National Coalition for Cancer Survivorship was formed by cancer survivors to offer support and effect progress against cancer through legislative efforts. They publish the *Cancer Survivor's Almanac*, a good reference for any cancer survivor. This book can be purchased from many stores, but if you order a copy from Barnes & Noble linking from NCCS's web site, Barnes & Noble will donate a portion of the proceeds to NCCS.

National Family Caregivers Association
10400 Connecticut Avenue, Suite 500
Kensington, MD 20895
(301) 942-6430
(800) 896-3650
http://www.nfcacares.org

The National Family Caregivers Association educates, supports, and empowers the millions of Americans who care for chronically ill, aged, or disabled loved ones through public awareness, advocacy, and programs targeted for caregivers. They publish the *Caregiver Survival Kit*, available through their web site. You can reach their counseling service, "Boomerang," Monday through Friday, EST, at (877) 712-4487.

National Network of Libraries of Medicine
National Library of Medicine
8600 Rockville Pike
Building 38, Room B1-E03
Bethesda, MD 20894
(800) 338-7657
http://www.nnlm.nlm.nih.gov

The National Network of Libraries of Medicine can tell you of the nearest medical library open to the public.

People Living Through Cancer, Inc.
323 Eighth Street, SW
Albuquerque, NM 87102
(505) 242-3263
email *cancerhope@aol.com*
http://members.aol.com/cancerhope

People Living Through Cancer, Inc., offers support groups, a telephone lifeline, and a lending library, and publishes the *Living Through Cancer* quarterly journal.

R. A. Bloch Cancer Foundation
4410 Main Street
Kansas City, MO 64111
(800) 433-0464
http://www.blochcancer.org

The R. A. Bloch Cancer Foundation offers telephone-based second medical opinions and one-on-one phone contact between cancer survivors.

Well Spouse Foundation
P. O. Box 801
New York, NY 10023
(800) 838-0879
email *wellspouse@aol.com*
http://www.sky.net/~dporter/wellsp.htm

The Well Spouse Foundation is a nonprofit, self-help group that offers support to those whose spouses are chronically ill with cancer or other life-threatening illnesses.

The Wellness Community
35 E. Seventh St., Suite 412
Cincinnati, OH 45202
(513) 421-7111
(888) 793-WELL
fax (513) 421-7119
email *help@wellness-community.org*
http://www.wellness-community.org

The Wellness Community was one of the first groups to offer positive emotional support to cancer patients and survivors. TWC has branches throughout the US. Check your local phone book for the chapter nearest you.

Reading and reference material

Books

The Alpha Book on Cancer and Living. Alameda, CA: The Alpha Institute, 1993.

Altman, Roberta, and Michael Sarg. *The Cancer Dictionary.* New York, NY: Facts On File, 1992. A good medical dictionary specifically for cancer survivors.

Brenner, David J., and Hall, Eric J. *Making the Radiation Therapy Decision.* Los Angeles: RGA Publishing Group, 1996.

Cancer Rates and Risks. Fourth edition. Bethesda, MD: The National Cancer Institute (NCI), 1996. Call (800) 4-CANCER for a free copy.

A Cancer Survivor's Almanac. The National Coalition for Cancer Survivorship, Barbary Hoffman, ed. Minneapolis, MN: Chronimed, 1996.

Crane, Judy B. *How to Survive Your Hospital Stay.* Westlake Village, CA: Center Press, 1997.

Cukier, Daniel, and Virginia McCullough. *Coping with Radiation Therapy: A Ray of Hope.* Los Angeles, CA: Lowell House, 1996.

Dollinger, Malin, Ernest Rosenbaum, and Greg Cable. *Everyone's Guide to Cancer Therapy.* Toronto, Ontario: Somerville House Books, 1997.

Drum, David. *Making the Chemotherapy Decision.* Los Angeles, CA: Lowell House, 1997.

Finn, Robert. *Cancer Clinical Trials: Experimental Treatments & How They Can Help You.* Sebastopol, CA: O'Reilly & Associates, 1999.

Friedman, Andrea, Thomas Klein, and Herman Friedman, eds. *Psychoneuroimmunology, Stress, and Infection.* New York: CRC Press, 1996.

Glaser, Ronald, and Janice Kiecolt-Glaser. *Handbook of Human Stress and Immunity.* New York: Academic Press, 1994.

Harpham, Wendy Schlessel. *After Cancer: A Guide to Your New Life.* New York: W.W. Norton & Co., 1994.

Harpham, Wendy Schlessel. *Diagnosis Cancer: Your Guide Through the First Few Months.* New York: W.W. Norton & Co., 1998.

Harpham, Wendy Schlessel. *When a Parent Has Cancer: A Guide to Caring for Your Children.* New York: Harpercollins, 1997.

Informed Decisions—The Complete Book of Cancer Diagnosis, Treatment and Recovery. The American Cancer Society. Murphy, G., L. Morris, and D. Lange, eds. New York: Penguin Group, 1997.

Inlander, Charles B., ed. *People's Medical Society Health Desk Reference: Information Your Doctor Can't or Won't Tell You.* New York: Hyperion, 1996.

Johnson, Judi, and Linda Klein. *I Can Cope: Staying Healthy With Cancer.* Minneapolis, MN: Chronimed, 1994.

Keene, Nancy. *Working with Your Doctor: Getting the Healthcare You Deserve.* Sebastopol, CA: O'Reilly & Associates, 1997.

Lerner, Michael. *Choices in Healing: Integrating the Best of Conventional and Complementary Approaches to Cancer.* Cambridge, MA: MIT Press, 1996.

McKay, Judith, and Nancee Hirano. *The Chemotherapy & Radiation Therapy Survival Guide.* Oakland, CA: New Harbinger Publications, 1998.

The Merck Manual. Seventeenth edition. Whitehouse Station, NJ: Merck, 1999. Available in either the paper version or at their web site (*http://www.merck.com*), this is a vast resource. Many public libraries have a copy of *The Merck Manual* in their noncirculating reference section. *The Merck Manual* is updated every few years.

Olson, Kaye. *Surgery and Recovery: How to Reduce Anxiety and Promote Healthy Healing.* Traverse City, MI: Rhodes and Easton, 1998.

Radiation Therapy and You: A Guide to Self-Help During Treatment. US National Cancer Institute. This 50-page booklet is available free from the US National Cancer Institute in Bethesda, MD by calling (800) 4-CANCER.

Rosenbaum, Ernest, and Isadora Rosenbaum. *Cancer Supportive Care: A Comprehensive Guide for Patients and Their Families.* Toronto, Ontario: Somerville House Publishing, 1998.

Schover, Leslie. *Sexuality and Fertility After Cancer.* New York: John Wiley & Sons, 1997.

Youngson, Robert, with the Diagram Group. *The Surgery Book: An Illustrated Guide to 73 of the Most Common Operations.* New York: St. Martin's Press, 1993.

Zakarian, Beverly. *The Activist Cancer Patient*. New York: John Wiley & Sons, 1996.

Zukerman, Eugenia, and Julie Ingelfinger. *Coping With Prednisone and other Cortisone-Related Medicines: It May Work Miracles, but How Do You Handle the Side Effects?* New York: St. Martin's Press, 1996.

Books for children

Clifford, Christine. *Our Family Has Cancer, Too!* Duluth, MN: Pfeifer-Hamilton Publishing, 1997.

Harpham, Wendy Schlessel. *Becky and the Worry Cup: A Children's Book About a Parent's Cancer.* New York: Harpercollins, 1997.

Kohlenberg, Sherry. *Sammy's Mommy Has Cancer.* Washington, DC: Magination, 1993. For preschoolers.

Trillin, Alice. *Dear Bruno*. New York: New Press, 1996. A cartoon book about adjusting to cancer; primarily, but not exclusively, for children.

Magazines

Coping
P.O. Box 682268
Franklin, TN 37068
(615) 790-2400

Living Through Cancer
323 Eighth Street, SW
Albuquerque, NM 87102
(505) 242-3263

Web sites

The ACOR cancer glossary contains a searchable dictionary of the most common cancer terms: *http://www.acor.org/glossary/index.html*.

Steve Dunn's CancerGuide is an excellent resource for those interested in researching their illness, particularly clinical trials: *http://www.cancerguide.org/sdunn_story.html*.

Cancer Supportive Care program, based on excerpts from the book, *Cancer Supportive Care: A Comprehensive Guide for Patients and Their Families* by Ernest H. Rosenbaum and Isadora Rosenbaum (Toronto, Ontario: Somerville House Publishing, 1998), is a good source of information for dealing with side effects: *http://www.cancersupportivecare.com*.

The Merck Manual web site is a vast resource of medical information geared to doctors, but generally useful to patients and caretakers: *http://www.merck.com*.

QuackWatch gives medical doctor Stephen Barrett's evaluation of cancer doctors practicing outside the mainstream: *http://www.quackwatch.com*.

Medical resources

Medical information targeted to special topics is available through the resources listed in these categories.

Drug and dosage information

Books

Physicians' Desk Reference 2000. Fifty-fourth edition. Montvale, NJ: Medical Economics Data, 2000. The *Physicians' Desk Reference (PDR)* is a compendium of information about drugs. It's now reprinted in versions that are easier for the general public to understand, but you might appreciate the detail in the original PDR: *http://www.pdr.net.*

Organizations

US Food and Drug Administration (FDA)
5600 Fishers Lane
Rockville, MD 20857
(301) 827-4420
(888) 332-4543
(800) 532-4440
http://www.fda.gov

The US Food and Drug Administration (FDA) offers multitudes of information about drugs. You can report adverse effects of drugs to the FDA via their MedWatch web site: *http://www. fda.gov/medwatch/how.htm.* See also their CDER listing, under "Clinical trials and investigational new substances," about gaining access to investigational new substances or importing drugs from other countries.

Internet

Many good web sites exist to provide you with drug information. All of the following have search engines:

- QuackWatch gives medical doctor Stephen Barrett's evaluation of those alternative remedies you've been hearing about: *http://www.quackwatch.com.*
- Glaxo's DoseCalc can be used to calculate your chemotherapy dose: *http://www.meds.com/ DChome.html.*
- Clinical Pharmacology Online is one of the most comprehensive sites, offering free, detailed information about drugs: *http://www.cponline.gsm.com.*
- Other sites that are less comprehensive than CPO, but still useful:
  - DrugInfoNet: *http://www.druginfonet.com*
  - HealthTouch: *http://www.healthtouch.com/level1/p_dri.htm*
  - RxMed: *http://www.rxmed.com/prescribe.html*
  - Mythos Pharmacy Online: *http://www.mythos.com/pharmacy*

Calculating body surface area is useful to verify your chemotherapy dose:

- Cornell University: *http://www-users.med.cornell.edu/~spon/picu/bsacalc.htm*
- Martindale's HS Guide: *http://www-sci.lib.uci.edu/HSG/Pharmacy.html*
- Medical College of Wisconsin: *http://www.intmed.mcw.edu/clincalc/body.html*

Resources for pain and other side effects

Cancer pain and the adverse effects of treatment are of great concern to most cancer patients.

Organizations

American Association of Sex Educators, Counselors, and Therapists (AASECT)
P.O. Box 238
Mount Vernon, IA 52314
(319) 895-8407
fax (319) 895-6203
email *AASECT@worldnet.att.net*
http://www.aasect.org

The American Association of Sex Educators, Counselors, and Therapists can refer you to a counselor if lung cancer or cancer therapy is affecting your sexuality or fertility.

American Association for Respiratory Care
11030 Ables Lane
Dallas, TX 75229
(972) 243-2272
fax (972) 484-2720 or (972) 484-6010
email *info@aarc.org*
http://www.aarc.org

The American Association for Respiratory Care can help you find a respiratory therapist and can furnish information on lung care, home oxygen therapy, and continuous positive airway pressure (CPAP).

American Cancer Society National Office
1599 Clifton Road NE
Atlanta, GA 30329-4251
(800) ACS-2345
http://www.cancer.org

The American Cancer Society has many programs to help cancer survivors with problems such as pain. Check your local phone directory for the office nearest you.

American Massage Therapy Association
820 Davis Street, Suite 100
Evanston, IL 60201-4444
(847) 864-0123
fax (847) 864-1178
http://www.amtamassage.org

The American Massage Therapy Association can share information with you regarding licensing of practitioners and names of licensed massage therapists near you.

American Society of Anesthesiologists
520 N. Northwest Highway
Park Ridge, IL 60068
(847) 825-5586
email *mail@asahq.org*
http://www.asahq.org

The American Society of Anesthesiologists maintains a database of patient education information regarding pain control.

American Society of Clinical Hypnosis
130 E. Elm Court, Suite 201
Roselle, IL 60172-2000
(312) 645-9810
fax (312) 645-9818
email *info@asch.net*
http://www.asch.net

The American Society of Clinical Hypnosis exists to "encourage and promote excellence in the use of hypnosis by qualified health and mental health professionals; to advance...standards of practice in hypnosis, and to advise others about the value, application and ethical use of hypnosis." They can advise you on finding hypnotists for pain control.

National Chronic Pain Outreach Association
7979 Old Georgetown Road, Suite 100
Bethesda, MD 20814-2429
(301) 652-4948

The National Chronic Pain Outreach Association educates families, patients, and caretakers about chronic pain and the choices of treatment.

Pulmonary Hypertension Association
850 Sligo Avenue, Suite 800
Silver Spring, MD 20907-8277
(800) 748-7274
email *candibleifer@earthlink.net*
http://www.phassociation.org

The Pulmonary Hypertension Association provides information for lung cancer survivors with PH and encourages research into the disorder.

Society of Reproductive Endocrinologists
c/o American Society for Reproductive Medicine
1209 Montgomery Highway
Birmingham, AL 35216
(205) 978-5000
fax (205) 978-5005

The Society of Reproductive Endocrinologists can help you if lung cancer treatment has impaired your ability to have children.

Additional web sites

- Cancer-Pain is an ACOR Internet-based discussion group for those with cancer-related pain. See also the earlier section "Support groups" and ACOR's site, *listserv.acor.org*.
- Acupuncture.com can refer you to a local acupuncturist and has information regarding state laws governing the licensing and practice of acupuncture: *http://www.acupuncture.com*.

Tests and procedures

These resources can help you learn how tests are done and what the results mean.

Books on how tests are done

Andrews, Maraca, and Michael Shaw. *Everything You Need to Know About Medical Tests*. Springhouse, PA: Springhouse, 1996. An excellent 691-page comprehensive reference written for the patient in a readable and respectful style.

Brodin, Michael B. *The Encyclopedia of Medical Tests*. New York: Simon and Schuster, 1997.

Pagana, Kathleen, and Timothy Pagana, eds. *Mosby's Diagnostic and Laboratory Test Reference*. St. Louis, MO: Mosby, 1992.

Stauffer, Joseph, and Joseph C. Segen. *The Patient's Guide to Medical Tests: Everything You Need to Know About the Tests Your Doctor Prescribes*. Fourth edition. New York: Facts on File, 1997.

Zaret, Barry L., Peter Jatlow, and Lee D. Katz, eds. *The Patient's Guide to Medical Tests*. Boston, MA: Houghton Mifflin, 1997.

Web sites on how tests are done

Each of these web sites has useful information on the patient's view of experiencing tests:

- The Biology Project: *http://www.biology.arizona.edu*
- ThriveOnline: *http://www.thriveonline.com*
- Mid-South Imaging & Therapeutics: *http://www.msit.com/patients.htm*

Normal values of tests

Finding the normal values of blood and urine tests to compare with your results can sometimes be difficult. These web-based resources show "normals" for many tests. Enter the test name and click the search button:

- The University of Michigan Pathology Laboratories Handbook: *http://po.path.med.umich. edu/handbook*
- CanCare: *http://www.health.sa.gov.au/cancare/REFERENCES/nvaltest.htm*
- The Merck Manual Online: *http://www.merck.com/pubs/mmanual*

Finding PET scanning facilities

Institute for Clinical PET (ICP)
1820 Jefferson Place NW
Washington, DC 20036
(202) 530-0990
fax (202) 833-1613
icpmail@aol.com
http://icppet.org

PET scanning has been studied for more than 30 years, but its use in the clinic is fairly new. Not all hospitals have PET scanners. For a list of PET centers, contact the Institute for Clinical PET (ICP).

Clinical trials and investigational new substances

Organizations

FDA Center for Drug Evaluation and Research
CDER Executive Secretariat (HFD-8)
5600 Fishers Lane
Rockville, MD 20857
(888) INFO-FDA [(888) 463-6332)]
http://www.fda.gov/cder/cancer/access.htm

The FDA can assist and direct you regarding federal regulations for obtaining investigational new drugs and for importing foreign drugs for single-patient use.

Books

Motulsky, Harvey. *Intuitive Biostatistics*. New York: Oxford University Press, 1995. This 385-page book can help you understand published results of clinical trials and can help you assess trial design if you're planning to enroll in a trial.

Web sites

The National Cancer Institute Clinical Trials web site is the most comprehensive way to locate trials of new substances and treatments. Only trials sanctioned by NCI are shown here: *http://cancernet.nci.nih.gov/prot/protsrch.shtml*.

Bruce Niebuhr's *Handbook of Clinical Trial and Epidemiological Research Designs*, January 1998, maintained at the University of Texas Medical Branch at Galveston, is a good technical description of clinical trials written from the practitioner's point of view, and consequently provides insights a patient might not otherwise find: *http://sahs.utmb.edu/pellinore/intro_to_research/clintrls.htm*.

Steve Dunn's CancerGuide is an excellent resource for learning how to assess clinical trials and how to research your illness. Steve is a ten-year survivor of metastatic kidney cancer: *http://www.cancerguide.org/sdunn_story.html*.

You can use CenterWatch to track new cancer treatment trials: *http://www.centerwatch.com*.

Verifying doctor and hospital credentials

The ABMS Public Education Program
47 Perimeter Center East, Suite 500
Atlanta, GA 30346
(800) 733-2267
http://www.certifieddoctor.org

The Official ABMS Directory of Board Certified Medical Specialists 1998. Thirtieth edition. 1997 Marquis Who's Who. This is a directory of board-certified physicians who have chosen to specialize in a particular area of medicine.

The American College of Surgeons
633 North Saint Clair Street
Chicago, IL 60611
(312) 202-5000
http://www.facs.org

The American College of Surgeons can verify whether your surgeon is board certified in a surgical specialty.

American Medical Association Directory of Physicians in the US. Chicago, IL: American Medical Association, 2000. This large reference, updated annually, provides a means to verify your doctor's credentials. The AMA's Physician Select web site also is an excellent means to check your doctor's education and board certification: *http://www.ama-assn.org*.

American Thoracic Society
1740 Broadway
New York, NY 10019
(212) 315-8700
fax (212) 315-6498
http://www.thoracic.org

The American Thoracic Society can help you locate a board-certified thoracic (chest) surgeon.

Center for Medical Consumers
237 Thompson Street
New York, NY 10012
(212) 674-7105
http://www.medicalconsumers.org/index.html

The Center for Medical Consumers provides information referrals to other organizations and maintains a medical consumer's library.

Consumer Health Information Research Institute
300 E. Pink Hill Drive
Independence, MO 64057
(816) 228-4595
fax (816) 228-4995
%20drenner@msn.net

The Consumer Health Information Research Institute provides an integrity index and a credibility of publication index.

Joint Commission on Accreditation of Health Care Organizations (JCAHO)
1 Renaissance Boulevard
Oakbrook Terrace, IL 60181
(630) 792-5000
http://www.jcaho.org

JCAHO is responsible for accreditation of hospitals. You can contact them if you have concerns about the quality of care you've received while hospitalized.

National Council Against Health Fraud
P.O. Box 141
Fort Lee, NJ 07024.
(201) 723-2955
wlondon@worldnet.att.net
http://www.ncahf.org

The National Council Against Health Fraud is a nonprofit volunteer health agency that tracks health fraud, misinformation, and quackery. It is private, nonpartisan, and nonsectarian, and its principals serve without compensation.

QuackWatch
http://www.quackwatch.com

QuackWatch gives the medical scientist's evaluation of alternative remedies. It also offers information on avenues of complaint for medical consumers to their local or federal government agencies: *http://www.quackwatch.com/02ConsumerProtection/complain.html*.

SearchPointe
http://www.searchpointe.com

SearchPointe is a fee-based service providing a single, private, nationwide source to medical consumers regarding physician education, license, and disciplinary action data.

Society for Surgical Oncology
85 West Algonquin Road, Suite 55
Arlington Heights, IL 60005
(847) 427-1400
fax (847) 427-9656
http://www.surgonc.org

The Society for Surgical Oncology can help you locate a board-certified thoracic (chest) surgeon who specializes in lung cancer.

***US News and World Report's* annual "Best Hospitals" edition**
2400 N Street NW
Washington, DC 20037-1196
(202) 955-2000
http://www.usnews.com

Document retrieval services

Document retrieval services can fax or mail you the full text of any published research paper for a fee. On the Internet, the Medline service providers Medscape, Helix, PhyNet, PDRnet. com, SilverPlatter, Ovid On Call, Infotrieve, PaperChase, and others offer full-text services. Do a web search on any of these names.

Medical information searches

Companies that will find medical information for you for a fee and are highly rated by Steve Dunn's CancerGuide (*http://www.cancerguide.org*) are:

The Health Resource, Inc.
933 Faulkner
Conway, AR 72032
(800) 949-0090
moreinfo@thehealthresource.com
http://www.thehealthresource.com
Minimum fee $125

Schine On-Line Services
39 Brenton Avenue
Providence, RI 02906
(800) FIND-CURE
email *schine@findcure.com*
http://www.findcure.com

Legal, financial, and insurance resources

Beyond the physical aspects of cancer lie its effects on our careers and finances. The following resources can offer guidance and aid.

Organizations that help

The Center for Medical Consumers

237 Thompson Street
New York, NY 10012
(212) 674-7105
http://www.medicalconsumers.org/index.html

The Center for Medical Consumers provides information referrals to other organizations and maintains a medical consumer's library.

American Consumer Credit Counseling, Inc.

24 Crescent Street
Waltham, MA 02453
(800) 769-3571
fax (781) 893-7649
help@consumercredit.com
http://www.consumercredit.com

American Consumer Credit Counseling can provide information and help with getting expenses under control.

Equal Employment Opportunity Commission

1801 L Street NW
Washington, DC 20507
(202) 663-4900
(800) 669-4000
http://www.eeoc.gov

The EEOC will help you if you have experienced unfair discrimination from an employer because of a cancer-related disability. (For other job-related problems caused by cancer, see the US Department of Justice and the Department of Labor.)

Federal Trade Commission

600 Pennsylvania Avenue NW
Washington, DC 20580
(202) 326-2222
http://www.ftc.gov

The Federal Trade Commission "enforces a variety of federal antitrust and consumer protection laws. The Commission seeks to ensure that the nation's markets function competitively, and are vigorous, efficient, and free of undue restrictions. The Commission also works to enhance the smooth operation of the marketplace by eliminating acts or practices that are unfair or deceptive. In general, the Commission's efforts are directed toward stopping actions that threaten consumers' opportunities to exercise informed choice." FTC can provide information about the federal Consumer Credit Protection Act, a landmark series of laws passed in 1968 to protect debtors.

Health Insurance Association of America (HIAA)
555 13th Street NW
Washington, DC 20004
(202) 824-1600
http://www.hiaa.org/index.html

Health Insurance Association of America (HIAA) has more than 250 members consisting of insurers and managed care companies. HIAA can supply booklets on disability income, health insurance, long-term care, medical savings accounts, and general insurance information, including a directory of state insurance departments.

Health Pages
100 Fifth Avenue, Tenth Floor
New York, NY 10011
(212) 366-4600
email *feedback@thehealthpages.com*
http://www.thehealthpages.com

Health Pages reports on ranges and norms of doctor's fees.

Lexis-Nexis
P.O. Box 933
Dayton, OH 45401-0933
(800) 227-4908
email *newsales@lexis-nexis.com*
http://www.lexis-nexis.com

For a fee, this group can send you a copy of any law or newspaper article. Fees are flat-rate, hourly, or per transaction.

Medical Information Bureau (MIB)
P.O. Box 105, Essex Station
Boston, MA 02112
(617) 424-3660
http://www.mib.com

The Medical Information Bureau (MIB) records all entries made by insurance companies about your health and, for an $8.50 fee, will send you a copy of this information. In some cases, the fee is waived—see their web site for all exceptions. If you find an error in these files, you can contact the MIB for the procedures necessary to correct errors.

National Association of Attorneys General
750 First Street NE, Suite 1100
Washington, DC 20002
(202) 326-6000
http://www.naag.org

The National Association of Attorneys General works to establish policy and maintains current information regarding tobacco settlements.

William M. Mercer, Incorporated
Social Security Information Services
462 South Fourth Avenue, Suite 1500
Louisville, KY 40202-3431
(800) 477-4541
social.security@us.wmmercer.com
http://www.wmmercer.com

The William M. Mercer Corporation publishes several guides to Social Security benefits and administration.

US Department of Justice
Employment Litigation Section
Civil Rights Division
P.O. Box 65968
Washington, DC 20035-5968
(202) 514-3831
fax (202) 514-1005, 1105
web@usdoj.gov
http://www.usdoj.gov

The US Department of Justice enforces the Americans With Disabilities Act and the Federal Rehabilitation Act. See also EEOC if you are disabled.

US Department of Labor Pension and Welfare Benefits Administration
200 Constitution Avenue NW
Washington, DC 20210
(202) 219-8776
(800) 998-7542
http://www.dol.gov/dol/pwba

The Pension and Welfare Benefits Administration (PWBA) protects the integrity of pensions, health plans, and other employee benefits for more than 150 million people. Their mission is to assist workers in getting the information they need to protect their benefit rights. HIPAA, COBRA, FMLA, and ERISA are enforced by USDOL.

US Department of Veterans Affairs
810 Vermont Avenue NW
Washington, DC 20420
(800) 827-1000
General web site *http://www.va.gov*
Agent Orange web site: *http://www.va.gov/pressrel/99fsao.htm*

The Department of Veterans Affairs provides care and financial assistance to those eligible for health care through the VA or disability benefits to lung cancer patients and survivors who were exposed to Agent Orange in Southeast Asia.

Books

Treanor, J. Robert, Dale R. Detlefs, and Robert J. Myers. *Mercer Guide to Social Security and Medicare 2000*. Louisville, KY: William M. Mercer, 2000.

Social Security Administration bulletins

Social Security benefits are available not just to retired people, but also to cancer patients and survivors who are disabled—see Chapter 17, *Finances, Employment, and Record Keeping*. The chief resource in this category is the 1997 Social Security Handbook, thirteenth edition: *http://www.ssa.gov/OP_Home/handbook/ssa-hbk.htm*.

Other, more specific SSA bulletins include:

- Social Security: What You Need To Know When You Get Disability Benefits (6/96; Pub. No. 05-10153)
- Social Security Disability Programs (5/96; Pub. No. 05-10057)
- A Guide to Social Security and SSI Disability Benefits for People with HIV Infection (6/95; Pub. No. 05-10020)
- How We Decide If You Are Still Disabled (4/96; Pub. No. 05-10053)
- How Social Security Can Help with Vocational Rehabilitation (9/94; Pub. No. 05-10050)
- Working While Disabled...How We Can Help (1/96; Pub. No. 05-10095)
- Red Book on Work Incentives for People with Disabilities (8/95; Pub. No. 64-030)

Web sites

A. M. Best's insurance company ratings can be seen online at *http://www.ambest.com/bestline/sales/ratings.html*.

Free treatment, drugs, travel, and lodging

Having cancer is bad enough. Paying for care can be prohibitive, particularly if you must pay in full for drugs or travel to a distant treatment center and stay for an extended period.

Free treatment

The National Cancer Institute in Bethesda, Maryland offers treatment free of charge to those who participate in NCI clinical trials. Free housing also is provided. Both US and foreign citizens are eligible. Call (800) 4-CANCER.

Free drugs

The FDA Investigational New Drug (IND) program, previously known as the Compassionate Use Program, is intended to provide drugs for those with serious illnesses who cannot afford payment. The Food and Drug Administration web site (*http://www.fda.gov*) explains regulations for obtaining investigational new drugs and for importing foreign drugs for single-patient use. Call (800) 532-4440.

You can also contact the drug manufacturer directly if you need an anticancer drug, but cannot afford it. Many have compassionate-use programs for this purpose. A partial list of pharmaceutical manufacturers who have such programs can be found at *http://www.cancersupportivecare. com/drug_assistance.html*.

International Aid, Inc.
17011 Hickory
Spring Lake, MI 49456
(616) 846-7490

International Aid might accept unused drugs you have for donation to those in other countries who cannot afford them.

Free air travel

Mercy Medical Airlift
National Patient Air Transport Helpline
(800) 296-1191
Patient Assistance Center
4620 Haygood Road, Suite 1
Virginia Beach, VA 23455
(888) 675-1405
fax (757) 318-9107
mercymed@erols.com
http://www.mercymedical.org

Mercy Medical Airlift's National Patient Air Transport Helpline (NPATH) helps cancer patients travel to distant health centers for care. Their Patient Assistance Center offers additional programs, such as Special-Lift and Child-Lift programs, to assist with transport of those needing care for pediatric or rare diseases.

Air Care Alliance
6202 South Lewis Avenue, Suite F2
Tulsa, OK 74136-1064
(918) 745-0384
(888) 662-6794
fax (918) 745-0879
AirCareAlliance@aol.com
http://www.aircareall.org

The volunteer pilots of Air Care Alliance help financially needy cancer patients travel to distant health centers for care.

Corporate Angel Network
Westchester County Airport
One Loop Road
White Plains, NY 10604
(914) 328-1313
http://www.corpangelnetwork.org

The Corporate Angel Network uses private corporate jets on regularly scheduled flights that are not full to transport cancer patients free of charge to distant health centers for care.

American Red Cross
430 17th Street NW
Washington, DC 20006
(202) 737-8300
http://www.redcross.org

The Red Cross can assist with emergency travel and communication for military personnel. Call (202) 728-6400 or their 24-hour line (202) 728-6401 to find the chapter nearest you or your destination.

Angel Flight for Veterans
4620 Haygood Road, Suite 1
Virginia Beach, VA 23455
(757) 318-7109
fax (757) 318-9107
angelflightveterans@erols.com
http://www.veterans-aeromedical.org

Angel Flight for Veterans provides free or reduced-rate medical transportation for veterans, active duty military personnel, and their families who need to travel long distances for medical evaluation, diagnosis, or treatment.

Mission Aviation Fellowship
Box 3202
Redlands, CA 92373
(909) 794-1151
MAF-US@maf.org
http://www.maf.org

Mission Aviation Fellowship supports air ambulance services and medical assistance in 57 countries.

Free land travel

The American Cancer Society regional offices in many cities have networks of volunteers who can provide transport by car to and from your treatment center. See their listing earlier in this appendix. Call your local office or (800) ACS-2345 or visit *http://www.cancer.org*.

Traveler's Aid International
1612 K Street NW, Suite 206
Washington, DC 20006
(202) 546-1127
travelers.aid@worldnet.att.net
http://www.travelersaid.org

Traveler's Aid International provides emergency travel and lodging for those in dire financial need. Check local phone books for contact information.

Free lodging

American Cancer Society Hope Lodge
http://www2.cancer.org/coe/index.cfm?key=crd

The American Cancer Society (ACS) sponsors Hope Lodges in many cities that provide free lodging for those who travel to receive cancer care. Their service is also offered to non-US citizens traveling within the US for medical care. Lodging is free and is provided on a first-come, first-served basis. Each Hope Lodge has kitchen and laundry facilities. Check your local phone book or use the web site above to submit a request for information.

National Association of Hospital Hospitality Houses (NAHHH)
P.O. Box 18087
Asheville, NC 28814-0087
(800) 542-9730
helpinghomes@nahhh.org
http://www.nahhh.org

The NAHHH can recommend hotels near hospitals with reduced room rates for cancer patients.

National Cancer Institute (NCI)
Bethesda, MD
(800) 4-CANCER
http://www.nci.nih.gov

The National Cancer Institute in Bethesda, MD will in some cases help pay for the travel and lodging expenses of those being treated at the NCI.

Ronald McDonald House Charities
One Kroc Drive
Oak Brook, IL 60523
(312) 836-7100
http://www.rmhc.com

Ronald McDonald Houses, sponsored by the McDonald's Corporation, offer free lodging not only to sick children, but also to pregnant women with high-risk pregnancies. Financial need may be a prerequisite for entry at some sites. A nominal fee of ten dollars a night may also be charged, but this fee may be waived if financial hardship is demonstrated.

Hospitals

Many hospitals have agreements with nearby hotels for reduced rates for patients and families. Contact the hospital's social worker or the admitting desk in advance of traveling for such information.

Cancer Centers

Some major cancer centers have outpatient lodging run by the institution for those requiring long-term follow-up care. Discuss these resources with the hospital admitting staff before you travel. The cost of having you and your family stay in such hospital-run facilities might be covered by your insurance policy.

Travel insurance with medical features

Before you travel for pleasure, you should verify your health policy's coverage for emergency medical care. A partial list of companies that offer such coverage can be found at *http://www.worldtravelcenter.com/eng/guides/policy_picker.cfm*, although this list does not imply our recommendation or endorsement.

End-of-life resources

Resources for increasing comfort and serenity in the last stage of life are included in this category.

Home and hospice care

Community Health Accreditation Program, Inc.
350 Hudson Street
New York, NY 10014
(800) 669-9656
http://www.chapinc.org

Community Health Accreditation Program, Inc., provides a list of accredited home care organizations.

National Association for Home Care
228 7th Street SE
Washington, DC 20003
(202) 547-7424
http://www.nahc.org

The National Association for Home Care represents all home health care agencies in the US. They offer publications on selecting home care.

National Hospice Organization
1700 Diagonal Road, Suite 300
Arlington, VA 22314
(703) 243-5900
(800) 658-8898
http://www.nhpco.org

The National Hospice Organization offers information on the goals of hospice care and how to choose a hospice.

Oley Foundation
214 Hun Memorial
Albany Medical Center A-23
Albany, NY 12208
(800) 776-OLEY
http://www.wizvax.net/oleyfdn

The Oley Foundation offers help with parenteral or enteral nutrition; that is, feeding by IV or stomach tube.

Olsten Health Services National Resource Center
175 Broadhollow Road
Melville, NY 11747
(800) 66-NURSE

The Olsten Health Services National Resource Center offers help with all home health care services.

Visiting Nurse Associations of America
3801 East Florida Avenue, Suite 900
Denver, CO 80210
(800) 426-2547
http://www.vnaa.org

The Visiting Nurse Associations of America provides skilled nurses, aides, and therapists for home care.

Reading material about dying

Basta, Lofty. *A Graceful Exit: Life and Death on Your Own Terms*. New York: Plenum Press, 1996.

Bernard, Jan, and Miriam Schneider. *The True Work of Dying*. New York: Avon Books, 1996.

Callanan, Maggie, and Patricia Kelley. *Final Gifts: Understanding the Special Awareness, Needs, and Communications of the Dying*. New York: Bantam Books, 1997.

Furman, Joan, and David McNabb. *The Dying Time: Practical Wisdom for the Dying and Their Caregivers*. Bell Tower, NY: Random House, 1997.

Groopman, Jerome. *The Measure of Our Days*. New York, NY: Viking (Penguin), 1997.

Humphry, Derek. *Final Exit: The Practicalities of Self-Deliverance and Assisted Suicide for the Dying*. Denver, CO: The Hemlock Society, 1997.

Kramp, Erin Tierney, Douglas H. Kramp, and Emily P. McKhann. *Living with the End in Mind; A Practical Checklist for Living Life to the Fullest by Embracing Your Mortality*. Three Rivers, CA: Three Rivers Press, 1998.

Kubler-Ross, Elisabeth. *Death: The Final Stage of Growth*. New York: Simon and Schuster, 1975.

Kubler-Ross, Elisabeth. *Living With Death and Dying*. New York: Simon and Schuster (Touch-stone), 1981.

Kubler-Ross, Elisabeth. *On Death and Dying*. New York: MacMillan Publishing, 1969.

Kubler-Ross, Elisabeth. *To Live Until We Say Good-bye*. New York: Simon and Schuster, 1978.

Lattanzi-Licht, Marcia, John Mahoney, and Galen Miller. *The Hospice Choice: In Pursuit of a Peaceful Death*. New York: Simon and Schuster (Fireside), 1998.

Nuland, Sherwin. *How We Die: Reflections on Life's Final Chapter*. New York: Alfred A. Knopf, 1993.

Ray, M. Catherine. *I'm With You Now: A Guide Through Incurable Illness for Patients, Families, and Friends*. New York: Bantam Books, 1997.

Weenolsen, Patricia. *The Art of Dying: How to Leave This World With Dignity and Grace, at Peace With Yourself and With Your Loved Ones*. New York: St. Martin's Press, 1996.

Books for children

Buscaglia, Leo. *The Fall of Freddie the Leaf*. New York: C. B. Slack, 1982.

Hitchcock, Ruth. *Tim's Dad: A Story About a Boy Whose Father Dies*. Springfield, IL: Human Services, 1988.

Holden, L. D. *Gran-Gran's Best Trick: A Story for Children Who Have Lost Someone They Love*. New York: Magination, 1989.

Krementz, Jill. *How It Feels When a Parent Dies*. New York: Alfred A. Knopf, 1981.

LeShan, Eda. *Learning to Say Goodbye: When a Parent Dies*. New York: Macmillan, 1976.

O'Toole, Donna. *Aarvy Aardvark Finds Hope: A Read Aloud Story for People of All Ages about Loving and Losing, Friendship and Hope*. Burnsville, NC: Celo Press, 1988.

Vigna, Judith. *Saying Goodbye to Daddy*. Morton Grove, IL: Albert Whitman, 1991.

White, E. B. *Charlotte's Web*. New York: Harper & Row, 1952.

Tests and Procedures

THIS APPENDIX LISTS TESTS AND PROCEDURES for lung cancer alphabetically. For each test, we describe what the test or procedure accomplishes, tell how to prepare for the test, detail how it is administered, relay how most people rank the test regarding pain, discuss recovery issues, and outline any risks.

Only the tests that are used most commonly for lung cancer patients are described here. Please see the *Notes* and Appendix A, *Resources*, for other resources that discuss tests.

Blood product transfusion

This outpatient procedure is a means of replenishing your red blood cell and platelet blood supply if surgery, chemotherapy, or radiation therapy has significantly lowered your red blood cell and platelet supply or has limited your bone marrow's ability to produce new blood cells.

Preparation

You should check the blood product brought to you for infusion to be sure it matches your blood type. Platelet matching may also become necessary after many platelet transfusions because the body gradually becomes sensitized to and attacks donated platelets. Be sure to tell the nursing staff if you have ever had an allergic reaction to donor platelets.

Method

An intravenous (IV) line is inserted into a vein in your forearm or into your central catheter, if you have one that can be used for transfusions. The blood product to be transfused is hung from an IV pole and is dripped into you over a period of about four hours. If you have chills, fever, or difficulty breathing during a transfusion, notify the nursing staff immediately; this may be the beginning of an allergic reaction.

Pain

If you have no catheter and an IV line is inserted into your vein, you may feel mild pain during its insertion.

Recovery

There are no recovery issues following transfusion. On the contrary, you can expect to feel much less tired almost immediately after red blood cells are infused.

Risks

There is a risk of serious allergic reaction if donated blood products are not properly matched to yours. There is a slight risk of infection at the site of IV insertion.

Blood tests

Various blood tests detect various conditions. Each blood test's purpose is discussed following the name of the test. All are outpatient procedures.

Preparation

Most blood tests require no preparation; however, some may require an overnight fasting diet or the cessation of certain medications for a few days. Always tell your doctor and the staff administering the test if you are taking any drugs, whether prescription or over-the-counter.

Method

Blood tests are performed by drawing blood into a syringe either from your venous access catheter (for which see "Catheter insertion (central catheter, central line)," later) or from the vein just inside your elbow. If you don't have a catheter and your veins have been damaged by chemotherapy, if they are hard to find, or if they roll, the technician (phlebotomist) may use a vein on the back of the hand or on the back of the lower forearm. A blood draw takes less than three minutes.

You can make your veins easier to access as follows:

- Lay a wet, warm cloth on the vein just before blood is drawn or ask to use a restroom to soak the forearm in warm water.
- Vigorously pump the muscles in that arm just before the draw.
- Hang the arm lower than the rest of the body for a few minutes just before the draw.
- Drink lots of fluids starting four hours before the blood draw.

Pain

Most people report minor pain or no pain during a blood draw. If, however, you are afraid of needles, of the pain of needles, or of the sight of blood, you are not alone. Here are a few tips for reducing fear and pain during a blood draw:

- Slap or rub the injection site just before the draw so that you will be less likely to feel the insertion.
- Ask for EMLA cream to use two hours before your appointment. Keep the site covered with an airtight bandage until your draw.
- Ask the phlebotomist, most of whom are quite skilled at reducing pain, to stretch the skin at the injection site.
- Look away while the blood is drawn.
- Think of someone who delights you and makes you smile.
- Ask the phlebotomist about his life, liking for the job, and so on.

Recovery

Most blood draws entail no recovery, but you may have slight, painless bruising at the injection site the following day, especially if your platelet count is low. Stretching the skin to make the blood draw less painful may increase the chance of bruising. Steady pressure on the injection site for a minimum of 60 seconds (more, if your platelet counts are low) directly after the needle is withdrawn facilitates clotting and can reduce the chance of bruising.

Risks

Unless you have blood that won't clot normally, there are only minor risks associated with a blood draw, such as the possibility of painless bruising.

Results

Normal values for blood tests are described in Appendix C, *Test Results*.

Specific blood tests

Alkaline phosphatase
> This product's value may be abnormal if liver function is affected by the tumor or if bone is being dissolved (for example, when calcium levels are out of balance).

Bilirubin
> As with other liver products, the level of this substance is a reflection of the tumor's effect on liver function.

Calcium
> Minerals and electrolytes are affected by kidney function and by the activity of certain lung tumors.

Carboxyhemoglobin (COHb)
> This test measures what percentage of red blood cells are bound to carbon monoxide.

Carcinoembryonic antigen (CEA)
> This product of tumor metabolism rises in the presence of certain types of lung cancer. It is meaningful only in concert with other findings and in the presence of certain symptoms.

Complete blood count (CBC)
> This test measures the three blood cell types and reports on their proportions, age, and other important parameters. Certain lung tumors are able to affect blood counts profoundly. During chemotherapy and radiation therapy, white blood cell counts can drop and make the patient susceptible to infections.

Creatinine (serum creatinine)
> This substance is an indication of how well your kidneys are working. Elevated creatinine levels might reflect the amount of dangerous toxins being released by the tumor as it breaks down, called tumor lysis syndrome, or the activity of tumors that produce hormone-like substances.

Electrolytes
> Levels of various minerals in the blood are sometimes a reflection of problems related to tumor metabolism or to chemotherapy. Levels of calcium, potassium, magnesium, iron, and other electrolytes can be modified by disease or by its treatment.

FISH
Fluorescence in situ hybridization: see ISH.

Flow cytometry
This method of examining tissue exploits two principles: first, cancer cells can be tagged with chemicals and be made to look different from normal cells. Second, these cells can be forced to flow single file through a narrow tube so they can be counted one at a time, much like schoolchildren returning from recess. The tagged cancer cells are counted as they pass through a light beam or other tool for detecting whatever tagging agent was used. In this manner, cells can be examined for very specific features indicating cancer, such as abnormal surface antigens.

Glucose
Both high and low blood sugar can be related to tumor metabolism.

Hormones
High or low levels of various hormones, such as gastrin, vasopressin, calcitonin, growth hormone, TSH, ACTH, HCG, and others can be a reflection of tumor activity.

5-HIAA
5-hydroxyindoleacetic acid is elevated in those with carcinoid syndrome.

ISH (in situ hybridization)
This test of the DNA contained in lung tumors uses such substances as fluorescent chemicals to mark damaged genes. The chemical consists of molecules constructed to match exactly the gene being sought, so ISH is not practical for broad screening for DNA damage. The probe untwists (denatures) the two strands of DNA and, when a match exists between the chemical probe and a gene, attaches itself to the one piece of DNA being sought: thus the term hybridization. Using a special microscope, the pathologist or geneticist can visualize the gene, its breakpoint, any crossing over with other genes on the same or other chromosomes, and so on, by viewing the visual effect produced (such as fluorescence in the case of FISH).

Lactate dehydrogenase (LDH)
High levels of LDH can correlate to disease activity.

Liver enzymes (SGOT, SGPT, ALT, AST)
Unusual amounts of liver enzymes correlate loosely with the presence and extent of liver disease and with liver function that is impaired for any reason.

PCO^2
The percentage of carbon dioxide (CO_2) in blood, usually arterial blood.

PO^2
The percentage of oxygen (O_2) in blood, usually arterial blood.

Polymerase chain reaction (PCR)
PCR can use many different source tissues as long as they contain genes and chromosomes (DNA). PCR is a method, not a test or substance. It involves taking a very small amount of genetic material and replicating it over and over so that enough exists to run tests that will require large amounts of genetic material.

Prostate-specific antigen (PSA)

This blood test can detect the activity of lung tumors that produce PSA, although it is not a specific test for lung cancer or even for prostate cancer.

Sodium

Low levels of sodium in blood indicate that kidney function has been affected by tumor metabolism, sometimes caused by secretion of antidiuretic hormone by the tumor.

Tissue polypeptide antigen (TPA)

Like CEA, this product of tumor metabolism rises in the presence of certain types of lung cancer. It is not accurate enough to use alone to track the progression or regression of cancer, but it is meaningful in concert with other findings and in the presence of certain symptoms.

Uric acid

As with creatinine, this substance reflects kidney function and possible effects of the tumor on the kidney, such as tumor lysis syndrome.

Bone scan (scintigraphy)

This outpatient test exploits the fact that some bone irregularities will absorb more of a substance than will healthy bone.

Preparation

A mildly radioactive agent, usually technetium-99, will be injected and you will be asked to return later, perhaps in three hours, for scanning. You will be encouraged to drink copious amounts of water to spread the agent from soft tissue into bone. Get comfortable after lying down on the table for the scan, because you must hold this position for up to an hour.

Method

Scanning is done by having the fully clothed patient lie on a table that has, above and below it, a camera that is sensitive to the energy emitted by the agent injected. It is important to hold still for duration of the film exposure. The table is fully open, not enclosed like an MRI machine, and you'll see the arm of the camera passing over your body, starting with your head and going toward your feet. The arm is about six inches wide and about as long as the table is wide. It moves slowly: a whole-body scan can take 30 or 40 minutes.

Pain

A slight sting may be felt when the scintigraphic agent is injected.

Recovery

There are no recovery issues associated with this test.

Risks

As with other imaging techniques, there are risks of false-positive and false-negative readings.

Results

Normal results generally show no suspicious lesions on the imaging medium, but normal results might vary depending on why the scan was performed. Results for detection of tumors may vary from patient to patient. Certain circumstances and certain drugs can result in findings on imaging studies that appear to be tumors, but are not. Suspicious lesions could be healed broken bones, bone loss, mineral deposition, or tumor invasion of bone. Follow-up testing, such as PET scanning or MRI, might be suggested.

Bronchoscopy

Bronchoscopy is a form of endoscopy, an outpatient procedure that uses a microscope and light source on a narrow flexible tube to examine, sample, or unblock tissue in the airways that otherwise would require an open surgery to access.

Bronchoscopy is sometimes not used on those who have:

- Difficulty breathing or are on a ventilator, because the risk of further compromising air intake with a bronchoscope and sedatives is too high. An exception is the patient who has difficulty breathing because of a narrowed airway, which might be correctable with bronchoscopy.

- Increased cranial pressure, because bronchoscopy can further increase cranial pressure.

- Cardiac arrhythmia, because bronchoscopy can worsen this condition.

Preparation

You might be asked to fast or restrict your diet for a number of hours or to forego certain medications, such as aspirin, for a day or more. You will be asked to bring someone with you to drive you home. Remove dentures, contact lenses, and jewelry, but retain hearing aids.

To reduce any pain or gagging the scope might cause, you will use a numbing spray and an anesthetic liquid gargle just before the procedure. Some medical centers might use a facial gas mask to deliver the numbing agent instead of a gargle or spray.

The doctor will inject a sedative into a vein of your forearm to relax you or make you sleep. She may use a syringe or an IV, which will remain in place until you are ready to go home. If she uses general anesthesia, she might use a gas mask to administer the anesthesia, but you might not notice it if the sedative has already taken effect. She may use a self-inflating blood pressure cuff on your upper arm and a rubber thimble for monitoring oxygen levels on your finger.

Method

You will be lying on your back, raised on pillows, or you'll be seated in a reclining chair. Your lung function will be supplemented with inhaled oxygen. Lights will be dimmed so that the doctor can see the images on the monitor.

Once the sedative and/or anesthesia has taken effect, the bronchoscope will be inserted into your mouth or nose. If you are awake, the medical staff might ask you to swallow, make sounds, or cough to assist them in placing the tube or to visualize certain tissues. If you are awake, do not try to talk. While the scope is being used, most likely you will be only vaguely aware that the procedure is underway, if you are at all awake. You are likely to gag and cough, but the sedative will make you feel as if it is happening to someone else.

The doctor will examine your lungs and bronchial tubes and might collect very small pieces of tissue and sputum to send to the pathology lab for testing. She might pass a needle through the lung into deeper nearby tissue, such as lymph nodes, a procedure called transbronchial lung biopsy. She might use instruments for clearing blockage or a saline wash called lavage to rinse cells out of the lungs for examination. She might use a fluoroscope (a large x-ray machine with a viewing screen) above your chest to show the bronchoscope's placement inside your airways.

Larry Coffman describes his bronchoscopies:

> I have had five bronchoscopies, all under general anesthesia. There was no reason for me to respond to the doctor verbally during these procedures. They were going in to take tissue samples and look around. I have told them I don't want to know when it goes in and I don't want to know when it comes out.

Recovery

It will take a half hour or more to awaken. The nursing staff will check your vital signs and your gag reflex for one to three hours to be sure all medications have worn off before you attempt to eat or drink. If your breathing has been compromised by lung disease, you will be watched especially carefully to be sure your pulmonary function is sound before you are allowed to leave. You will be instructed to spit out your saliva instead of swallowing it, to avoid smoking for at least 24 hours, and to avoid clearing your throat or coughing for several hours. No matter how alert you feel, you should not drive for at least eight hours after having had a sedative.

For a few days after having a bronchoscopy, fatigue, achiness, swelling and pain in your throat, difficulty swallowing, hoarseness, and dry mouth are common.

Pain

Some people report a panicked feeling of being unable to breathe during bronchoscopy, a strong urge to cough, or a sore throat afterward.

Risks

There are low to moderate risks of the following associated with bronchoscopy: puncture of a bronchial tube or lung, infection at the sedative injection site, infection from an improperly disinfected bronchoscope, slight or copious bleeding from the lungs, pneumonia arising from accidental introduction of foreign material, and spasms of the airway that reduce pulmonary function.

If a biopsy or brushing is done, a slight chance exists of collapsed lung or of pneumothorax—air escaping through a small opening in the lung into surrounding tissue.

If after bronchoscopy you have pain, fever, difficulty breathing, blood in sputum, such cardiac symptoms as chest tightness, or lumps under the skin near the chest, call your doctor immediately.

Results

Normal results vary depending on why bronchoscopy was done. It is possible to have normal results on bronchoscopy even when a tumor is present in the lung if the tumor is occluded, lying beneath healthy tissue, or otherwise out of sight or reach of the bronchoscope.

Catheter insertion (central catheter, central line)

This procedure can be inpatient or outpatient. A central catheter or line is a flexible tube that is threaded into a very large vein near your heart. Its presence in a large vein dilutes chemotherapy drugs amidst a large volume of blood and thus makes chemotherapy safer; moreover, depositing chemotherapy drugs near your heart will distribute them more quickly and more evenly to all parts of your body than is possible when chemotherapy is infused directly into an arm vein. Using a central catheter can eliminate damage to arm veins during chemotherapy and can eliminate somewhat painful penetration of arm veins for blood testing and for administering other drugs. Figure B-1 shows various types of catheters.

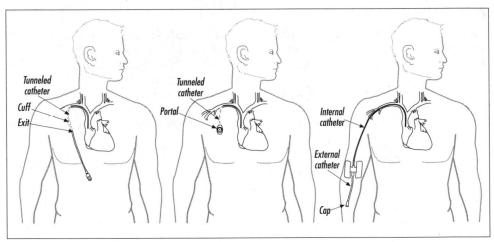

Figure B-1. Types of catheters

Preparation

You need to decide whether a catheter is the right choice for you. If you have symptoms of superior vena cava syndrome (SVCS), for instance, your surgeon might recommend against catheter insertion. You will also need to decide whether to get an external catheter (with tubing emerging from the skin) or a subcutaneous or internal catheter (under the skin). Your oncologist might have strong opinions on this topic.

Advantages

Some advantages of catheter use are:

- Chemotherapy is safer when diluted by lots of blood.
- Chemotherapy is spread throughout the body more quickly and evenly with a central catheter.

- Vein damage is minimal or nonexistent.
- Some models can be used for blood transfusions.
- Some models can be used for hemapheresis, the collecting of stem cells for stem cell rescue.
- Blood gases can sometimes be measured via a central venous access catheter.
- Certain types of intravenous feeding can be accomplished via a central catheter, but not via arm veins.
- With an external catheter, there are no needle sticks that hurt.
- With an internal catheter, cleaning is not necessary.

Drawbacks

Some drawbacks of catheter use are:

- Surgery is required to install a central catheter.
- External catheters must be cleaned and flushed daily or tri-weekly and must be kept dry.
- Infections can lodge in a catheter. Their treatment may entail use of very strong antibiotics with risky side effects, such as permanent vertigo, or may require surgical removal—with a third surgery for reinsertion at a later date.
- The external types that emerge from the skin of the neck or chest can make the patient feel unsightly.
- The types that do not emerge from the skin still require somewhat painful skin penetration to access the port.
- Central catheters can break and travel through the vein to your heart.
- Central catheters can kink and make drug infusion difficult.

Method

You may be given the choice of a local or a general anesthetic. If you choose a general anesthetic, preparation for and recovery from this procedure may be more complex. On the other hand, some who choose a local anesthetic report that they can feel deep pain during the procedure. See Chapter 10, *Experiencing Hospitalization*, for a description of preparation for general anesthesia.

You will be asked to dress in a hospital gown and will be taken to a surgical suite. After the anesthetic takes effect, two areas—both on the chest or one on the chest and one on the neck—will be cleansed and two incisions will be made. The surgeon will access the large vein near the heart through one of these incisions. He will thread the central line through the large vein until it rests near your heart. He will thread the other end beneath your skin and, for an internal port, secure it there. For an external port, he will threaded the line through the surface of the skin, with an anchor just below the surface.

Kathleen Houlihan describes her catheter insertion:

> On Monday afternoon, they surgically installed a "port" under the skin near my clavicle. It's a round device with a rubber-like top and a catheter that goes to a large vein. Now whenever they need vein access, e.g. for chemotherapy, they poke a needle through the skin (deadened with an anesthetic cream first) into the

rubber part of the port, and they're all linked up. They can use if for drawing
blood, too, and the same needle can stay in for up to a week, if there are multiple
reasons they need vein access.

Recovery

See Chapter 10 for recovery issues after general anesthesia.

You will be taught how to clean and flush your port if you have chosen an external catheter. Redness, swelling, or bleeding that persists at the incision site should be reported to your doctor.

Pain

Some people report that, for several weeks following implantation, they experience pain when moving their arms or when lying in a certain position. Some who elect local anesthesia report feeling pain deep in the body during the procedure.

Risks

See the section called "Drawbacks." In addition, surgery entails such risks as accidental penetration of a major vein, uncontrolled bleeding, and the slight risks associated with anesthesia.

Chest x-ray

See "X-rays (radiographic studies)."

CT scan (computed tomography, "CAT" scan)

An outpatient procedure, computed tomography is a series of many very narrow x-rays taken at many varying depths of tissue and from different angles around your body. These x-ray images are then analyzed and reassembled by a computer into an image of your internal organs. CT scans differ from traditional x-ray imaging in that x-ray imaging can't readily distinguish organs that are lying behind other organs. Imagine looking at several veils hanging one behind the other, each painted with a different design. Imagine how difficult it might be to discern the design on the farthest veil. CT scans, on the other hand, are able to delineate even those organs that are obscured by other tissue.

Preparation

You may be asked to fast overnight, to use a laxative, or to purchase and drink a contrast agent if a CT scan of your abdomen and/or pelvis is planned.

Your studies may require an iodine-based contrast agent. Be sure to tell your doctor and the staff doing the test if you have thyroid disease or are allergic to iodine in seafood or other sources; they can substitute a non-ionizing version of the contrast agent. Because the iodine contrast agent used may cause a sensation of heat, skin flushing, or rapid heartbeat, be sure to tell the technician if you have heart disease, high blood pressure, or any other health concerns in addition to being a lung cancer survivor.

If you have internal staples from a previous surgery or pieces of metal embedded in your body from a previous injury, tell the technician. They represent no danger to you during the scan, but may appear on the film as unexplained phenomena.

CT scanners are open, doughnut-shaped machines that generally do not cause patients to feel claustrophobic.

Method

CT scans are performed while you are lying in a carefully chosen position that has been aligned with the machine. It is important to maintain the position that was chosen until the technician says you can relax. Most CT scan sessions include a fast, initial pass with no contrast agent, followed by a second, slower scan with a contrast agent. The first scan images the entire body to use as a frame of reference for the rest of the scanning. During the first scan, you'll feel the table you're lying on move smoothly through the doughnut-hole opening of the machine, without stopping and starting.

While the second, slower scan is underway, you may be asked to hold your breath briefly over and over. Some scanning machines take ten to twenty minutes to scan, depending how much of the body is being scanned. During this time, the contrast agent is pumped into your vein. The part of you being scanned is positioned inside the doughnut hole, which is about twelve inches thick. You'll feel the table you're lying on move slowly through the machine a few centimeters at a time, stopping and starting. Some people prefer taking a nap at this point.

Newer scanners can do the entire scan very quickly, in about twenty seconds. For these machines, you may have to hold your breath for the entire twenty seconds, and if a contrast agent is injected, it will be pushed rapidly into your vein. This quick administration of the contrast agent may cause stronger feelings of heat and faster heartbeat, sensations that are not considered an allergic reaction. You will feel the table you're lying on move smoothly through the doughnut hole of the machine without stopping and starting.

For some studies of the stomach or bowels, you may be required to drink a contrast agent just before the scan is taken or as it is being done.

Pain

CT scans are painless; however, when a contrast agent is used, it is injected into a vein, perhaps causing minor discomfort—see "Blood tests." As mentioned above, the iodine contrast agent that is used may cause a sensation of heat, skin flushing, or rapid heartbeat.

Recovery

If you have had a study that required drinking a contrast agent, you may experience gas, diarrhea, or constipation for one to three days afterward. Drinking large amounts of water will hasten the removal of the contrast agent from the digestive tract. If you have had a contrast agent injected, you may have a harmless and temporary discoloration of the urine or skin for several days afterward. If you are sensitive to iodine or have a thyroid condition, you may feel fatigue for several days after receiving an iodine-based contrast agent.

Risks

A CT scan, if repeated over and over for many years, may deliver enough radiation to body tissue to cause health problems later in life, such as lung, thyroid, or breast cancers. However, as CT scanning technology has improved, the amount of radiation delivered has decreased.

Results

Normal results vary, depending on why the scan was performed. Results for detection of tumors are not quantifiable because they vary from patient to patient and might be more meaningful when older scans are compared to latest ones. Certain circumstances and use of certain drugs can result in findings on imaging studies that appear to be tumors, but are not. Your radiologist will evaluate your scans using factors specific to your case. Follow-up testing, such as PET scanning or MRI, might be suggested.

Electrocardiogram (ECG, EKG, stress EKG, treadmill EKG, thallium EKG, Holter EKG)

An electrocardiogram (ECG or EKG) captures electrical impulses generated by your heart and records them as continuous waves. This can be done in several ways: for a few minutes while you are lying down; continuously, as you wear a Holter heart monitor for 24 hours; as part of increasingly strenuous exercise until your target heart rate is approximated; or with injected thallium for subsequent visualization of heart and lung tissue via gamma camera.

Preparation

For all types of ECG, five to fifteen disc-shaped electrodes will be attached to your chest, arms, and legs with an adhesive. This might require skin cleansing or clipping of hair. Tell the medical staff if you are allergic to adhesives, such as that used on Band-Aids, or if you are taking any medications. Leave jewelry at home; wear loose-fitting clothing that will allow access to chest, arms, and legs.

- If you will be having a thallium scan, do not wear clothing with metal fasteners, such as zippers or bra strap length adjusters or hooks.
- If you will be wearing a Holter monitor for 24 hours, bathe before the test, because you will not be able to do so while the monitor is attached.
- If you are having a treadmill stress ECG, wear athletic shoes.

Method

Each test differs in its administration:

- For a resting ECG, the monitor is turned on and a recording is done for five minutes or less.
- For a Holter monitor session, the monitor is attached and you are sent home with instructions for recording the times of symptoms over the next 24 hours. These times will be matched to information recorded by the monitor.
- For a stress ECG, a resting ECG is done first, followed by a second ECG during rapid breathing. These are done to establish norms for cardiac behavior related to breathing, but not exercise. Finally, increasingly strenuous treadmill or cycling exercise is undertaken, with

blood pressure and ECG readings every two to three minutes until your target heart rate—a pulse reading of 220 minus your age—is reached, or until you're breathless, tired, or experiencing pain. Typically this takes fifteen to thirty minutes, but the very fit, such as marathon runners, might require a much longer testing session to reach their target heart rate.

- For a thallium ECG, a stress ECG is undertaken as described above, then stopped at a specific point so that thallium can be injected. The stress ECG is resumed and completed. You can stroll, nap, read, or visit the cafeteria for a few hours afterward while the thallium is absorbed into heart tissue. Finally, you lie beneath a gamma camera that moves close to, but not on, your chest, recording thallium particles as they decay.

Pain

The strenuous exercise of a treadmill or cycle ECG might cause discomfort for some people. If exercise is causing you chest pain or other symptoms of heart attack, you must tell the staff and stop the test, even if your target heart rate has not been achieved.

Slight pain is associated with the injection of thallium.

Recovery

Report any chest pain or unusual symptoms to your doctor at once.

Do not bathe with hot water for one hour after an exercise ECG because you might become dizzy.

Risks

There is a risk that heart problems will become apparent or acute during a stress (treadmill or bicycle) ECG. The medical staff will be with you at all times during the test and will stop the test if you report pain or if the ECG shows abnormal heart activity. There is a slight risk of injury associated with getting on or off a moving treadmill. The staff will help you with this maneuver. If you are allergic to adhesive, a rash might develop at the sites where electrodes are attached. There is virtually no incidence of allergic reaction to injected thallium. A very small risk of infection at the site of injection is possible following a thallium EKG. A very low amount of radiation exposure is associated with thallium injection. There is no risk of electric shock. The machine to which electrodes send signals from your skin does not emit electricity.

Results

There is no such thing as a completely normal EKG. Your cardiologist will interpret what a specific finding might mean in your case. Follow-up testing, such as a MUGA scan or angiogram, might be recommended.

Endoscopy

See "Bronchoscopy."

Flow cytometry

See "Blood tests."

GI series

See "X-rays (radiographic studies)."

ISH (in situ hybridization)

See "Blood tests."

Lumbar puncture

See "Spinal tap (lumbar puncture)."

Lung diffusion testing (diffusing capacity)

This test measures the amount of carbon monoxide taken up by the lungs. Because carbon monoxide (CO) is more readily absorbed by blood from the lungs than is oxygen, certain critical pulmonary functions regarding gas exchange can be measured with this test.

Preparation

Avoid heavy meals and smoking for four to six hours before the test. You might be asked either to use or avoid certain medications, such as bronchodilators, beforehand.

Method

You'll be asked to inhale a gas that contains a known amount of carbon monoxide, hold your breath for ten seconds, then rapidly exhale. The amount of CO remaining in the exhaled gas reveals how much was absorbed by your pulmonary bloodstream. The mouthpiece will fit snugly against your mouth, and noseclips will be used to prevent the escape of air through the nose.

Pain

No pain is experienced during this test. The sensation of breathing through a mouthpiece might be uncomfortable.

Recovery

No recovery events are anticipated following this test.

Risks

No risks are associated with this test.

Results

See Appendix C. Results vary depending on age, weight, height, race, level of exercise, and amount of lung tissue remaining. Your pulmonologist will assess the images and interpret their meaning in view of your specific circumstances. Follow-up testing, such as PET scanning or biopsy, might be suggested.

Lung volume tests

See "Spirometry and other lung volume tests," "Pulmonary ventilation/perfusion scan (V/Q scan)," "Lung diffusion testing (diffusing capacity)," and Appendix C.

Mammography (mammogram, breast x-ray)

Women who have had radiation therapy for lung cancer should have regular mammograms because this group of women faces a risk of breast cancer that's significantly higher than that faced by the general population.

Preparation

If you are still having menstrual periods, schedule your mammogram for the ten days following the first day of your period. This will lessen the chance that your breasts will be tender and will give a more accurate x-ray result. Avoid caffeine, chocolate, and other foods that may contribute to breast tenderness for several days prior to your mammogram.

Request an appointment that includes a patient/doctor consultation directly following the x-ray session so you can discuss immediately with the doctor any unusual results and have repeat x-rays or ultrasound, if warranted. Otherwise, if the results are questionable, you may have to wait several highly stressful days, or even longer, for the staff to find an opening in their schedule for repeat testing or for the doctor's availability.

Tell the technicians and the radiologist that you are a lung cancer survivor.

Directly before the mammogram, remove all aluminum-based antiperspirants and all metallic jewelry. Be sure the technician is aware of moles, scars, or other skin characteristics that may appear questionable on the films.

You will be asked to remove all clothing from the waist up and to replace them with a gown. While the mammograms are being performed, however, the gown must be partially removed to facilitate placing the breast above the photographic plate.

Method

Mammography is usually done while the woman is standing with the breast resting against a warmed, flat surface that contains a photographic plate. The technician will measure the density of the breast tissue and slowly lower a matching plate from above until the breast is somewhat compressed. While you are holding that position carefully, she will step behind a radiation shield and activate the x-ray machine for about three seconds.

Usually, the technician takes two x-rays of each breast, each from a different angle, to maximize the amount and location of tissue imaged. It is particularly important to capture the tissue high against the chest wall, approaching the collarbone, because breast tissue extends beyond what we traditionally refer to as the breast. Using equipment commonly available today, tissue compression remains necessary to ensure good visualization of all breast tissue.

You will be asked to wait, wearing the gown, until the films are developed to ensure that films of high clarity were obtained. If unclear, the studies must be repeated. If unusual features are present on one of the films, the x-ray may be redone using a small compression paddle to highlight a particular area of breast tissue. Alternately, ultrasound may be used to re-image the breast in an attempt to distinguish benign fluid-filled cysts from other lesions.

Pain

Many women report discomfort, minor pain, or moderate pain during breast compression. Some women report a great deal of pain. If you have had previous breast surgery or breast implants, you may experience pain that is qualitatively or quantitatively different from that experienced by other women.

Recovery

Many women report a bruise-like pain or a discharge from the nipple for a day or two. Report these aftereffects to your oncologist and your primary care doctor.

Risks

Some researchers believe that the accumulated dose of radiation delivered to breast tissue over a lifetime may increase a woman's risk of getting breast cancer. This, of course, must be weighed against the risk of failing to detect a breast cancer. The risk associated with bruising or discharge from the nipple is thought to be minor or absent.

Results

Results for detection of tumors vary from patient to patient and might be more meaningful when older mammograms are compared to the latest. Suspicious lesions usually are scanned with ultrasound or biopsied to rule out or confirm malignancy. Follow-up testing, such as PET scanning, might be recommended.

MRI (magnetic resonance imaging)

This outpatient test uses large magnets and radio waves to cause the different atoms that make up our cells to vibrate at different speeds. A computer then maps the different speeds into an image of the body part being examined. MRI is better than a CT scan for imaging soft tissue, such as cartilage or the brain.

Preparation

You will be asked to lie on a table that moves in and out of the tunnel-shaped MRI machine. The body part being scanned may be positioned within a basket-like brace to help keep the position chosen by the technician.

MRI machines make hammering noises because the magnets are being repositioned constantly while the images are generated. The technician will supply you with disposable earplugs.

A contrast agent may be injected for imaging certain organs. Imaging the brain, for example, is sometimes facilitated by injecting a very safe contrast agent called Gadolinium. Ask the technician about the risk associated with the agent being used and tell him if you have any allergies or problems with blood clotting.

Some people find enclosed MRI machines claustrophobic. Other MRI models have an open gazebo-like design to reduce claustrophobia, with the magnets overhead supported on pillars. Yet others are made of clear plastic. While images from open models may be distinct enough for diagnosing knee problems, for example, they might not be detailed enough for mapping the brain.

If you're claustrophobic, there are several things that will help, such as knowing that there is a speaker inside the machine so that the technician can hear you if you ask for help, and that you, in turn, can hear him. There is also a hand-held beeping summons that you can press if you feel tense. Most facilities have a sound system and will let you choose the music. You might also notice that relaxing photographs have been taped to the inside of the machine. Fans circulate fresh air into the tunnel at all times. It's also possible that, unless your head is being imaged, only part of your body will be within the machine and your head may not. Most relaxing of all may be the thought that this is seventeen million dollars of technology, and for one hour, it's all yours.

Some people, on the other hand, report that the MRI experience is comforting, like a return to the womb. In fact, a friend reports that he likes to have an MRI because it's the only place where nobody can interrupt his thinking.

If you still feel that claustrophobia will be a serious problem, ask your doctor whether a sedative would interfere with the imaging process.

Method

An initial scan to set benchmarks is done rapidly using no contrast agent. A second scan for finer detail is then repeated at slower speed. If a contrast agent is to be used, it is injected into a vein in the arm before the second scan. Although sound is muted by earplugs, you will hear hammering noises that vary in speed and pitch. While being scanned, one must remain as still as possible, but breathing is not restricted as it sometimes is during a CT scan.

A scan of the knee or brain, for example, takes about forty minutes. After scanning is complete, there is a five- to ten-minute wait while the computer analyzes and maps the signals generated by the magnets. The technician will check the resulting images to be sure they are readable.

Pain

The imaging process is painless, although you may feel a slight sting or warmth during injection if a contrast agent is used.

Recovery

If a contrast agent is used, temporary changes might occur in the color of skin, urine, or feces.

Risks

There may be risks of an allergic reaction associated with specific contrast agents: ask your doctor or the technician. As always, there is a very slight risk of infection at the injection site and a risk of minor, painless bruising at the injection site.

Results

Normal results vary depending on why the scan was performed. Results for detection of tumors vary from patient to patient and might be more meaningful when prior scans are compared to the latest. Certain circumstances and certain drugs can result in findings on imaging studies that appear to be tumors, but are not. Follow-up testing, such as PET scanning, might be suggested.

Needle biopsy (fine-needle aspiration, CT-guided needle biopsy, percutaneous needle biopsy)

Needle biopsy might be used as a means of diagnosing lung cancer that has spread to other organs, such as the liver. Organs commonly examined using needle biopsy are the thyroid, kidney, liver, lymph nodes, breast, uterine cervix, pancreas, salivary gland, spinal fluid, and bone marrow.

Lung biopsy performed during bronchoscopy is discussed under "Bronchoscopy."

Preparation

You may have to fast for twelve hours before the procedure if a sedative or general anesthetic will be used or if the tissue being biopsied is part of the digestive system. You might need to give blood or urine samples prior to the biopsy. Bring comfortable clothing to wear afterward and plan on not being able to walk or drive alone after a sedative or general anesthetic is used.

Method

You will lie flat on a table for most such biopsies. The doctor will clean the skin and inject a local anesthetic. Alternatively, you might have a sedative or general anesthetic given by injection or by inhalation, or, if a fine-needle biopsy through the skin is planned, no anesthetic might be used. Directly before the biopsy, you might have a CT scan, ultrasound, or x-ray to image the area of interest, and the assistant might use ink or dye to target the skin above. Depending on the organ being examined, you may have to regulate your breathing or hold quite still during the biopsy. The doctor makes a tiny incision and inserts the biopsy needle through the incision. For kidney biopsies, she might first use a guide needle. She then draws (aspirates) a small amount of tissue into the syringe, withdraws the needle, applies pressure to halt bleeding, applies a bandage—no stitches are required—and sends the tissue to the pathology lab for analysis.

Pain

A slight sting from injected anesthetic or fine-needle biopsy is common. Depending on which organ is biopsied, you may feel pressure; a brief, sharp pain; a dull, deep ache; or cramping. For liver or other digestive tract biopsies, you may feel pain in the shoulder. Tenderness or bruising may exist at the site of the biopsy and within any intervening muscle tissue for three to seven days. Some physicians prescribe Tylenol or Tylenol/Codeine combinations for the aftereffects.

Recovery

Following kidney biopsies you may have to lie on your back for 12 to 24 hours, and you may note red blood in your urine for 24 hours.

Risks

Risks of organ failure while under general anesthesia; of infection; of bleeding, internal or external, at the site of the puncture; or of injury to adjacent organs exist. For kidney biopsies, blood in the urine may persist beyond twenty-four hours and should be reported to your doctor.

Results

Normal results are the absence of tumor cells in aspirated tissue examined under the microscope or subjected to other tests. Follow-up testing, such as PET scanning, might be suggested.

PCR (polymerase chain reaction)

See "Blood tests."

PET scan (positron emission tomography)

This outpatient test exploits the fact that some tumors will metabolize more of certain substances than will healthy tissue. The metabolic substance, often glucose, but perhaps ammonia, water, methionine, or another drug, is first coupled to a radioactive substance that gives off energy that can be detected by specialized equipment.

PET scanning has been studied for more than 30 years, but its use in the clinic has emerged only since the 1990's. Not all hospitals have PET scanners. For a list of PET centers, contact the Institute for Clinical PET (ICP) at (202) 530-0990 or visit *http://icppet.org*.

Preparation

You might have to fast for several hours prior to the scan. You might also have to temporarily discontinue some medications prior to the scan. After lying down on the table, get comfortable because you must hold this position for a while. Wear warm, comfortable clothing because the room that houses this equipment usually must be kept cool. The procedure might take as long as two or three hours.

Method

A technician injects the metabolic substance into a vein in the forearm or into your catheter, then withdraws the needle. A wait of 40 minutes or so is common while tissue absorbs the injected substance.

The equipment might scan for over an hour. Usually, you lie fully clothed on a table that will move back and forth through the doughnut-shaped sensing equipment, similar to a CT scanner. It is important to hold still when asked to do so. Some patients are embarrassed to note that, although they are fully clothed, the computer-assembled image on the screen is of the naked body.

Pain

A slight sting may be felt when the metabolic agent is injected.

Recovery

There are no recovery issues associated with this test. Allergic reactions are very rare.

Risks

As with other imaging techniques, there are risks of false-positive and false-negative readings with radiolabeled agents. An amount of radiation exposure equivalent to about two chest x-rays is associated with the radioactive agents used. You won't have to stay away from others later to avoid exposing them to radioactivity, as is necessary after receiving injections of some other isotopes.

Results

Normal results indicate no unusual or unexplained uptake of the radiolabeled agent, but in some cases, results are not straightforward; they must be interpreted by a radiologist in concert with patient history and earlier scans.

Port insertion

See "Catheter insertion (central catheter, central line)."

Pulmonary function tests

See "Spirometry and other lung volume tests," "Pulmonary ventilation/perfusion scan (V/Q scan)," "Lung diffusion testing (diffusing capacity)," and Appendix C.

Pulmonary ventilation/perfusion scan (V/Q scan)

This is a two-part test performed to determine pulmonary capacity. Both injection and inhalation of one or more mildly radioactive agents are done to visualize circulation of air and blood in the lungs with a special camera.

Preparation

Remove dentures; wear clothing with no metal zippers or fasteners. A chest x-ray usually is performed either directly before or after these two tests.

Method

- Perfusion. A technician injects into an arm vein natural body protein, albumin, that has been joined to a mildly radioactive element, technetium-99. Directly afterward, you lie on a table beneath a scanner that contains a movable gamma camera. The camera detects technetium-99 particles as they decay, which shows how well your blood is circulated by and within your lungs.

- Ventilation. You lie upon a table and wear a mask that allows you to inhale a mixture of air and a mildly radioactive agent, perhaps technetium-99 or xenon-133, that can be detected with a gamma camera as you inhale and exhale.

For both of these studies, you must lie still while being scanned.

Pain

The mask worn for the ventilation study might cause feelings of claustrophobia or an inability to breathe in some people. Some people might feel minor pain with the injection of technetium-99 into an arm vein for the perfusion study.

Recovery

No special recovery events are expected to occur with these tests.

Risks

Very low risks include low radiation exposure associated with the radioactive agents, a small risk of infection at the site of injection, and a small chance of an allergic reaction to the injected compound.

Results

See Appendix C. The results of a V/Q scan vary depending on age, weight, height, race, level of exercise, remaining lung tissue, and other patient-specific factors. Your pulmonologist will assess the images and determine what they mean in your case. He might order follow-up testing, such as PET scanning or an MRI.

Radioimmunoscintigraphy

A SPECT scan is a type of radioimmunoscintigraphy.

This outpatient test exploits the fact that some tumors will attract and retain more of a substance than will healthy tissue. This homing agent is first coupled to a radioactive substance that gives off energy that can be detected by specialized equipment.

Your doctor will choose a radioimmunoscintigraphic agent that works best for the type of tumor you have. Agents often used today for detecting microscopic lung cancer are radioactive isotopes coupled with monoclonal antibodies—proteins secreted by white blood cells and made en masse in the laboratory.

Preparation

An enema or laxative may be necessary the day before the test. After lying down on the camera table, get comfortable because you must hold this position for about one hour.

Method

The technician injects the radioactive agent into a vein in the forearm and then withdraws the needle. Depending on the agent used, you might have to return for scanning in 2, 4, 24, 48, or 72 hours, or a combination of these times. No second injection is required before the second scan.

Scanning usually occurs by having the fully clothed patient lie above or below a camera table that is sensitive to the energy emitted by the agent injected. It is important to hold still for the duration of the film exposure. Some patients are embarrassed to note that, although they are fully clothed, the computer-assembled image on the screen is of the naked body.

Depending on the scintigraphic agent used, this procedure may be performed using a camera that is sensitive to the emission of a single photon (a photon is a piece of an atom). This is called a SPECT (single photon emission computed tomography) scan and works on the principle that the radioactive agent makes your tissue more visible to the camera. If the substance emits gamma rays, a gamma camera might be used; it is similar to a shield that moves back and forth in half circles, starting at the top of the body and working down. It moves close to the body, but does not touch it.

Kathleen Houlihan tells about her imaging scan:

> Wednesday morning we had breakfast early and went for my NeoTect scan injection at 8:00AM, and went back for the scan about 9:30. I was lying on a table and had to hold still with my arms over my head for 30 minutes. That's a lot harder than it sounds, especially for my restricted-range radiated shoulder. I was ready to quit after about five minutes. My husband Holt came and supported my arm on the radiated side, and the technician ended up supporting the other arm, and somehow I made it through the whole half hour.

Pain

A slight sting may be felt when the scintigraphic agent is injected.

Recovery

There are no recovery issues associated with this test.

Risks

As with other imaging techniques, there are risks of false-positive and false-negative readings with scintigraphic agents. A very low amount of radiation exposure is associated with the radioactive agents used. You won't have to stay away from others later to avoid exposing them to radioactivity, as is necessary after receiving injections of some other isotopes. Because many of these agents are manufactured using white blood cell antibodies from mice, they may cause an allergic reaction in humans, although allergic reactions are rare.

Results

Normal results indicate no unusual or unexplained uptake of the radiolabeled agent.

SPECT scan

See "Radioimmunoscintigraphy."

Spinal tap (lumbar puncture)

This outpatient test collects a sample of cerebrospinal fluid (CSF) that surrounds the spine and brain. For lung cancer, CSF usually is examined for the presence of cancer cells, but it also may be collected for many other reasons, such as identifying opportunistic organisms that may gain a foothold during chemotherapy.

Preparation

No physical preparation is necessary.

Method

You will be asked to lie on your side with your knees pulled up to your chest and your chin down on your collarbone during the drawing of the fluid, which takes only a few minutes. The technician cleans the area around your lower spine and injects a local anesthetic. After the anesthetic has taken effect, the doctor inserts a needle between two bones of your backbone (lumbar vertebrae) to tap the fluid that lies under the membrane that surrounds your spinal column. Once the needle is inserted, you must hold very still in the curved position to avoid spinal damage. The physician draws spinal fluid into the syringe, removes the needle, applies brief pressure to stop bleeding, and applies a small bandage.

Pain

Some people report a brief, sharp pain as the needle enters the membrane. Others report pronounced pressure until the needle is properly positioned. Some people report severe headache after the procedure, especially if they were not able to lie flat for the six or eight hours recommended.

Recovery

You must lie flat for six to eight hours after this procedure to allow your body to replace and redistribute spinal fluid surrounding the spine and the brain. This posture prevents headache.

Risks

A serious risk of spinal damage or paralysis exists if movement during the procedure displaces the needle. Slight risks exist of infection at the injection sites or of bleeding into the spinal column. Risk of headache exists, especially if the patient does not lie flat for several hours after the procedure.

Results

A normal result is cerebrospinal fluid that does not contain the substance for which testing is being done.

Spirometry and other lung volume tests

These tests measure the amount of air taken in, held, and expelled by the lungs in one breath. Usually they are repeated several times over a few minutes, using both normal and forceful breathing.

A man preparing for diagnostic surgery describes his presurgical testing:

> *I had to go in to get lung capacity tests to see if I would have enough lung capacity to undergo the operation—they want to make sure you'll be able to keep breathing. You huff and blow and all that. I had pretty good lung capacity, so the surgery was scheduled.*

Preparation

Avoid heavy meals and smoking for four to six hours before the test. You might be asked to either use or avoid certain medications, such as bronchodilators, beforehand. Wear loose clothing and sit straight or stand during these tests.

Method

- Spirometry, FVC, FEV. Exhale into the spirometer, which offers no resistance to breathing, but measures the speed and volume of air that passes through it, known as forced vital capacity (FVC) and forced expiratory volume (FEV), in one second. A mouthpiece might be used, which will fit snugly against your mouth, and noseclips might be used to prevent the escape of air through the nose.

- Match Test. Using a deep breath, a forceful exhalation, and an open (not pursed) mouth, try to blow out a lighted match held six inches from your mouth.

- Forced expiratory time (FET). Exhale your deepest breath as fast and completely as possible with your mouth wide open. Count the number of seconds it takes for you to exhale the air. Repeat three times; note the fastest time.

- Peak expiratory flow rate (PEFR). Breathe in as deeply as possible. Blow into the peak expiratory flow monitor's mouthpiece as hard and fast as possible. Do this three times; record the highest flow rate.

- Maximum ventilatory volume (MVV). Using rapid in-and-out breaths, blow as hard and as fast as possible into the mouthpiece of a spirometer for fifteen seconds. Count the number of breaths as you go. Multiply this number by four to determine the number of breaths for one minute.

Pain

No pain is experienced during these tests, but dizziness or shortness of breath might result from rapid, forceful breathing.

Recovery

No recovery events are anticipated following these tests.

Risks

No risks are associated with these tests.

Results

See Appendix C.

Sputum cytology

This test examines phlegm that is suctioned or deliberately expelled from your lungs. It can in some cases, detect cancerous cells being shed by a tumor, but this test is not accurate enough to be used alone as a screening or diagnostic tool.

Preparation

You'll be asked to have this outpatient test, or to collect sputum at home, in the early morning. You might be instructed to drink lots of fluids up to twelve hours beforehand or to avoid food or drink for twelve hours before, to brush your teeth and to gargle with a mouthwash. If you collect sputum at home, you'll be given a sterile container to collect sputum and instructions for handling it.

Method

A saline aerosol mist is administered as a spray or inhalant for five to fifteen minutes.

If you're collecting sputum at home, this saline aerosol will loosen phlegm to enable you to cough samples out of the lung. Be sure the material you collect is thick mucus, not thin saliva.

If this test is being done in the clinic, saline aerosol is administered, and you will be asked to breathe oxygen through a mask. A tube called a catheter will be inserted into your nose or mouth to suction material for evaluation. After a few seconds of suction, the tube is removed.

Pain

Some pain or discomfort might be associated with insertion of the suction tube into the nose and throat.

Recovery

No recovery is associated with this test, although you might have a sore throat afterward if a suction tube was used.

Risks

No physical risks are associated with this test. There is a possibility that precancerous or cancerous cells will be detected in sputum originating in a lung tumor that cannot be found. This might be either a false positive result or a very early tumor, the location of which is undetectable using the technology available today.

Results

Normal results are the absence of cancerous cells or suspicious white blood cells in sputum. Follow-up imaging studies, bronchoscopy, or tissue biopsy might be recommended.

Sonogram (ultrasound, sonography)

An outpatient procedure, sonography creates a map of how your body structures appear when sound waves echo from them. The sonography equipment includes a wand that generates sound waves and a microphone for sensing the echoes the sound waves generate. A computer reformats the wave signals into a picture of body organs on a screen.

Bone interferes with sonography, so scanning the brain with this equipment is not successful using the equipment readily available today.

Color Doppler ultrasound is specialized sonography that can detect the speed and direction of blood flow within the body, called the Doppler shift. The computer maps the differences as different colors. This is useful because some tumors commandeer a large blood supply, and this excessive blood supply may be visible and meaningful using color Doppler ultrasound.

Ultrasound might be used in conjunction with bronchoscopy; see "Bronchoscopy."

Preparation

For a pelvic sonogram, you may be asked to drink large quantities of water because the urinary bladder acts as a window for sound waves when the bladder is very full. If prostate tissue will be biopsied during transrectal sonogram, an antibiotic may be required for several days prior, and an enema is necessary about four hours beforehand.

Method

You will be lying on a table while the technician gently presses a wand called a transducer over your body. Depending on what body part is being imaged, you may be asked to remove certain items of clothing and to wear a sheet in their place. The technician will first apply warmed gel to your skin to make the wand move smoothly. He may ask you to tilt your body and to maintain the tilt with your muscles, or he may place pillows under you. For transrectal ultrasound, you may be asked to lie on your side with your knees pulled up to your chest.

For transvaginal or transrectal ultrasound, the technician will apply warm gel to a specially shaped wand and ask you to insert it comfortably into your vagina or rectum. Once it is in place, she will guide it from side to side to visualize the uterus, ovaries, prostate, or rectum. This specialized wand is quite long, which means that the technician's hands are not very close to your private body parts, and, being covered by a sheet, you probably won't feel that your body is overly exposed to a stranger.

If prostate tissue is to be sampled via transrectal sonography, a needle rapidly enters and exits the prostate gland through the wall of the rectum to collect tissue for analysis.

If you are having pelvic sonography along with a second sonographic scan, ask the technician to do the pelvic scan first so that you can empty your bladder.

Pain

Most sonography procedures are not painful, but having to maintain a very full bladder for a pelvic sonogram is uncomfortable.

If prostate tissue is sampled during a transrectal sonogram, slight pain or pressure may be felt as the needle rapidly enters and exits the prostate gland through the wall of the rectum.

Risks

There are no known risks associated with most sonography procedures, except for biopsy of prostate tissue during ultrasound, which entails a slight risk of continued bleeding.

Recovery

There are no recovery issues following sonography if biopsy was not performed. If prostate tissue was sampled, blood in the stool or semen may persist for a few days after the procedure.

Results

Normal results vary depending on why the scan was performed. Results for detection of tumors vary from patient to patient and might be more meaningful when prior scans are compared to the latest. Certain circumstances and certain drugs can result in findings on imaging studies that appear to be tumors, but are not. Follow-up testing, such as CT scanning, PET scanning, or MRI, might be suggested. More specific sonography, such as color Doppler imaging, might be recommended.

Stent placement

Stents are placed within an airway to correct narrowing caused by disease or scarring. Most stents are placed using a CT-guided bronchoscope; see "Bronchoscopy."

Stress EKG

See "Electrocardiogram (ECG, EKG, stress EKG, treadmill EKG, thallium EKG, Holter EKG)."

Thoracentesis

See "Needle biopsy (fine-needle aspiration, CT-guided needle biopsy, percutaneous needle biopsy)."

Ultrasound (ultrasonography, sonogram)

See "Sonogram (ultrasound, sonography)."

V/Q scan

See "Pulmonary ventilation/perfusion scan (V/Q scan)" and Appendix C.

X-rays (radiographic studies)

X-ray imaging may be used early in the diagnostic process to detect unusual masses and determine the extent of disease, although x-ray studies in the absence of a biopsy cannot positively diagnose lung cancer. During treatment, x-rays can be used to track tumor shrinkage and to detect other secondary conditions caused by tumor growth, such as blockage of the ureters, the tubes descending from the kidney to the bladder. After treatment, radiographic studies of the chest may be done to monitor the lungs for possible spread of disease.

X-ray imaging is diagnostic and differs from x-radiation therapy in that it delivers much lower doses of radiation to tissue. X-ray studies are an outpatient procedure.

Preparation

You may be asked to fast overnight, to use a laxative, to purchase and drink a contrast agent, or to drink copious amounts of water, if x-ray imaging studies of your kidneys are planned.

If your studies will require an iodine-based contrast agent, as is used for certain x-ray studies of the kidneys, be sure to tell your doctor and the staff doing the test if you have thyroid disease or are allergic to iodine in seafood or other sources. A non-ionizing version of the contrast agent can be substituted.

If you have internal staples from a previous surgery or pieces of metal embedded in your body from a previous injury, tell the technician. They represent no danger to you during the x-ray session, but may appear on the film as unexplained phenomena.

Method

X-rays are taken while you are sitting, standing, or lying in a carefully chosen position that has been aligned with the x-ray machine. It is important to maintain the position that was chosen and to remain very still until the technician says you can relax.

For some studies of the stomach or bowels, you may be required to drink an additional amount of contrast agent while the x-rays are being taken. For some bowel studies, an enema may be administered to fill the lower bowel with a contrast agent, such as barium or barium and air.

Pain

X-ray studies are painless; however, if a contrast agent, such as dye, is needed, it may be injected into a vein and may causing minor discomfort—see "Blood tests." Some studies require positioning of the body that may be temporarily uncomfortable if, for example, you suffer from back pain. If you are having a barium enema, ask the technician to let you remove the nozzle of the enema yourself when the test is complete to reduce the chance of rectal discomfort.

Recovery

If you have had a study that required barium in the stomach, small intestine, or large intestine, you may experience gas, diarrhea, or constipation for one to three days afterward. Drinking large amounts of water will hasten the removal of the contrast agent from the digestive tract and will reduce the chance of barium's forming an obstruction. If you have had a contrast agent injected, you may have a harmless and temporary discoloration of the urine or skin for several days afterward. If you are sensitive to iodine or have a thyroid condition, you may feel fatigue for several days after receiving an iodine-based contrast agent.

Risks

X-ray studies, if repeated over and over, may deliver enough radiation to body tissue to cause health problems later in life, such as lung, thyroid, or breast cancers. Barium used as a contrast agent in the gastrointestinal tract can cause an impaction if not cleared by drinking copious amounts of water after the test.

Results

Normal results vary depending on why the x-ray was performed. Results for detection of tumors vary from patient to patient and might be more meaningful when prior x-rays are compared to the latest. Certain circumstances and certain drugs can result in findings on radiographic studies that appear to be tumors, but are not. Follow-up testing, such as CT scanning, PET scanning, MRI, or biopsy, might be suggested.

Test Results

THE FOLLOWING TABLES WILL PROVIDE YOU with approximate quantitative information about certain test results. Test results can be influenced by many things, such as how blood was drawn and stored, whether the patient exercised recently or was dehydrated, who administered the test, how equipment was calibrated, medications taken by the patient, and so on.

For blood or urine tests, your lab will display its own norms alongside your test results. These norms may differ from other sources, because each lab recalculates their norms as their data accumulates.

Pulmonary function tests (PFTs) measure the capacity of the lung to exchange oxygen for carbon dioxide and other gases. Results of many pulmonary function tests, including spirometry, vary significantly based on age, race, weight, height, activity level, and the laboratory performing the tests. A measurement 20 percent higher or lower than a given laboratory's normal values might be interpreted as abnormal, but assuming so is dangerous in the absence of comprehensive patient information. This means that you should be cautious when interpreting test results that you find in your medical records. You should ask your oncologist or surgeon for a full explanation of PFT results.

Only the most common tests are included in the following table. Neuroendocrine tumors, however, can affect a wide range of body systems and might require other blood or urine tests. See one of the books on testing recommended in Appendix A, *Resources*, or see the Health-Central web site, which includes many tests and detailed descriptions of them, at *http://www. healthcentral.com.*

Complete blood counts in normal adults

Test Name	Low Normal	High Normal
White cell count (WBC), × 10⁹/liter blood	3.9	11.3
White cell differentials (percents)		
Polys	42	78
Bands	0	4
Lymphocytes	15	45
Monocytes	0	12
Eosinophils	0	7
Basophils	0	2
Atypical lymphocytes	0	4
Platelet count (PLT), × 10⁹/liter blood	140	450
Mean platelet volume (MPV)	6.3	10.3

Test Name	Low Normal	High Normal
Mean corpuscular volume, fl/red cell (MCV)	80.0	100
Mean corpuscular hemoglobin, pg/red cell (MCH)	26.4	34.0
Mean corpuscular hemoglobin conc., g/dl red cells (MCHC)	31.0	36.0
Red cell distribution width (RDW), CV (%)	11.5	14.5

Red cell counts by gender

Test Name	Men		Women	
	Low	High	Low	High
Red cell count (RBC) x10^{12} /liter blood	4.52	5.90	4.1	5.10
Hemoglobin (HB) g/dl blood	14.0	18.0	12.3	15.3
Hematocrit (HCT)	0.40	0.52	0.36	0.45

Other blood or urine tests

Test Name	Low Normal	High Normal
Direct bilirubin, mg/dl (Bili)	0	0.4
Total bilirubin, mg/dl (Bili)	0	1.0
Blood urea nitrogen, mg/dl (BUN)	8	25
Calcitonin pg/mL	0	10
CEA ng/ml	0	3.0–5.0
Cholesterol	130	200
Cortisol in blood at 8 AM mcg/dl	6	23
Cortisol in urine mcg/24 hr	10	100
Creatinine, mg/dl (CRT)	0.6	1.5
Calcium mg/dl (Ca)	8.5	10.5
Chlorine mEq/l (Cl)	95	100
Insulin mcU/ml	5	20
Potassium, mEq/l (K)	3.5	5.0
Phosphate mg/dl (P)	2.5	4.5
Sodium, mEq/l (Na)	135	145
Magnesium, mEq/l (Mg)	1.5	2.5
Erythrocyte Sedimentation Rate mm/hr (ESR)	0	20
Glucose, mg/dl	65	100
Lactate Dehydrogenase u/l (LDH)	100	190
Albumin gm/dl (Alb)	3.5	5.0
Alkaline Phosphatase (AlkP) u/l	50	135
(ALT, formerly SGPT) u/l	5	40
(AST, formerly SGOT) u/l	10	50

Test Name	Low Normal	High Normal
Thyroid TSH	0.5	5.0
Thyroid free T4	1	4
Uric acid, mg/dl	2.5	8.0

Pulmonary function tests

Tests of lung volume include:

- Four primary lung test volumes, quantified using spirometry:
  - Vt, the volume of air entering with each breath; normally 350 to 500 mL when you are at rest.
  - IRV, the inspiratory (inhalation) reserve volume, the amount of air you can draw in after Vt.
  - ERV, the expiratory (exhalation) reserve volume, the amount of air you can force out after a normal exhalation.
  - RV, the residual lung volume, as lungs do not completely collapse with each breath. RV cannot be directly measured.
- Lung capacities derived from the four primary volumes:
  - FRC, functional residual capacity, equals ERV + RV
  - IC, inspiratory capacity, equals Vt + IRV
  - VC or TVC, vital capacity or total vital capacity, equals Vt + IRV + ERV
  - TLC, total lung capacity, equals Vt + IRV + ERV + RV or VC + RV
  - RV:TLC, respiratory volume to total lung capacity ratio
- Other lung volume tests include:
  - FEF, forced expiratory flow
  - FET, forced expiratory time
  - FEV, forced expiratory volume
  - FEV1, forced expiratory volume in one second
  - FEF25–75, the average FEF during the midportion (25–75 percent) of FVC
  - FVC, forced vital capacity
  - FEV1:FVC, forced expiratory volume in one second to forced vital capacity ratio
  - Minute ventilation, equal to Vt times respiratory rate per minute
  - MVV, maximum ventilatory volume
  - PEFR, peak expiratory flow rate
  - Flow volume loops, a graph of inhalation and exhalation during spirometric breathing tests
  - Match test, a measure of force of exhalation

Pulmonary tests other than volume testing include:

- Pulmonary ventilation/perfusion scan (V/Q scan), an imaging study with no quantified normal values
- ABG, arterial blood gases
    - Arterial oxygen (PO_2); normal value 70 to 100 mm Hg, depending on age
    - Arterial carbon dioxide (PCO_2); normal value 37 to 44 mm Hg, depending on age
- Carboxyhemoglobin, a measure of carbon monoxide binding to red blood cells. Normal value is under 10 percent.
- Lung diffusion testing (diffusing capacity, including DLCO, diffuse capacity of lungs for carbon monoxide).

Many pulmonary test results vary depending on age, weight, height, race, level of exercise, remaining lung tissue, and other patient-specific factors. Your pulmonologist will assess the images and determine what they mean in your case. For examples of normal test results, see:

- Johns Hopkins University Pulmonary Function Lab results calculator: *http://www.med.jhu.edu/pftlab/pfthome.html*
- Virtual Hospital: *http://www.vh.org/Providers/ClinRef/FPHandbook/Chapter03/06-3.html*
- The Merck Manual of Diagnosis and Therapy search engine, in which you can enter the keyword "pulmonary": *http://www.merck.com/pubs/mmanual*
- The HealthAnswers.com search engine, into which you should enter the key phrase "pulmonary function tests": *http://www.healthanswers.com/Centers/Body*

For a list of terms used in respiratory testing, see MedRemote's respiratory terms dictionary at *http://www.mtdesk.com/lstresp.shtml*, or the Merck Manual of Diagnosis and Therapy, which contains a search engine in which you can enter the keyword "pulmonary": *http://www.merck.com/pubs/mmanual*.

Chemotherapy Drugs and Regimens

THIS APPENDIX, ALONG WITH THE TREATMENT CHAPTERS, can help answer questions you might have about the drugs being given to you and how they work. The tables included below show all chemotherapy regimens and drugs that have been used recently for lung cancers. Please see the treatment chapters for either SCLC or NSCLC or visit the NCI's web site (*http://cancernet. nci.nih.gov/pdq/pdq_treatment.shtml*) to ascertain which treatments are currently recommended by the NCI.

In the past, drug names often were abbreviated to three letters, such as VCR for vincristine. The oncologic community is moving away from this practice in order to avoid confusion about which drugs are given.

Three tables are provided below.

Single drug names, abbreviations, trade names, and modes of action are supplied in the first table.

Multi-drug regimen acronyms and their component drugs for both NSCLC and SCLC are shown in the last two tables. Most often an acronym is assembled from either:

- The first letters of the generic names of the drugs used
- The first letters of the abbreviations for the drug names, such as V, used for etoposide (VP-16)
- Less often, the first letters of the registered trade names, such as Adriamycin for doxorubicin

Your doctor may alter doses and schedules to suit your circumstances. Consequently, dose amounts and schedules are not given below unless needed to distinguish one regimen from another.

Common drug names and abbreviations

The following table lists in alphabetic order the FDA-approved drugs, their abbreviations, trade names, and modes of action. For drugs in clinical trials for lung cancer and not yet approved by the FDA for any other use, see Chapter 23, *The Future of Therapy*.

Generic Name, Abbreviation	Trade Names	Mode of Action and Comments
Carboplatin (CBDCA)	Paraplatin	Alkylating agent similar to cisplatin, but 45 times less toxic
Cisplatin (CDDP)	Platinol	Idiosyncratic alkylating agent
Cyclophosphamide (CTX)	Cytoxan or Neosar	Alkylating agent
Cytoxan	—	See cyclophosphamide
Doxorubicin (DOX)	Adriamycin, Doxil, Rubex	Topoisomerase inhibitor
Docetaxel	Taxotere	See paclitaxel
Erythropoietin, Epoietin alfa (EPO)	Epogen, Procrit	Biological therapy; colony stimulating factor; stimulates formation of red blood cells
Etoposide (VP-16)	Toposar, VePesid	Topoisomerase inhibitor
Filgrastim (G-CSF)	Neupogen	See granulocyte colony stimulating factor
5-fluorouracil (5-FU)	Adrucil, Efudex, Fluoroplex	Incorporated into RNA in place of uracil, causing malfunction of protein synthesis; as continuous infusion, a thymidylate synthase inhibitor
Gemcitabine	Gemzar	Antimetabolite closely related to cytarabine
Granulocyte colony stimulating factor (G-CSF)	Neupogen	Biological therapy; colony stimulating factor that stimulates growth of white blood cells
Granulocyte-macrophage colony stimulating factor (GM-CSF)	Leukine	Biological therapy; colony stimulating factor that stimulates growth of white blood cells and macrophages
Hydrocortisone (HC)	A-hydroCort, Cortef, Hydrocortone Hytone, Locoid, Pandel, Solu-Cortef, Westcort	Corticosteroid immune suppressant
Hydroxorubicin	Adriamycin	See doxorubicin
Ifosfamide (IFF)	Ifex	Alkylating agent
Irinotecan	Camptosar	Topoisomerase inhibitor (soluble metabolite of camptothecin)
Lomustine (CCNU)	CeeNU	Alkylating agent, nitrosourea family
Mesna	Mesnex	Chemoprotectant against hemorrhagic cystitis; used against ifosfamide and cyclophosphamide
Methotrexate or amethopterin (MTX)	Methotrexate	Antimetabolite
Methylprednisolone (SOL)	Medrol, A-methaPred, Depo-Medrol, Solu-Medrol, SOL	Immune suppressant
Mitomycin (MMC)	Mutamycin	Atypical alkylating agent, cell cycle-phase nonspecific, obtained from the fungus Streptomyces caespitosus
Paclitaxel	Paxene, Taxol	Tubulin binding agent, but mechanism different from vinca alkaloids

Generic Name, Abbreviation	Trade Names	Mode of Action and Comments
Prednisone (Pred)	Deltasone, Orasone, Prednisone	Immune suppressant
Prednisolone	Econopred, Hydeltrasol, Inflamase, Pediapred, Pred Forte, Pred Mild, Prelone	Immune suppressant
Procarbazine (PCB)	Matulane	Alkylating agent
Sargramostim (GM-CSF)	Leukine	See granulocyte-macrophage colony stimulating factor
Taxotere	—	See docetaxel and paclitaxel
Thrombopoietin (TPO)	(Still in clinical trials)	Biological therapy; man-made copy of a natural body substance that stimulates the production of platelets
Topotecan	Hycamtin	Topoisomerase inhibitor (soluble metabolite of camptothecin)
Vinblastine (VLB)	Velban, vinblastine	Vinca alkaloid; tubulin binding agent
Vincristine (VCR)	Oncovin	Vinca alkaloid; tubulin binding agent
Vinorelbine	Navelbine	Vinca alkaloid; tubulin binding agent

NSCLC drug regimens

Acronym	Drugs Included
CAMP	Cyclophosphamide (CTX), doxorubicin (Adriamycin), methotrexate (MTX), procarbazine (PCB)
CAP	Cyclophosphamide (CTX), doxorubicin (Adriamycin), cisplatin (CDDP)
CBDCA+VP-16	Carboplatin (CBDCA), etoposide (VP-16)
CDDP + VP-16	Cisplatin (CDDP), etoposide (VP-16)
FED	Cisplatin (CDDP), etoposide (VP-16), fluorouracil (5-FU)
—	Cisplatin (CDDP), gemcitabine
—	Carboplatin (CBDCA), paclitaxel
—	Cisplatin (CDDP), paclitaxel
MACC	Methotrexate (MTX), doxorubicin (Adriamycin), cyclophosphamide (CTX), lomustine (CCNU)
MVP	Mitomycin (MITC), vinblastine (VLB), cisplatin (CDDP)
NVB-30	Vinorelbine (NVB) 30 mg/m2 IV weekly
NVB-15	Vinorelbine (NVB) 15 mg/m2 IV weekly
NVB-30+CDDP	Vinorelbine (NVB) 30, cisplatin (CDDP)
NVB-15+CDDP	Vinorelbine (NVB) 15, cisplatin (CDDP)
PVP-16	Cisplatin (CDDP), etoposide (VP-16)
VIP(ICE)-2	Ifosfamide (IFF) with MESNA, cisplatin (CDDP), etoposide (VP-16)

SCLC drug regimens

Acronym	Drugs included
CAE	Cyclophosphamide (CTX), doxorubicin (DOX), etoposide (VP-16)
CAV	Cyclophosphamide (CTX), doxorubicin (DOX), vincristine (VCR)
CAVE	Cyclophosphamide (CTX), doxorubicin (DOX), vincristine (VCR), etoposide (VP-16)
CAV/EP	Cyclophosphamide (CTX), doxorubicin (DOX), vincristine (VCR)/etoposide (VP-16), and cisplatin (CDDP)
CEV	Cyclophosphamide (CTX), etoposide (VP-16), vincristine (VCR)
—	Cyclophosphamide (CTX), methotrexate (MTX), lomustine (CCNU)
—	Cyclophosphamide (CTX), methotrexate (MTX), lomustine (CCNU), vincristine (VCR)
—	Single-agent etoposide (VP-16)
EC	Etoposide (VP-16), cisplatin (CDDP), 4000-4500 cGy chest radiation therapy
ECV	Etoposide (VP-16), cisplatin (CDDP), vincristine (VCR), 4500 cGy chest radiation therapy
EP	Cisplatin (CDDP), etoposide (VP-16)
PET	Cisplatin (CDDP), etoposide (VP-16), paclitaxel
VIP(ICE)-1	Ifosfamide (IFF) with MESNA, cisplatin (CDDP), etoposide (VP-16)

Experimental Prognostic Markers

TUMORS PRODUCE MANY SUBSTANCES that are sought for use as diagnostic and prognostic tools. The few known to be of prognostic use are discussed in Chapter 6, *Prognosis*. Those under study are included here because they might appear on your pathology reports. To date, none of these substances are meaningful in the absence of other prognostic information.

Tumor markers

Some of the tumor markers listed here overlap the genetic anomalies discussed in the section "Genetic characteristics." This is so because the proteins encoded and released by damaged genes can act as tumor markers, particularly if they are detectable in blood.

For SCLC, increases in the following investigational tumor markers appear to be associated with worse prognosis, but further study is needed:

- Carcinoembryonic antigen (CEA)
- Neuron-specific enolase (NSE)
- Thymidine kinase[1]
- Creatine kinase[2]
- Tissue polypeptide antigen (TPA)
- Ferritin
- Protein-bound carbohydrates (fucose, mannose, galactose)
- Urinary polyamines (putrescine, spermidine)
- Neuroendocrine products (cortisol, gastrin-releasing peptide (GRP), and calcitonin)

For NSCLC, the following tumor markers are in some studies associated with worse prognosis, but further study is needed:

- Cyfra 21-1 above 3.5 nanograms per milliliter[3]
- Increased EGF
- Increased VEGF
- Loss of the A antigen from tumor cells (blood type A or AB)
- Presence of NCAM (NKH1)
- Presence of NSE
- Increased Cyclin-D1[4]

- Expression of Factor VIII in stage I[5]
- Expression of CD-44 in stage I[6]
- Lack of the Lewis Y antigen in stages I, II, or IIIA[7]
- Increased PCNA-LI[8]
- Expression of uPA[9]
- CEA in pleural effusion
- Increased SCC in squamous cell type
- Increased levels of orosomucoid
- Increased levels E-cadherin
- Increased stromelysin-3
- Decreased plasminogen activator inhibitor 2
- Increased cathepsin B
- Increased Ki-67 protein

Genetic characteristics

There have been many studies for lung cancer that attempt to draw a statistical correlation between certain kinds of genetic damage within a cancer cell and its outcome for the patient.

NSCLC genetic traits

For NSCLC, these genetic errors are thought to worsen prognosis, but further study is needed:

- Damaged or missing p53 gene
- Damaged RAS genes
- For squamous cell subtype, gain or loss of an entire chromosome
- Deletion of the short arm of chromosome 3 (3p)
- Loss of RB genes
- Overexpression of Her2 gene
- Overexpression of L-MYC and c-MYC genes[10]
- Expression of p185neu in stage III[11]

SCLC genetics characteristics

For SCLC, these genetic changes are known, but their correlation to prognosis is not fully delineated:

- Damaged or missing short arm of chromosome 3 (3p)[12]
- Changes in the short or long arms of chromosome 5 (5p, 5q),[13] especially genes at 5q21 and 5q33-35[14]
- Loss of long arm of chromosome 5 (5q)
- Damaged or missing long arm of chromosome 13 (13q)[15]
- Loss of short arm of chromosome 17 (17p)

- Overexpression of the MYC or MYCN genes
- Increased MDR1 gene expression
- Loss of TGF-bII gene expression
- Loss of RB gene
- Damaged or missing p53
- Overexpression of the dmin gene
- Overexpression of the hsr gene

Notes

Chapter 2, *Diagnosis and Staging*

1. R. Ginsberg, "Continuing Controversies in Staging NSCLC: An Analysis of the Revised 1997 Staging System," *Oncology* (Jan 1998): 12(1).

2. F. A. Shepherd et al., "Importance of Clinical Staging in Limited Small-cell Lung Cancer: a Valuable System to Separate Prognostic Subgroups," *Journal of Clinical Oncology* 11, no. 8 (Aug 1993): 1592–7.

3. P. Dumont et al., "Bronchoalveolar Carcinoma: Histopathologic Study of Evolution in a Series of 105 Surgically Treated Patients," *Chest* 113, no. 2 (Feb 1998): 391–5.

4. J. Austin et al., "Missed Bronchogenic Carcinoma: Radiographic Findings in 27 Patients with a Potentially Resectable Lesion Evident in Retrospect," *Radiology* 185 (1992): 115.

Chapter 5, *What is Lung Cancer?*

1. See *http://www-seer.ims.nci.nih.gov/Publications/CSR1973_1996/overview/overview1.pdf*.

2. See *http://www.cancer.org/cancerinfo/load_cont.asp?ct=26*.

3. See *Cancer Rates and Risks*, NCI, 4th ed., 1996.

4. Donald Shopland, "Cigarette Smoking as a Cause of Cancer," *Cancer Rates and Risks*, NCI, Fourth ed., 1996.

5. A. J. Sasco and H. Vainio, "From in Utero and Childhood Exposure to Parental Smoking to Childhood Cancer: a Possible Link and the Need for Action," *Human Experimental Toxicology* 18, no. 4 (Apr 1999): 192–201.

6. Please note that SEER chart XV-16 contains higher incidence rates for both races than chart XV-3.

7. Gonghuan et al., "Smoking in China: Findings of the 1996 National Prevalence Survey," *Journal of the American Medical Association* 282 (Oct 1999): 13.

8. N. Krieger, "Social Class, Race/Ethnicity, and Incidence of Breast, Cervix, Colon, Lung, and Prostate Cancer Among Asian, Black, Hispanic, and White Residents of the San Francisco Bay Area, 1988–92," *Cancer Causes and Control* 10, no. 6 (Dec 1999): 525–37.

9. G. D. Smith et al., "Adverse Socioeconomic Conditions in Childhood and Cause Specific Adult Mortality: Prospective Observational Study," *British Medical Journal* 316, no. 7145 (30 May 1998): 1631–5.

10. B. Marshall, "Socioeconomic Status, Social Mobility and Cancer Occurrence During Working Life: a Case-control Study Among French Electricity and Gas Workers," *Cancer Causes and Control* 10, no. 6 (Dec 1999): 495–502.

11. M. R. Law and J. K. Morris, "Why Is Mortality Higher in Poorer Areas and in More Northern Areas of England and Wales?" *Journal of Epidemiology and Community Health* 52, no. 6 (Jun 1998): 344–52.

12. S. D. Stellman and K. Resnicow, "Tobacco Smoking, Cancer and Social Class," *IARC Scientific Publications* 138 (1997): 229–50.

13. W. J. Gauderman and J. L. Morrison, "Evidence for Age-Specific Genetic Relative Risks in Lung Cancer," *American Journal of Epidemiology* 151, no. 1 (1 Jan 2000): 41–9.

14. S. T. Mayne et al., "Familial Cancer History and Lung Cancer Risk in United States Nonsmoking Men and Women," *Cancer Epidemiology, Biomarkers and Prevention* 8, no. 12 (Dec 1999): 1065–9.

15. A. Andersen et al., "Work-related Cancer in the Nordic Countries," *Scand J Work Environ Health* 25, Suppl 2 (1999): 1–116.

16. L. Carpenter and E. Roman, "Cancer and Occupation in Women: Identifying Associations Using Routinely Collected National Data," *Environ Health Perspect* 107, Suppl 2 (May 1999): 299–303.

17. E. Lynge et al., "Organic Solvents and Cancer," *Cancer Causes Control* 8, no. 3 (May 1997): 406–19.

18. Baumgartner et al., "Occupational and Environmental Risk Factors for Idiopathic Pulmonary Fibrosis: a Multicenter Case-Control Study," *American Journal of Epidemiology* 152, no. 4: 307–315.

19. T. Naoe et al., "Molecular Analysis of the T(15;17) Translocation in De Novo and Secondary Acute Promyelocytic Leukemia," *Leukemia* 11, Suppl 3 (Apr 1997): 287–8.

20. Note that one reviewer felt some of these were speculative.

21. H. Wiebelt and N. Becker, "Mortality in a Cohort of Toluene Exposed Employees (Rotogravure Printing Plant Workers)," *Journal of Occupational and Environmental Medicine* 41, no. 12 (Dec 1999): 1134–9.

22. B. Ritz et al., "Chemical Exposures of Rocket-Engine Test-Stand Personnel and Cancer Mortality in a Cohort of Aerospace Workers," *Journal of Occupational and Environmental Medicine* 41, no. 10 (Oct 1999): 903–10.

23. K. Nakachi et al., "Risk Factors for Lung Cancer Among Northern Thai Women: Epidemiological, Nutritional, Serological, and Bacteriological Surveys of Residents in High- and Low-Incidence Areas," *Japanese Journal of Cancer Research* 90, no. 11 (Nov 1999): 1187–95.

24. F. E. Speizer et al., "Prospective Study of Smoking, Antioxidant Intake, and Lung Cancer in Middle-Aged Women (USA)," *Cancer Causes and Control* 10, no. 5 (Oct 1999): 475–82.

25. K. Wakai et al., "Risk Modification in Lung Cancer by a Dietary Intake of Preserved Foods and Soyfoods: Findings from a Case-Control Study in Okinawa, Japan," *Lung Cancer* 25, no. 3 (Sep 1999): 147–59.

26. R. Sankaranarayanan et al., "A Case-Control Study of Diet and Lung Cancer in Kerala, South India," *International Journal of Cancer* 58, no. 5 (Sep 1994): 644–9.

27. F. Nyberg et al., "Dietary Factors and Risk of Lung Cancer in Never-Smokers," *International Journal of Cancer* 78, no. 4 (9 Nov 1998): 430–6.

28. X. D. Wang and R. M. Russell, "Procarcinogenic and Anticarcinogenic Effects of Beta-Carotene," *Nutrition Reviews* 57, no. 9 pt 1 (Sep 1999): 263–72.

29. M. C. Alavanja, "Estimating the Effect of Dietary Fat on the Risk of Lung Cancer in Non-smoking Women," *Lung Cancer* 14, Suppl 1 (Mar 1996): S63–74.

30. S. T. Mayne et al., "Dietary Beta Carotene and Lung Cancer Risk in U.S. Nonsmokers," *Journal of the National Cancer Institute* 86, no. 1 (5 Jan 1994): 33–8.

31. J. L. Chan et al., "Cancer Risk in Collagenous Colitis," *Inflammatory Bowel Disease* 5, no. 1 (Feb 1999): 40–3.

Chapter 6, *Prognosis*

1. S. R. Harris and U. P. Thorgeirsson, "Tumor Angiogenesis: Biology and Therapeutic Prospects," *In Vivo* 12, no. 6 (Nov-Dec 1998): 563–70.

2. A. E. Fraire, "Prognostic Significance of Histopathologic Subtype and Stage in Small Cell Lung Cancer." *Human Pathology* 23, no. 5 (May 1992): 520–8.

3. S. X. Jiang et al., "Large Cell Neuroendocrine Carcinoma of the Lung: a Histologic and Immunohistochemical Study of 22 Cases," *American Journal of Surgical Pathology* 22, no. 5 (May 1998): 526–37.

4. J. Watine et al., "Do Blood Cell Counts Have an Independent Prognostic Value in Primary Lung Cancer?" *Hematologic Cell Therapy* 40, no. 3 (Jun 1998): 99–106.

Chapter 8, *Treating Non-Small Cell Lung Cancer*

1. PORT Meta-analysis Trialists Group, "Postoperative Radiotherapy in Non-Small Cell Lung Cancer: Systematic Review and Meta-Analysis of Individual Patient Data from Nine Randomised Controlled Trials," *Lancet* 352, no. 9124 (1998): 257–63.

Chapter 15, *Stress and Stress Reduction*

1. W. Neuhaus, et al., "A Prospective Study Concerning Psychological Characteristics of Patients with Breast Cancer," *Archives of Gynecology and Obstetrics* 255, no. 4 (1994): 201–9.

2. R. Schwarz and S. Geyer, "Social and Psychological Differences Between Cancer and Non-cancer Patients: Cause or Consequence of the Disease?" *Psychotherapy and Psychosomatics* 41, no. 4 (1984): 195–9.

Chapter 16, *Getting Support*

1. Ellen E. Schultz, "If You Use Firm's Counselors, Remember Your Secrets Could Be Used Against You," *Wall Street Journal*, 26 May 1994.

Chapter 20, *Clinical Trials*

1. See trials MSKCC-95021A4 and NCCTG-984652, for example.

Chapter 23, *The Future of Therapy*

1. S. A. Rummel et al., "Role of a Small Molecular Weight Phosphoprotein in the Mechanism of Action of CI-994 (N-acetyldinaline)," *International Journal of Cancer* 62, no. 5 (4 Sep 1995): 636–42.

Appendix E, *Experimental Prognostic Markers*

1. A. J. Vangsted, "Serological Tumor Markers for Small Cell Lung Cancer and Their Therapeutic Implications," *APMIS* 102, no. 8 (Aug 1994): 561–80.

2. A. Usui et al., "Creatine Kinase BB and Neuron Specific R-Enolase as Biomarkers for Lung Cancer," *Gan No Rinsho* 33, no. 14 (Nov 1987): 1763–70.

3. T. Hirashima et al., "Prognostic Significance of CYFRA 21-1 in Non-Small Cell Lung Cancer," *Anticancer Research* 18, no. 6B (Nov-Dec 1998): 4713–6.

4. M. Caputi et al., "Prognostic Role of Cyclin D1 in Lung Cancer. Relationship to Proliferating Cell Nuclear Antigen," *American Journal of Respiratory Cell Molecular Biology* 20, no. 4 (Apr 1999): 746–50.

5. T. A. D'Amico et al., "A Biologic Risk Model for Stage I Lung Cancer: Immunohistochemical Analysis of 408 Patients with the Use of Ten Molecular Markers," *Journal of Thoracic and Cardiovascular Surgery* 117, no. 4 (Apr 1999): 736–43.

6. ibid.

7. F. Tanaka et al., "Lewis Y Antigen Expression and Postoperative Survival in Non-Small Cell Lung Cancer," *Annals of Thoracic Surgery* 66, no. 5 (Nov 1998): 1745–50.

8. A. M. Lavezzi et al., "Prognostic Significance of Different Biomarkers in Non-Small Cell Lung Cancer," *Oncol Rep* 6, no. 4 (Jul-Aug 1999): 819–25.

9. M. Volm et al., "Relationship of Urokinase and Urokinase Receptor in Non-Small Cell Lung Cancer to Proliferation, Angiogenesis, Metastasis and Patient Survival," *Oncol Rep* 6, no. 3 (May-Jun 1999): 611–5.

10. Moore et al., Chapter 29, *Lung Cancer: Principles and Practice*, 1996, eds. Pass, Harvey, et al..

11. M. Thomas et al., "Trimodality Therapy in Stage III Non-Small Cell Lung Cancer: Prediction of Recurrence by Assessment of p185neu," *European Respir Journal* 13, no. 2 (Feb 1999): 424–9.

12. R. Ullmann et al., "Unbalanced Chromosomal Aberrations in Neuroendocrine Lung Tumors as Detected by Comparative Genomic Hybridization," *Human Pathology* 29, no. 10 (Oct 1998): 1145–9.

13. R. Ullmann et al., *Human Pathology* 29, no. 10 (Oct 1998): 1145–9.

14. S. Hosoe, "Search for the Tumor-Suppressor Gene(S) on Chromosome 5q, Which May Play an Important Role for the Progression of Lung Cancer," *Nippon Rinsho* 54, no. 2 (Feb 1996): 482–6.

15. R. Ullmann et al., *Human Pathology* 29, no. 10 (Oct 1998): 1145–9.

Glossary

THIS GLOSSARY LISTS only terms specific to lung cancers. Guides to pronunciation are included.

For a comprehensive glossary of cancer medical terminology, see Altman and Sarg's *The Cancer Dictionary*. For more general medical terms, any one of several inexpensive medical dictionaries available in bookstores and libraries should suffice. You can also access ACOR's glossary of cancer terms at *http://www.acor.org/glossary/index.html*.

Blood, urine, and pulmonary function tests are defined in Appendix B, *Tests and Procedures*.

But first: Unusual phrases

There are a few specific words and phrases that may be jarring because they mean something different in medicine than they do in everyday usage:

Anecdotal
> When used in a medical context does not mean a funny story. It means a single case report not yet substantiated by studies using large numbers of people.

Impressive or not impressive
> When used in a medical context does not mean anything derogatory. Not impressive means that, when the patient was examined, a particular feature did not strike the examiner as overwhelmingly unusual. For instance, after palpating your abdomen, the doctor may note in your medical record that your liver was "not impressive." This means it did not feel enlarged and that you did not report pain when she pressed on it.

Morbid or morbidity
> Do not mean that you're neurotic. They simply mean illness and are somewhat the opposite of mortality. You might read, for example, that a treatment resulted in 20 percent low-level morbidity but only 2 percent mortality. Likewise, comorbidity means the illnesses a person has in addition to cancer, such as high blood pressure or diabetes.

"The patient denies . . ."
> Does not mean that the doctor thinks you're lying. It's just used as the opposite of "the patient reports . . . ." For instance, your medical record might read, "The patient reports frequent morning cough, but denies the presence of dark phlegm."

Pathologic
> In the context of tissue studies means the study of the appearance of healthy cells, cancerous cells, and affected organs. It does not mean mental or emotional illness, such as would be meant by the phrase "pathological liar" or the word psychopath.

Tolerable
Is a word often used by medical staff to describe the side effects of treatment. Your idea of what is tolerable may be much lower than their definition, because medicine defines a tolerable side effect as one that can be ameliorated with supportive care and that does not result in permanent organ damage. But for you, these side effects might be intolerable, and if so, you should say so.

X terms dx, hx, rx, tx
Mean diagnosis, history, prescription, and treatment.

Lung cancer terminology

Adenocarcinoma (AD in oh kar sih NO mah)
A subtype of non-small cell lung cancer.

Adenosquamous carcinoma (AD in oh SKWAH mus)
A subtype of non-small cell lung cancer.

Adenopathy (ad en AH path ee)
The enlargement of lymph glands. Its presence in a lung cancer survivor, especially in the chest, might suggest the spread of cancer to the lymphatic system.

Adhesion (ad HEE shun)
Scar tissue that forms after surgery or radiotherapy.

Adjuvant therapy (ADD ju vant)
Chemotherapy or radiotherapy used before, during, or after surgery to improve the chance for cure.

Adrenal glands (ad REE nel)
Two glands that sit atop each kidney and release hormones for balancing salt levels and reacting to stress. Certain lung cancers can invade the adrenals; this can result in symptoms caused by unusual hormone levels.

Alopecia (owl uh PEA she uh)
Hair loss.

Alveolus (al VEE oh lus, plural alveoli)
The smallest unit of the lung, positioned at the very end of lung tissue, responsible for exchanging oxygen for carbon dioxide and for balancing amounts of other gases in the circulatory system.

Anhidrosis (ann high DROH sis)
Absence of sweat.

Antiangiogenic (ann tee ann gee oh GEN ik)
Interfering with the growth of blood vessels.

Apoptosis (app uh TOE sis; a pup TOE sis)
Orderly cell death characterized by slow dissolving and reuse of cell parts by neighboring tissue. Some chemotherapy drugs induce apoptosis; others cause cell lysis or bursting.

Arterial blood gas volume
A measure of the gases in an artery that indicates how well the lungs are working.

Atelectasis (at el EK te sis)
A partially or totally collapsed lung.

Ascites (ah SIGH teez)
A collection of fluid in the abdominal cavity.

BAC
Bronchioloaveolar carcinoma, a subtype of NSCLC.

Brachytherapy (brack ee THERE ah pea)
Placing a source of radiation very near a tumor to kill it. See also "Interstitial radiotherapy."

Breastbone
The sternum, a vertical bone that runs from collarbone to abdomen, to which the front ends of the ribs are attached.

Bronchial carcinoma (BRON ke al kar sih NO ma)
A general name for all lung cancers.

Bronchial-sleeve resection
Removal of part of one bronchial tube with reattachment (anastomosis) of the remaining ends.

Bronchioloalveolar (bronk yole al VEE ah larr)
See "Bronchoalveolar (bronk oh al VEE ah larr) carcinoma (BAC)."

Bronchoalveolar (bronk oh al VEE ah larr) carcinoma (BAC)
A subtype of non-small cell lung cancer that can at times grow slowly.

Bronchogenic carcinoma (bron ko GEN ik kar sih NO ma)
A general name for all lung cancers

Bronchorrhea (bronk a REE uh)
A cough producing large amounts of phlegm.

Bronchoscopy (bron KOS keh pea)
Viewing and biopsy of the bronchial tubes with an endoscope called a bronchoscope.

Bronchus (BRAHN kus, plural bronchi)
Two tubes that branch from the trachea and enter the lungs; the main airways into the lungs.

Bronchial tree
The branches from the main bronchi that penetrate the lungs to deliver air to minute lung tissue responsible for gas exchange.

Bulky disease
Any tumor that measures greater than 10 centimeters in any dimension. Bulky disease can be in the lung or in the lymph nodes, for example.

Calcitonin (kal sih TOE nin)
A parathyroid hormone that controls the release and uptake of calcium between bone and blood.

Cancerized field
See "Field cancerization."

Carcinoma in situ (kar sih NO ma in SEE tyoo ; in SIGH tyoo)
A tumor that is still confined to the innermost layer of the lung where it first arose.

Carina (ke RYE nuh; ke REE nuh)
Cartilage that supports the airway where the two bronchi join into the trachea.

Centigrey or cGy
A measurement of radiation dose absorbed by the body.

Cervicotomy (Ser vih KOT eh mee)
A surgical incision into the chest near the collarbone.

Cervical mediastinoscopy
The insertion of an endoscope through an incision near the collarbone to examine the mid-chest, especially its lymph nodes.

Cilia (SIL ee uh)
Minute hairlike components of the lung that wave continuously in an upward direction to remove mucus from the lung. Often in smokers the cilia are immobile.

Clavicle
The collarbone.

Clubbing
A swelling of the fingertips or toes that can be associated with pulmonary disease, including lung cancer.

Combined small cell carcinoma
Small cell lung cancer combined with cancerous squamous and/or glandular components.

Diaphragm
A horizontal muscle that separates the chest cavity from the abdomen and is an integral part of the push-pull mechanism of breathing.

Differentiation (diff er en she A shun)
The process of cells maturing and developing for a particular task. Cancer cells that fail to differentiate often are characterized as very aggressive, not functional for their organ type, and hard to identify as belonging to a particular type of tissue.

Diffusion capacity
A measure of how well the lungs take in air to exchange oxygen for carbon dioxide and other gases.

Distal (DISS tul)
The portion of the lung that is farthest from the mouth.

Dysphagia (dis FAJ ee yuh)
Difficulty swallowing.

Dyspnea (DISP nyuh)
   Difficulty breathing.

Echocardiography (ek oh card dee AH grah fee)
   An ultrasound of the heart to determine its health.

Emphysema
   A loss of elasticity in the lungs that results in an inability to exchange oxygen for carbon dioxide and other gases.

Endocarditis (en doe car DIE tiss)
   An inflammation of one of the sacs that surround the heart.

Endoscopy (en DOSS keh pea)
   Any of several surgeries utilizing an endoscope. See "Thoracoscopy," "Mediastinoscopy."

Extensive-stage SCLC
   Small cell lung cancer that has spread to distant organs; see also "Limited-stage SCLC." Unlike NSCLC, SCLC is not staged at levels I through IV.

Field cancerization
   The observation that some lung tumors arise in broad areas of lung tissue that all contain damaged DNA. One explanation is that substances that trigger damage to DNA do so in sweeping areas, not just in single cells, as may happen with other solid tumors, such as colorectal cancers.

Gamma knife (GAMM uh)
   See "Stereotactic radiosurgery."

Grey or Gy
   A measurement of radiation dose absorbed by the body.

Hemoptysis (hih MAP tih sis)
   Coughing blood.

Hilum (HIGH lem)
   The area on the lung where the bronchial tubes, blood vessels, and nerves enter.

Hormone
   A substance released by a gland to trigger a reaction in another organ. Some forms of lung cancer modify levels of certain hormones, either directly by producing the hormone or invading the gland, or indirectly by changing the body's chemistry sufficiently to affect hormone production. These hormone changes can cause uncomfortable symptoms.

Horner's syndrome
   A collection of symptoms that can be caused by some forms of lung cancer. See Chapter 1, *Symptoms of Lung Cancer.*

Hypercalcemia (high per kal SEE me uh)
   An excess of calcium in the blood, caused by illness that triggers the release of calcium from bone. Some types of cancer, including some lung cancers, cause hypercalcemia as a side effect of the tumor's production of the parathyroid hormone calcitonin, or from tumors that have traveled to and destroyed bone.

Hyponatremia (high poe nay TREE me eh)
   Too little salt in the blood. See "Hormone."

Infiltrating, infiltration
> Lung cancer cells that have invaded other organs or single cells that have broken loose from the tumor and infiltrated the lymph nodes outside the lung in the midchest (mediastinum). See also "Invasion."

Infiltrating lymphocytes
> White blood cells called lymphocytes are sometimes found very near to or within lung tumors or in lung fluid. It is thought that the immune system is attempting to kill the tumor with these lymphocytes. Some lung cancers are confused with lymphomas and vice versa when, during diagnosis, lymphocytes are found in sputum or in bronchoscopic biopsies.

Intercostal space (in ter KOS tul)
> For lung cancer, the space between the ribs.

Interstitial radiotherapy (in ter STISH ul)
> Implanting a very small seed or capsule containing a radioactive substance within a tumor to kill it.

Invasion
> Lung cancer cells that have advanced beyond the very earliest growth stages (carcinoma in situ) acquire the ability to invade other organs, nearby and distant.

Karnofsky
> See "Performance status."

Lambert-Eaton myasthenic syndrome
> A collection of symptoms, including muscle weakening, that can be caused by some forms of lung cancer. See Chapter 1.

Larynx
> The voice box.

Leukocyte (LU ko site)
> A general term for all white blood cells.

Limited-stage SCLC
> Small cell lung cancer that is limited to one lung and its lymph nodes; it has not spread to distant organs. See also "Extensive-stage SCLC." Unlike NSCLC, SCLC is not staged at levels I through IV.

Lobe
> One major section of one lung. The right lung has three lobes, but the left has just two to accommodate other left-side organs, such as the heart.

Lobectomy (low BECK toe me)
> Removal of one lobe of either lung.

Lymph node
> A kidney-bean-shaped swelling along a lymphatic duct, responsible for filtering lymphatic fluid of foreign substances. The body has hundreds of lymph nodes; healthy nodes vary in size from very tiny to almond-size, depending on their position and function. Many are located between the lungs.

Lymphadenectomy (lim fa den EK toe me)
Removal of all lymph nodes and lymphatic vessels draining the lung as part of lung cancer surgery.

Mediastinal pleura (me dee ah STY nal ploor eh)
The lining of the inner chest between the lungs.

Mediastinum (me dee ah STY num)
The area of the chest between the lungs and behind the breastbone that houses the heart, some major blood vessels and nerves, and a collection of lymph nodes.

Mediastinoscopy (me dee ass tih NAHS koe pea)
An examination of the midchest between the lungs using a small camera inserted through a small incision.

Mesothelioma (mezz oh theel ee OH mah)
A type of cancer that grows on the outer surface of the lung. It is often mistakenly called lung cancer by those unfamiliar with its characteristics. Mesothelioma is often, but not always, linked to inhalation of fibers of the mineral asbestos.

Metachronous (meh TAH crow nis)
Second tumors that occur independently some time after the primary tumor, not as a result of spread of the first tumor, which is called metastasis.

Metastasis (me TASS te sis)
The spread of cancer to other tissues.

Micrometastasis (MY krow me TAS te sis)
Less than 2 millimeters of detectable cancer at a site other than the original tumor.

Miosis (my OH sis)
A constricted pupil in the eye.

Mucin (MYEW sin)
See "Solid adenocarcinoma with mucin."

Mucositis (myew koe SIGH tis)
An inflammation of the mucous membranes. Any mucus-producing tissue from the mouth to the anus can develop mucositis.

Myelopathy
Damage to the nervous system, sometimes caused by radiotherapy.

Nebulize (NEB yew lies)
To reduce to a fine spray or to atomize.

Neoadjuvant therapy
Chemotherapy or radiotherapy used before surgery to shrink a tumor.

Neuropathy (nyoor AH pah thee)
Damage to the nervous system causing numbness, pain, tingling, or any other neurologic symptom, such as dizziness, blurred vision, or cognitive impairment (e.g., memory loss or slowed thinking).

Neutropenia (nu trow PEA nee uh)
   The condition of having abnormally low numbers of one type of white blood cell called neutrophils.

NSCLC
   Non-small cell lung cancer.

Oat cell
   An older name for small cell lung cancer.

Occult disease
   Cancer not detectable by visual exam or by testing strategies, such as imaging studies.

Overall survival
   The total amount of time that a patient survives following treatment, including recurrences of disease that were successfully retreated. A broader category than event-free survival with no recurrence of disease.

Palliation (pal ee A shun)
   The relief of pain without an intent to cure disease.

Pancoast syndrome
   A collection of symptoms that can be caused by some forms of lung cancer. See Chapter 1.

Papillary (PAP ill airy; papp ILL ah ree)
   A subtype of non-small cell lung cancer.

Parietal (pe RYE uh tull)
   Relating to the walls of a cavity.

Parietal pleura
   A layer of tissue that surrounds the lungs and lines the inside of the chest.

Partial response
   A tumor's response to treatment that is fifty percent smaller or more, but still remains. It's not unusual to see a partial response on imaging halfway through treatment and a total response by the end of treatment.

Pathologic fracture
   A broken bone caused by weakening owing to chemical changes created by the tumor.

PCA, PCI
   Patient-controlled analgesia, patient-controlled infusion. Both refer to pumps that allow a patient to self-administer pain killing drugs after surgery.

-penia (PEEN yuh)
   A suffix denoting abnormally low numbers of blood cells: leukopenia, erythropenia, thrombocytopenia, or neutropenia.

Performance status
   A measure of how well the patient can do everyday things, such as eating, bathing, and walking. Karnofsky is one such scale; ECOG and Zubrod are others. Many clinical trials specify a particular level of performance status as an entry requirement. Some forms of lung cancer have a better outcome if performance status remains high.

Perfusion scan
A test that measures how well the lungs take in air to exchange oxygen for carbon dioxide and other gases.

Pericardial effusion (pair ee KAR dyul ef FYUH shun)
Collection of fluid in the sac that surrounds the heart.

Pericardiocentesis (pair eh kar dyo sen TEE sis)
Insertion of a narrow needle with a large reservoir through the chest wall for one-time drainage of the heart sac via suction aspiration.

Pericardiotomy (pair eh kar dy OTT uh mee)
Opening of the sac containing the heart to release and drain accumulated fluid. Temporary drains are installed to remove any remaining fluid over the following days or weeks.

Pericarditis (pair eh kar DYE tiss)
An inflammation of the sac that surrounds the heart.

Pericardium (pair eh KAR dee um)
A sac that surrounds the heart to protect and cushion it.

Peripheral neuropathy
Numbness, tingling, or pain in the hands or feet, often associated with vincristine or platinum-based chemotherapies.

PFT
Pulmonary function tests.

Photodynamic therapy
Use of three components: a drug that sensitizes cells to light, a light source (usually a laser), and oxygen, to kill tumor cells on the surface of the inside of the airways.

Platelet
A blood cell called a thrombocyte, important in blood clotting.

Pleura (PLOOR ah)
The two membranes, parietal pleura and visceral pleura, that line the chest wall and cover the lungs. Between the pleura is fluid that cushions the lungs and aids in breathing.

Pleural effusion (PLOOR el eh FYEW shun)
A leakage of fluid into the space between the lungs and the chest wall.

Pleurectomy (ploor EK toe mee)
Surgery that removes the two sacs encompassing the lung.

Pleurodesis (ploor oh DEE sis)
Sclerotherapy involving injecting a substance that will cause scarring in the tissue layers between which fluid has been collecting. Scarring causes the two layers (pleura) to adhere, which discourages the collection of fluid.

Pleuroperitoneal shunt (ploor eh pair eh teh NEE al)
Insertion of tubing (under anesthesia) that will transfer fluid from the pleural space into the abdominal space called the peritoneal cavity, where it is absorbed and processed by the body. Fluid is transferred to the peritoneal cavity via a pump.

Pneumonectomy (new mon NECK tuh mee)
Surgery to remove one lung.

Pneumothorax
An accumulation of air escaped from the lung into the pleural space in the chest or beneath the skin (sometimes distant from the lung) as a result of disease, accidental injury, or a surgical procedure.

Posterolateral (poss tier oh LAT er al)
On the side near the back.

Precision dissection
A very minimal "lumpectomy" of deep diseased lung tissue, using sealing techniques, such as laser or cautery to close blood and lymphatic vessels after the tumor is removed.

Primary tumor
The original tumor. Metastases may spread from certain malignant primary tumors.

Prophylactic cranial irradiation (PCI)
Irradiation of the brain to prevent future metastases. See also whole brain irradiation in Chapter 7, *Types of Treatment.*

Proximal (PROX i mull)
The portion of the lung that is closest to the mouth.

Pulmonary artery
The blood vessel that returns oxygen-depleted blood to the lungs.

Pulmonary function tests
Any of a number of tests, such as lung diffusion testing (diffusing capacity), spirometry, FVC, FEV, match test, forced expiratory time (FET), peak expiratory flow rate (PEFR), maximum ventilatory volume (MVV), pulmonary ventilation/perfusion scan (V/Q scan), or other lung volume tests that are intended to determine how well one's lungs are functioning. See Appendix B for more information.

Pulmonary vein
The blood vessel that carries oxygen-replenished blood from the lungs to the heart for dispersal throughout the body.

Radiation port
The carefully delineated area of the body at which external beam radiotherapy is directed and the internal tissues that receive the radiation dose.

Radiation recall
The recurrence of side effects at the site of previous irradiation. See Chapter 13, *Adverse Effects of Treatment,* "Recall sensitivities."

Radiosensitizing drugs
Drugs that make radiotherapy more effective in killing tumors. See Chapter 7.

Resection
Surgery that removes all or part of an organ.

SCLC
Small cell lung cancer.

Scar carcinoma
  A subtype of lung cancer that creates a scarlike buckling on the outside of the lung near the tumor.

Sclerotherapy (sklair oh THAIR ah pea)
  Causing scarring deliberately as a means to halt or cure certain conditions. See "Pleurodesis."

Seeding
  (1) The tendency of tumor cells to spread along surgical lines if the tumor is accidentally cut open while still in the body. (2) The implantation of radioactive particles into a tumor to kill it; see "Interstitial radiotherapy."

Segmentectomy (seg men TEK tuh mee)
  Removal of a segment of one lobe of one lung, its blood supply, and nearby lymph nodes and vessels.

SIADH
  Syndrome of inappropriate antidiuretic hormone. A collection of symptoms that can be caused by some forms of lung cancer. See Chapter 1.

Solid adenocarcinoma with mucin
  A subtype of non-small cell lung cancer (NSCLC). For more details, see Chapter 2, *Diagnosis and Staging*.

Spirometry (spih ROM eh tree)
  The measure of the amount of air that the patient can inhale and expel from the lungs.

Split-lung function study
  A test of each lung's capacity separate from the other.

Sputum (SPYEW tum)
  Mucus brought from the airways, usually by coughing.

Squamous cell carcinoma (SKWAM us)
  A subtype of non-small cell lung cancer, also called epidermoid carcinoma.

Stable disease
  One or more tumors still visible on imaging that are not growing.

Staging
  A measurement of how far cancer has spread from the original tumor. For lung cancer and most other cancers, staging is meaningful in prognosis.

Stenosis (steh NO sis)
  A narrowing of a body canal such that the substance it normally carries cannot pass readily through it. Stenosis can occur in the airways following lung cancer treatment or as a result of disease.

Stent, stenting
  A brace to hold a canal open so that air or liquid can pass through it. Stents can be used to hold airways, veins, or kidney ureters open, for example.

Stereotactic radiosurgery
  The administration of a one-time dose of radiation to a carefully targeted filed that is aligned to a frame made to fit the patient and used as a reference point for targeting.

Compare to the Cyberknife, which requires no frame because it uses the skeleton as a reference, and to fractionated stereotactic radiosurgery, which spreads the dose over several to many sessions.

Sternotomy (ster NAH tuh mee)
Gaining access to the chest by surgically separating the ribs from the breastbone.

Sternum (STER num)
See "Breastbone."

Stridor (STRIDE er)
A harsh vibrating sound heard when the airways are blocked.

Subclavian vein
A large vein behind the collarbone (clavicle) sometimes used to administer IV drugs.

Superior sulcus (SUL cuss)
The groove in the upper chest where the airways and blood supply pass through supportive chest tissue.

Superior vena cava (VEE nuh KAY vah)
A large vein in the chest near the lungs that drains blood from the head and neck.

Supraclavicular (soo prah klah VIK you lar)
Above the collarbone.

Synchronous (SINK run us)
Synchronous tumors are tumors that appear at the same time. See "Metachronous."

T-Tube
A plastic tube inserted into an airway to keep it open.

Thoracentesis (thor eh sen TEE sus)
Inserting a narrow needle with a large reservoir through the chest wall for one-time drainage via suction aspiration.

Thoracoscopy (thor eh KOSS koh pea)
An examination of the chest with a small camera through a small incision into the chest.

Thoracostomy (thor eh KOSS toe mee)
See "Tube thoracostomy."

Thoracotomy (thor eh KOT oh mee)
A surgical incision into the chest.

Thorax
The part of the body above the abdomen, but below the neck.

Thrombosis
A blood clot that blocks a blood vessel.

TNM
Three measures of tumor spread—Tumor size, lymph Nodes affected, and Metastatic (distant) sites involved—that are used to stage lung cancer and many other cancers at levels I through IV.

Torsion (TOR shin)
A twisting of an organ out of its normal position.

Trachea (TRAY kee uh)
The windpipe.

Transthoracic needle aspiration
A means of retrieving tissue for biopsy by inserting a fine needle through the skin of the chest. This technique is an alternative to bronchoscopy or a larger surgery.

Tube thoracostomy (thor ah KOSS te me)
Temporary implantation of a chest tube to drain away fluid continuously.

VATS
Video-assisted thoracic surgery, a less invasive surgical technique that utilizes a camera to guide various surgical tools, principally an endoscope called a thoracoscope.

Watch and wait, watchful waiting
Close medical monitoring without anticancer treatment, often for months, until disease warrants treatment because symptoms become troublesome or disease is too extensive. Some slow-growing lung tumors are treated with watchful waiting.

Wedge resection
Surgery to remove a wedge of tissue from one lobe of one lung. This surgery usually is done only for early-stage disease or isolated tumors.

Whole brain irradiation
A radiologic treatment used to prevent the spread of certain lung cancers to the brain.

Zubrod
See "Performance status."

Index

anxiety (continued)
    fear as cause of, 226
    physical causes of, 225–226
    symptoms of, 225
    vs. worry, 225
appetite changes, 181
ARDS (acute respiratory distress
        syndrome), 179
arm/leg motion, unsteady, 10
arterial thrombosis, 11
artery/vein syndromes, 11
asbestos, 82
assessing unproven remedies, 380
attending physicians, 142

B

balance, loss of, 10
bankruptcy, 287–288
bargaining for outcome, 100
biofeedback, 234–235
biological therapies, 118–120
    anti-growth factor, 118
    colony stimulating factors, 119–120
    cytokines, 119
    monoclonal antibodies, 119
    research trends in, 386–387
    stem cell support, 120
    tumor vaccines, 120
    See also non-small cell cancer; small
        cell cancer
biopsies
    fine needle aspiration (needle
        biopsy), 24, 454–455
    and thoracotomy, 26–27
biopsy tissue samples, storage of, 292
bladder damage, 181–182
blame, 42
bleeding, 182
blinded trials, 329
blood
    bloody/dark phlegm, 2
    cell counts, 23, 189, 205
    clots, 10, 179, 182
    sugar levels, 15
    syndromes, 10–11
    tests/procedures, 437–441
    values, 24, 96–97, 466–468
board certification, 45, 52

body fluid (sputum) analysis, 19, 461
bone damage, 183
bone growth, 10, 15
bone marrow
    biopsy, 24
    transplantation, 393
bone pain, 179
bone scans, 20, 441–442
bowel, pseudo-obstruction of, 13
bowel changes, 183
bowel perforation, 7
brachytherapy, 117, 322
brain death, 357
breast growth in men, 10, 15
breathing problems, 2, 6, 179, 183–185
bronchial-sleeve resection/lobectomy,
        106
bronchioloalveolar carcinoma
        (BAC), 97–98
bronchitis, recurrent, 2
bronchorrhea, 2
bronchoscopy, 21, 442–444
bruising, 179

C

cachexia, 15
calcitonin, excess secretion of, 15
calcium, blood levels of, 10, 14
cancer counselors, 270
cancer organizations, 366, 409–410,
        412–416
cancer prevention, 388
cancers
    causes of, 81–82
    non-lung, and predisposition to
        lung cancer, 84
carboplatin, 124, 133, 321
carcinoid syndrome, 15
carcinoid tumor, 29
cardiothoracic surgeon, 45
cardiovascular changes, 193
case-control trials, 330
catheter
    insertion, 444–446
    removal, 302
cerebellar degeneration, 10, 13
changing doctors, 69
    See also interacting with medical
        personnel

J

jaundice, 6, 195
joint pain/swelling, 196

K

kidneys
    damage, 196
    function test, 23

L

lactate dehydrogenase, 23
Lambert-Eaton myasthenic syndrome
    (LEMS), 13
large cell carcinoma, 28
laser therapy, 120–121
late effects. *See* adverse effects of
    treatment
laughter, 239
learning about illness and treatments,
    238
leukocyte therapy, 400
leukopenia, 196–197
licensed practical nurses (LPNs), 141
life insurance, 284–285
limited-stage small cell cancer, 132
liver
    biopsy, 24
    dysfunction, 197–198
    function test, 23
lobar torsion, 179
lobectomy, 106
lomustine, 133, 322
loneliness, 309–310, 323
long-term care insurance, 285
long-term disability insurance, 285–286
lumbar puncture, 24, 459
lumps (various sites), 7–8
lung cancer, overview, 71–85
    causes, known/possible, 82–85
    distinguished from other cancers,
        72–73
        factors linked to development,
            75–80
    incidence/trends of, 73–74
    lungs, function of, 71–72
    in never-smokers, 74–75

resources, 409–412
statistics, 73–74
See also non-small cell cancer; small
    cell cancer
lungs
    collapse, 179
    damage, 198
    gas exchange, measures of, 26, 450
lung-sparing surgeries, 106–107
lung volume tests, 26, 451, 459–460
lungs, function of, 71–72

M

magnetic resonance imaging (MRI), 20,
    452–454
malaise, 198
managed care. *See* health insurance
massage therapy, 239
matrix metalloproteinase inhibitors, 114
mediastinoscopy, 21
medical dictionaries, 363
medical libraries, 372
medical research papers, 367–368
medical textbooks, 373–374
Medicare/Medicaid/MediGap, 284
meditation, 239–240
Medline/PubMed, 368–372
memorial services/burial/cremation, 360
memory loss, 198
menopause, 216–217
mental slowness, 39
metabolic imbalances, 199
metastasis
    distant, as staging definition, 29, 33
    sites of, 7
    symptoms, 7–9
methrotrexate, 133, 322
methylation, 400
military (VA) disability income,
    289–290
mitochondrial DNA, 404
mitomycin, 124, 321
molecular oncology, 405
monoclonal antibodies, 119, 161, 400
mouth changes, 199–200
MRI, 20
mucositis, 199–200
mucus production, 2

muscle cramps/spasms, 200
music/song, 241
myelopathy, 13
myopathy, 12

N

nail changes, 200–201
nausea, 179, 201–202
NCI-designated comprehensive cancer
centers, 49
needle aspiration, 24
nephrotic syndrome, 15
nerve damage, 179
nervous system syndromes, 13
neuroendocrine tumors, 97
neurotoxicity, 202–203
neutropenia, 203
never-smokers, lung cancer in, 74–75
new therapies, 383, 407
and genetic basis of cancer, 81–82
possible future trials, 403–406
research trends in, 384–389
trials of new drugs/techniques,
390–403
See also clinical trials
nipples, discharge of milk from, 15
non-fractionated stereotactic
radiosurgery, 168
non-small cell cancer
and clinical trials, 126–129
prognosis
blood values, 97
histology, 96
staging exceptions, 94–95
tumor grade, 95
recurrence of, 321
staging, 29–43
abbreviations used with, 33
definitions of terms, 30–33
and prognosis, 94–95
stages in, 34
TNM staging definitions,
30–33
symptoms
in tumor-free organs
(paraneoplastic
syndromes), 9–10

treatment by stage
chemotherapy drugs used,
124–125
occult tumors, 125
Stage 0 through Stage IV,
125–129
treatment options
biological therapies, 124
chemotherapy, 123–124
elimination of fluid in chest,
124
inhalation therapy, 124
photodynamic therapy,
123–124
radiotherapy, 123–124
surgery, 122–123
See also biological therapies;
chemotherapy; prognosis;
radiotherapy; surgery
nonbacterial thrombotic endocarditis,
11
nonhealing wounds, 203
nonspecific immune-modulator therapy,
400–401
normal values (blood tests), 466–469
notes, 477–480
numbness, 6, 203
nursing staff, 63–64, 141
nutrition, 242

O

occult carcinoma, 34
occupation as risk factor, 79–80
odors, 203
oncologists, 45
oncology nurses, 63–64
oral therapy, 159
osteomalacia, 12

P

packing for hospitalization, 138–140
paclitaxel, 124, 133, 321–322
pain
as adverse effect of treatment,
203–205
control of, 17–18

surgery, specific kinds of
endoscopic procedures, 105–106
extended/distant sites, 109
extended/en bloc, 107–109
full lung removal, 107
partial lung removal (lung-sparing),
106–107
See also new therapies; non-small
cell cancer; small cell
cancer
swallowing, difficulty in, 2
sweats/sweating, 13, 190
swelling of face/arms/neck, 6
symptoms, 1–16, 99
of distant spread (metastasis), 7–9
in organs near lungs, 5–7
and prognosis, 99
pulmonary, 2–5
regression of, at end of treatment,
301
in tumor-free organs
(paraneoplastic
syndromes), 9–15
vs. syndromes, 2
wide variation in, 1–2
syndromes. *See* symptoms

T

taste changes, 181
teaching fellows, 142
telomerase inhibitors, 405–406
tests and procedures
communicating results of, 18
experiencing, 437–465
follow-up at end of treatment,
297–300
interpreting results of, 379–380
list of, 437–465
resources, 422–423
results of (tables), 466–469
See also diagnosis; *specific names of
tests*
thirst, 211
thoracentesis, 24, 463
thoracic surgeon, 45
thoracotomy, 26–27, 104
thorascopic surgery, 21, 402
throat changes, 199–200

thrombophlebitis, 11
thyroid-stimulating hormone, excess, 15
tibulin binding agents, 115
tissue engineering, 406
TNM staging definitions, 30–33
abbreviations used with, 33
M: distant metastasis, 33
N: regional lymph nodes, 32–33
T: primary tumor, 30–32
tobacco industry settlements, 286
tobacco smoke. *See* smoking
topoisomerase inhibitors, 115, 402
topotecan, 115
transbronchial needle aspiration, 24
travel for care, 47, 287, 431–433
treatment centers/hospitals
choosing, 49–52
importance to diagnosis, 37
insurance issues, 47
as research resources, 366
types of
community clinical oncology
programs, 51
cooperative groups, 51
free care/clinical trials, 52, 347,
431
NCI-designated comprehensive
cancer centers, 49
university hospitals, 50–51
See also hospitalization
treatment teams
checking credentials of, 52–53,
424–426
finding doctors, 46–47
finding oncologists/surgeons,
47–49
importance of, 1, 44
insurance issues, 47
non-medical considerations, 56
oncologists, types of, 45
questions before choosing, 53–56
surgeons, types of, 45
ways to search for, 48–49
See also hospitalization; interacting
with medical personnel
treatment types, overview, 102–120
See also chemotherapy;
radiotherapy; surgery
triplex molecules, 406

About the Author

Lorraine Johnston first became involved with the cancer patient community in 1993 while researching and advocating for family members. She is the wife of a 10-year lymphoma survivor and the daughter of a 25-year lymphoma survivor. Several of her family members have had gastric cancers and many have been smokers. In the years since her husband's diagnosis, Lorraine has been involved in a number of support groups that offer emotional and practical support to cancer survivors.

In the course of her support group efforts, Lorraine has been interviewed about the best ways to find reliable medical information by the *Philadelphia Inquirer*, National Public Radio's *Marketplace* program, WebMD, Gail Allen's *Lifelines* radio program on KDWN in Las Vegas, and Martha Griswold's *Access Unlimited* radio program on KPFK radio in Los Angeles. She attempts to dispel the myth that access to sound medical information is cloaked in secrecy and that medical literature is impossible to interpret. Using her lifelong love of biology and her degree in life sciences, she helps cancer survivors accurately evaluate the material they locate.

Lorraine's years of study included many courses in psychology, but she found that nothing in her educational background adequately prepared her for facing the terror and heartbreak of cancer. One of her chief interests is helping newly diagnosed and long-term survivors feel less lonely and afraid as they confront their diagnoses and weigh their options.

Lung Cancer: Making Sense of Diagnosis, Treatment, and Options is Lorraine's third book. Her first book was *Non-Hodgkin's Lymphomas: Making Sense of Diagnosis, Treatment, and Options*. Her second was *Colon and Rectal Cancer: A Comprehensive Guide for Patients and Families*. She is currently working on patient advocacy projects, including fundraising for cancer causes and cohosting Internet discussion groups for patients and survivors.

Colophon

Patient-Centered Guides are about the experience of illness. They contain personal stories as well as a combination of practical and medical information. The faces on the covers of our Guides reflect the human side of the information we offer.

The cover of *Lung Cancer* was designed by Kristen Throop of Combustion Creative. The warm colors and quilt-like patterns are intended to convey a sense of comfort. The use of repetitive patterning was inspired by tile work seen by the designer on a recent trip to Turkey. The layout was created on a Macintosh using Quark 4.0. Fonts in the design are: Berkeley, Coronet, GillSans, Minion Ornaments, Throhand, and Univers Ultra Condensed. The design was built with tints of three PMS colors.

The interior layout for the book was designed by Melanie Wang, based on a series design by Edie Freedman and Alicia Cech. The interior fonts are Berkeley and Formata. Anne-Marie Vaduva prepared the text using FrameMaker 5.5.6. Illustrations that appear in this book were created by Robert Romano and Jessamyn Read using Macromedia Freehand 9 and Adobe Photoshop 6.

Ann Schirmer was the production editor and proofreader for *Lung Cancer*. Paulette Miley copyedited the text, and Claire Cloutier, Sarah Jane Shangraw, and Rachel Wheeler provided quality control. Kate Wilkinson wrote the index. Interior composition was done by Ann Schirmer.